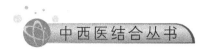
中西医结合丛书

中西医结合医学英语

（第二版）

主　编　郭云良　　倪同上　　扈国杰

副主编　刘天蔚　葛科立　徐颖婕　李宏国

编　委　张　睿　王婷婷　翟　丽　刘英娟

　　　　朱　琳　李　珊　季亚清　王潇璐

　　　　王　悦　李义召　程保合　叶学敏

U0333295

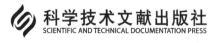
科学技术文献出版社
SCIENTIFIC AND TECHNICAL DOCUMENTATION PRESS

·北京·

图书在版编目（CIP）数据

中西医结合医学英语 / 郭云良，倪同上，扈国杰主编. —2版. —北京：科学技术
文献出版社，2018.10（2019.12重印）
ISBN 978-7-5189-4742-3

Ⅰ．①中… Ⅱ．①郭… ②倪… ③扈… Ⅲ．①中西医结合—英语—研究生—教材
Ⅳ．① R2-031

中国版本图书馆 CIP 数据核字（2018）第 185070 号

中西医结合医学英语（第二版）

策划编辑：孙江莉	责任编辑：宋红梅	责任校对：文 浩	责任出版：张志平

出　版　者	科学技术文献出版社
地　　　址	北京市复兴路15号　邮编 100038
编　务　部	（010）58882938，58882087（传真）
发　行　部	（010）58882868，58882870（传真）
邮　购　部	（010）58882873
官 方 网 址	www.stdp.com.cn
发　行　者	科学技术文献出版社发行　全国各地新华书店经销
印　刷　者	北京虎彩文化传播有限公司
版　　　次	2018 年 10 月第 2 版　2019 年 12 月第 2 次印刷
开　　　本	787×1092　1/16
字　　　数	501千
印　　　张	22.75
书　　　号	ISBN 978-7-5189-4742-3
定　　　价	98.00元

版权所有　违法必究

购买本社图书，凡字迹不清、缺页、倒页、脱页者，本社发行部负责调换

Foreword to the Second Edition

There are several differences including historical origin, cultural deposits, social environment, religious faith and so on between traditional Chinese medicine (TCM) and Western medicine, which lead to some advantages and disadvantages themselves at many aspects of theoretical basis, research method, and diagnosis and treatment systems, so it is important to develop integrative medicine with the ideas of inheritance, innovation, integration, development and modern medical techniques.

Adhering to the equal emphasis on TCM and Western medicine is the basic principles and policies of our national medicine and health. For more than half a century, TCM and integrated medicine have entered a new era with the rapid development of modern medical technology, which leads to more frequent exchanges of theory and technique. *The Law of the People's Republic of China on Traditional Chinese Medicine* released in 2016 stressed adhering to develop integrative medicine.

Integrative medicine is important for both Chinese and Western medical students. This textbook aims to make graduates to learn modern medical knowledge in English language, exchange and spread TCM internationally, so that they will combine Chinese and Western medicine to realize an integrative medicine in scientific meaning.

This revision aims to culture and exercise reading and writing abilities for graduates of integrative medicine. On the basis of maintaining the style of the original teaching materials, we reduced some contents of pure TCM and pure Western medicine, and added the new study progress of integrative medicine, such as Artemisinin, Ligustrazine, Berberine, Astragaloside, Laminarin, Buyang Huanwu Tang, Angong Niuhuang Wan, Liuwei Dihuang Wan, etc.. We also increased vocabulary on integrative medicine to help graduates' applying abilities.

After the revision, it could satisfy the graduates of integrative medicine, and be a reference book for associated discipline's researchers.

We gratefully acknowledge Qingdao University Medical College and the Affiliated Hospital of Qingdao University Medical College for supporting to publish this book.

There may be weaknesses in the book due to the limited level of the editors, and we thank you for your comments.

EDITORS

2018.8

再版前言

中西两种医学体系在历史渊源、文化底蕴、社会环境、宗教信仰等方面均存在差异，在理论基础、研究方法、诊疗体系等方面各有优势和不足。因此，以传承、创新、融合、发展的思路，利用现代医学技术促进结合医学的发展具有重要的现实意义。

坚持中医、西医和中西医结合并重，历来是国家医药卫生的基本方针政策。半个多世纪以来，随着现代医学技术的快速发展，中医学和中西医结合医学也步入了一个崭新的时代，中西医学的理论、技术、方法交流更加频繁。2016年发布的《中华人民共和国中医药法》强调指出，要坚持中西医结合发展的道路。

西医学生不懂中医是很大的不足，中医学生不懂西医也将寸步难行。本教程旨在使中西医结合专业研究生通过英语语言工具获取西医学的知识，以专业英语为桥梁，进行国际交流，传播中医。从而使中医和西医专业知识糅为一体，相互借鉴、取长补短，实现真正意义上的中西结合医学。

本次修订旨在培养和锻炼中西医结合专业研究生的英语阅读理解能力和写作（汉译英）能力。因此，在保持原教材风格的基础上，减少了纯中医和纯西医的内容，增加了中西医结合的新进展，例如，青蒿素、川芎嗪、小檗碱、黄芪甲苷、昆布多糖、补阳还五汤、安宫牛黄丸、六味地黄丸等中西医结合应用研究进展。此外，还增加了中西医结合专业名词的中英对照内容，供研究生在翻译和写作时参考。

修订以后，全书内容由浅入深、循序渐进，从医学科普知识，逐渐深入到专业论文的翻译和写作，最终使研究生具备顺利阅读和翻译（双向翻译）本专业英文文献的能力。本书可满足中西医结合相关专业研究生的需要，也可供相关专业研究人员参考使用。

在编写过程中，青岛大学医学部及其附属医院给予了支持，在此表示感谢。

由于编者水平有限，书中难免存在不足之处，恳请读者指正。

编　者

2018.8

FOREWORD

Since the founding of People's Republic of China in 1949, the government has been paying high attention to traditional Chinese medicine (TCM) and pushing it developed to combine with Western medicine closely, and found a new discipline: Integrative Chinese-Western Medicine (Integrative Medicine).

Integrative medicine is important for both Chinese and Western medical students. This textbook aims to make graduates to learn modern medical knowledge in English language, exchange and spread TCM internationally, so that they will combine Chinese and Western medicine to realize an integrative medicine in scientific meaning.

This textbook consists of 18 chapters and each chapter consists of 4 parts. The first part is mainly about Western medicine to culture English-Chinese and Chinese-English translating abilities for graduates from undergraduates of TCM, while the second part is mainly about integrative medicine to exercise those abilities for undergraduate from modern medicine. The third part is an original article of integrative medicine to exercise graduates' reading and writing abilities, while the fourth part is Chinese-English vocabulary of TCM to help applying abilities.

This textbook involves Chinese medical theories of yin and yang, five elements, syndrome differentiation for treatment, meridians and collaterals, acupuncture and moxibustion, pushing and grasping, formula of traditional Chinese medicine and prescriptions, etc.. And modern medicine includes the basic knowledge of human system, the mechanism, diagnosis and treatment for major diseases, etc.. It could satisfy the graduates of integrative medicine, and might provide a reference book for associated discipline's researchers.

We thank Dr. Long Shaohua, Li Xiaodan, Zhao Li, Bao Hong, Hao Zhimin, He Xinze, Jiang Wen, Gao Yuanyuan, Sun Binbin and Zhang Kaitai for editing this book.

We also thank Qingdao University Medical College and the Affiliated Hospital of Qingdao University Medical College for supporting to publish this book.

There will be weaknesses under correction, and we thank you for your comments.

EDITORS

2013.8

前　言

20世纪中叶新中国成立以来，我国政府对中医学给予了高度的重视，极大地推动了中医学的发展，并将中医学和西医学有机结合，形成了一门新的科学体系——中西结合医学。

西医学生不懂中医是很大的不足，中医学生不懂西医也将寸步难行。本教程旨在使中西医结合专业研究生通过英语语言工具获取西医学的知识，以专业英语为桥梁，进行国际交流，传播中医。从而使中医和西医专业知识糅为一体，相互借鉴、取长补短，实现真正意义上的中西结合医学。

本书共有18章，每章包括四部分。第一部分主要为西医内容，以培养和锻炼本科为中医专业的研究生的英语阅读理解（英译汉）能力和写作（汉译英）能力。第二部分主要为中西医结合内容，着重于培养和锻炼本科为西医专业的研究生的阅读理解能力和英语写作能力。第三部分系一篇中西医结合研究论文，培养和锻炼学生的专业阅读和写作能力。第四部分为中西医结合专业名词的中英对照，以便使研究生在翻译和写作时能正确应用。

本书中医内容包括阴阳五行、八纲辨证、经络俞穴、针灸推拿、中药方剂等。西医内容包括各器官系统的基础知识，主要疾病的病因、发病机制和诊疗方法等。内容由浅入深、循序渐进，从医学科普知识，逐渐深入到专业论文的翻译和写作，最终使研究生具备顺利阅读和翻译（双向翻译）本专业英文文献的能力，可满足中西医结合相关专业研究生的需要，也可供相关专业研究人员参考使用。

除编写委员会外，参加编写的人员还有：龙少华、李晓丹、赵丽、包红、郝志民、贺新泽、姜文、高媛媛、孙彬彬、张开泰等。

　　在编写过程中，青岛大学医学院及其附属医院给予了支持，在此表示感谢。

　　由于编者水平有限，书中难免存在不足之处，恳请读者指正。

编 者

2013.8

目 录
Contents

Chapter 1　Bone

Section 1　Fracture and Osteoporosis

A fracture can be more than just a broken bone. It may be a warning sign of osteoporosis or porous bone, a medical condition that weakens bone by making it more porous and less dense. Bone density is one of the factors that determine bone strength, so individuals with low bone density have a higher risk for fracture and refracture.

Osteoporosis causes bones to become weak and brittle — so brittle that a fall or even mild stresses such as bending over or coughing can cause a fracture. Osteoporosis-related fractures most commonly occur in the hip, wrist or spine. Bone is living tissue that is constantly being broken down and replaced. Osteoporosis occurs when the creation of new bone doesn't keep up with the removal of old bone. It was reported that osteoporosis is a contributing factor in as many as 1.5 million fractures each year, including about 300 000 hip fractures, 700 000 vertebral (spine) fractures, 250 000 wrist fractures and 300 000 fractures at other sites.

The risk of a serious fracture can double after a first fracture in certain high-risk groups. Additionally, many patients, particularly those who suffer hip fractures, are at high risk for premature death or loss of independence after the fracture. In fact, one out of four people who have an osteoporotic hip fracture will need long-term nursing home care; half of those who experience osteoporotic hip fracture are unable to walk without assistance; those who experience the trauma of osteoporotic hip fracture have a 24% increased risk of dying within one year following the fracture. So it is essential for identifying osteoporosis early and initiating treatment.

Recent data indicates that osteoporosis should not just be concern for aging white women, but occurs in all racial groups. (1) Hispanic women may be among those at highest risk of osteoporosis with 13%~16%. As many as 49% of Mexican-American women 50 years of age or older have low bone density. (2) Although the rate of hip fracture is lower in Asian-American women, the rate of vertebral fractures is about equal between Asian-American and Caucasian women. (3) About 10% of African women over 50 years have osteoporosis.

An additional 30% have low bone density. About 80%~95% of all fractures experienced by African-American women over age 64 are related to osteoporosis.

Hormone levels: Osteoporosis is more common in people who have too much or too little of certain hormones in their bodies. Examples include: (1) Sex hormones. Lowered sex hormone levels tend to weaken bone. The reduction of estrogen levels in women at menopause is one of the strongest risk factors for developing osteoporosis. Men experience a gradual reduction in testosterone levels as they age. Treatments for prostate cancer that reduce testosterone levels in men and treatments for breast cancer that reduce estrogen levels in women are likely to accelerate bone loss. (2) Thyroid problems. Too much thyroid hormone can cause bone loss. This can occur if your thyroid is overactive or if you take too much thyroid hormone medication to treat an underactive thyroid. (3) Other glands. Osteoporosis has also been associated with overactive parathyroid and adrenal glands.

Men should also be concerned about osteoporosis. Approximately 1/8 of men will have an osteoporotic fracture. Men with a history of hypogonadism, thyroid dysfunction, long-term steroid therapy, high alcohol consumption or low physical activity are especially at risk. 1/3 of all hip fractures experienced by men are related to osteoporosis, and 1/3 of these men will die within the first year after the fracture.

A fracture in adulthood does not always mean an individual has osteoporosis. However, every adult who suffers a fracture should discuss the need for bone density testing with a physician. If one's bone density is low, he may need additional medical tests. Medical conditions other than osteoporosis can cause low bone density.

Symptoms: There typically are no symptoms in the early stages of bone loss. But once your bones have been weakened by osteoporosis, you may have signs and symptoms that include: back pain, caused by a fractured or collapsed vertebra; loss of height over time; a stooped posture; a bone fracture that occurs much more easily than expected.

Complications: Bone fractures, particularly in the spine or hip, are the most serious complication of osteoporosis. Hip fractures often are caused by a fall and can result in disability and even an increased risk of death within the first year after the injury. In some cases, spinal fractures can occur even if you haven't fallen. The bones that make up your spine (vertebrae) can weaken to the point that they may crumple, which can result in back pain, lost height and a hunched forward posture.

Although there is no specific cure for osteoporosis, diet and lifestyle changes can reduce the risk of re-fracture. People should also discuss medical therapy with their physician. Even individuals without osteoporosis should follow these four simple guidelines: (1) Make sure get enough calcium and vitamin D in diet. The National Academy of Sciences recommends 400~800 units of vitamin D and 1000~1500 mg of calcium per day. (2) Participate in activities that will strengthen bone and muscle. Regular exercise is one of the best things to prevent one's osteoporosis. Weight-bearing exercises like walking, jogging and tennis and low-impact exercise classes are best for building and maintaining strong bones. (3) Because falls are the most common cause of fractures, some balance activities could reduce the risks. The benefits of tai chi which can decrease falls among older individuals by 47% in particular have been documented. (4) Once a broken bone occurred, a bone density test and other steps to reduce the risk of a second fracture should be done.

Prevention: Good nutrition and regular exercise are essential for keeping your bones healthy throughout your life. Protein is one of the building blocks of bone. And while most people get plenty of protein in their diets, some do not. Vegetarians and vegans can get enough protein in the diet if they intentionally seek suitable sources, such as soy, nuts, legumes, and dairy and eggs if allowed. Older adults may also eat less protein for various reasons. Protein supplementation is an option.

Body weight: Being underweight increases the chance of bone loss and fractures. Excess weight is now known to increase the risk of fractures in one's arm and wrist. As such, maintaining an appropriate body weight is good for bones just as it is for health in general.

Calcium: Men and women between the ages of 18 and 50 need 1000 milligrams of calcium a day. This daily amount increases to 1200 milligrams when women turn 50 and men turn 70 years old. Good sources of calcium include: low-fat dairy products, dark green leafy vegetables, canned salmon or sardines with bones, soy products, such as tofu, calcium-fortified cereals and orange juice.

If you find it difficult to get enough calcium from your diet, consider taking calcium supplements. However, too much calcium has been linked to kidney stones. Although yet unclear, some experts suggest that too much calcium especially in supplements can increase the risk of heart disease. The Institute of Medicine recommends that total calcium intake, from supplements and diet combined, should be no more than 2000 milligrams daily for people older than 50 years old.

Vitamin D: Vitamin D improves your body's ability to absorb calcium and improves bone health in other ways. People can get adequate amounts of vitamin D from sunlight, but this may not be a good source if you live in a high latitude, if you're housebound, or if you regularly use sunscreen or avoid the sun entirely because of the risk of skin cancer.

Scientists don't yet know the optimal daily dose of vitamin D for each person. A good starting point for adults is 600~800 international units (IU) a day, through food or supplements. For people without other sources of vitamin D and especially with limited sun exposure, a supplement may be needed. Most multivitamin products contain 600 ~ 800 IU of vitamin D. Up to 4000 IU of vitamin D a day is safe for most people.

Exercise: Exercise can help you build strong bones and slow bone loss. Exercise will benefit your bones no matter when you start, but you'll gain the most benefits if you start exercising regularly when you're young and continue to exercise throughout your life.

Combine strength training exercises with weight-bearing and balance exercises. Strength training helps strengthen muscles and bones in your arms and upper spine, and weight-bearing exercises — such as walking, jogging, running, stair climbing, skipping rope, skiing and impact-producing sports — affect mainly the bones in your legs, hips and lower spine. Balance exercises such as tai chi can reduce your risk of falling especially as you get older.

Swimming, cycling and exercising on machines such as elliptical trainers can provide a good cardiovascular workout, but they're not as helpful for improving bone health.

Section 2　Nomenclature in TCM

Correctly naming a discipline can directly portray the object of study, clearly point out its essence, and presage its future development. Carefully naming an independent discipline may provide the breakthrough necessary to establish its independence. Given the importance of nomenclature, the terminology being applied to the various branches of traditional Chinese medicine (TCM) is disconcerting. Current usage of such terms as Chinese Medicine, Oriental Medicine, Herb, Herbology or Herbal Medicine and Acupuncture are improper. The present article aims to discuss these terms and definite their meaning more precisely.

1　Regarding Chinese Medicine

The traditional medicine of China is the classical medicine of China and is distinguishable from modern Chinese medicine. TCM is a medical science guided by traditional Chinese medical theories, and includes natural product medication, acupuncture, moxibustion, massage, plaster, steam bath, etc. as modalities in the treatment and prevention of disease.

TCM is called Zhongyixue (phonetic transcription of Chinese character, the same below) in Chinese. The Chinese characters Zhongyixue and Zhonghua Yixue are both translated literally into the English words Chinese medicine. However, to refer to TCM as Chinese medicine has two shortcomings. First, Chinese medicine fails to convey the rich tradition associated with TCM; and second, this translation leads to confusion by not distinguishing between TCM and modern Chinese medicine. Examples of the confusion associated with the global term Chinese medicine include the following. Currently, some books and journals published in English include Chinese medicine in their titles; however, they are concerned only with TCM. On the other hand, another journal entitled *Chinese Medical Journal* is concerned only with modern Chinese medicine. Although Chinese medicine in the above titles suggests that they contain similar material, the material in fact is quite different. In addition, some institutions with the name Chinese medicine in fact are concerned only with TCM, not modern Chinese medicine. Finally, an organization named *Chinese Medical Association* is a society involved only with modern medicine in China. The subject material of Chinese medicine as used above differs so extensively that TCM and modern Chinese medicine must have a distinguished nomenclature.

Medicine in the broadest sense should include both modern medicine and traditional medicine. However, the term Medicine typically refers only to modern medicine. The word traditional is often used to distinguish traditional medicine from (modern) medicine. For these reasons, Zhongyixue should be translated into English according to its precise definition, traditional Chinese medicine. This translation conveys both the traditional and the Chinese aspects of the discipline, and distinguishes it from modern Chinese medicine.

2　Regarding Oriental Medicine

Another vague, ambiguous term is oriental medicine. Oriental medicine in English publications is usually synonymous with traditional medicine of China, Japan, Korea, Vietnam, etc.. Actually, all of these disciplines are various branches of TCM which according to relevant literature originated in China. Moreover, in Japanese, traditional medicine is called Hanfang, which can be translated into TCM. The term oriental medicine probably originated to distinguish it from western occidental medicine which is usually associated with modern medicine since it originated in the west. Although the oriental or occidental qualifier may be convenient in dialogue to emphasize the origin of particular aspects of medicine, such use is detrimental because of its ambiguity. The use of the oriental qualifier has at least two shortcomings: (1) it fails to express its original meaning of traditional medicine in China, and (2) it is also fails to recognize the existence of modern medicine in the east. The use of the occidental qualifier bears the same kind of shortcomings. It does not convey the difference between occidental traditional medicine and modern medicine. If medicine was referred to as occidental medicine as currently is done with oriental medicine, differentiation of modern and classical Western medicine such as Hippocratic medicine in 6 BC ~ 4 BC or American Indian folk medicine would be compromised. Though the classical medicine in the west has gradually withered away, it existed in history and needs to be distinguished just as traditional Chinese medicine needs to be distinguished from modern Chinese medicine.

Difference in the nature of medicine in the west and the east has been dissolving for a long time. Currently only differences in tradition and degree of development distinguish the two. With time, the disparity in development between western and eastern medicine will become smaller and smaller, leaving only tradition as a distinction. Since the essence of oriental medicine is traditional Chinese medicine, its true colors of TCM should be restored.

To name disciplines of medicine by using the oriental or the occidental qualifier can not directly portray the object of study, clearly point out its essence, or presage its future prospects of growth. Neither differentiates traditional medicine and modern medicine in either the west or the east. If the word oriental is necessary to precede traditional medicine in the east, it can only be named traditional oriental medicine to differentiate (modern) medicine in the east. This reason is the same as that the naming of TCM is differentiated with (modern) medicine in China.

3　Regarding Herb, Herbology or Herbal Medicine

Traditional Chinese materia medica (TCMM) is a branch of TCM, which studies the theory and application of medication based on theories of TCM. TCMM differs extensively from herbal medicine. The relationship between the two is somewhat akin to the difference between folk medicine and natural product pharmacy in the US. It is improper to use TCMM synonymous with the terms herbology or herbal medicine. In China, TCMM is an officially recognized branch of TCM with standardized medication procedures documented in the state pharmacopoeia or equivalent books. Herbal medicine, however, is folk medicine, and is not officially recognized in the state pharmacopoeia. The two procedures are much different with TCMM having a systematic theory as guidance for its practice while the latter is employed entirely without theory. In TCMM medicines are derived mainly from plants, but animals and minerals provide additional sources. The materials are prepared and refined using well established procedures. The English phrase herbal medicine generally refers to folk medicine, and in most cases the crude herb or crude extract is used. Animal products and minerals are generally not included in definitions of herbal medicine.

For the above reasons, to translate Chinese word Zhongyao — TCMM into herb, herbology or herbal medicine is improper on either the basis of the definition of TCMM or the English meaning of the world herb.

4　Regarding Acupuncture

The science of acupuncture and moxibustion is a branch of TCM which prevents and treats diseases by puncturing specific points on the body with needles, or the burning or warming of the points by applying heat via ignited moxa wool or roll. These procedures are important external therapies of TCM. The term acupuncture is derived from the Latin words acus which means surgical needle, and puncture, which means to puncture. Moxibustion can be defined as the burning, warming, fumigating, or placing hot compression on certain points for the treatment or prevention of diseases. The two therapies are commonly applied in combination, and are also typically used as compound word acupuncture-moxibustion (acumoxibustion — Chinese sound Zhenjiu, which literally means Needling-moxibustion).

In the literal sense, acupuncture refers to a method of needling (i.e. Chinese words Zhenci) or a therapy of needling (i.e. Chinese words Zhenci Liaofa); however, science of acupuncture and moxibustion is also a discipline (i.e. Chinese words Zhenjiuxue), a branch of TCM. When using the term acupuncture we should make clear whether we are referring to its meaning as a method, a therapy or a scientific discipline. The use of the term acupuncture without distinguishing among these three meanings leads to a confusion that could be eliminated by restricting and refining the use of the term. In this light, it is proposing that when using acupuncture to refer to the discipline, we should use the term acupunctology (i.e. acupuncture plus -ology). This term should become the standard through international scientific meetings. It is assumed that acupunctology in the broad sense could cover moxibustion and such similar therapies in the same field.

In summary, the present study suggests that the current use of Chinese medicine, Oriental medicine, herb, herbology or herbal medicine and acupuncture as terms representing disciplines of TCM and its branches is either improper or indistinct. Without more attention to concisely defining these terms, many individuals consider that TCMM is a folk herbology, and acupuncture as only a therapeutic method. Under such conditions, TCM is demoted to folk medicine; the science of TCMM to herbology or herbal medicine; the doctor of TCM to herbalist; the science, acupunctology to the therapy acupuncture; and the acupunctologist to the acupuncturist. The present study is a call to recognize TCMM and acupuncture as scientific branches of TCM with appropriate translations to reflect their scientific nature and separate them from folk therapies.

Section 3   Research Article

Zhuangjin Xugu decoction enhances fracture healing in rats by augmenting the expression of BMP-7 and NPY

[Abstract] This study aimed to investigate the effects of Zhuangjin Xugu decoction (ZJXG decoction) on healing of femoral fracture in rats. Femur fractures were generated in fifty male adult Wistar rats by cutting femur transversely at middle point. ZJXG decoction was administered orally after surgery for $7 \sim 14$ d. The healing process was analyzed by X-ray and hematoxtlin-eosin (HE) staining in rats of sham group, control group and treatment group. The expression of bone morphogenetic protein-7 (BMP-7) and neuropeptide Y (NPY) in fibroblasts and osteoblasts in callus was evaluated by immunohistochemical assay. The serum levels of BMP-7 and NPY were detected by enzyme linked immunoabsorbent assay (ELISA). X-ray imaging analysis indicated that the fibrous callus tissue at the femoral fracture-end increased and the fracture line became fuzzy at $7 \sim 14$ d following treatment with ZJXG decoction, compared to the control group. HE staining showed that the fibrous-granular tissue at the fracture-end changed gradually to fibrous, cartilaginous and osseous callus tissues. Immunostaining and ELISA results showed that BMP-7 and NPY in the fibroblasts and osteoblasts of callus and their serum levels increased significantly $7\sim14$ d following treatment with ZJXG decoction, compared to the control group. It is concluded that ZJXG decoction could enhance the fracture healing by up-regulating the expression of BMP-7 and NPY in fibroblasts and osteoblasts of callus in rats.

Keywords: ZJXG decoction; fracture; callus; X-ray; pathology; BMPs; NPY; rats

1　Introduction

Most fractures are caused by a bad fall or automobile accident. Healthy bones are extremely tough and resilient and can withstand surprisingly powerful impacts. As people age, two factors make their risk of fractures greater: weaker bones and a greater risk of falling. Children, who tend to have more physically active lifestyles than adults, are also prone to fractures. People with underlying illnesses and conditions that may weaken their bones have a higher risk of fractures. Examples include osteoporosis, infection, or a tumor. As mentioned earlier, this type of fracture is known as a pathological fracture. Stress fractures, which result from repeated stresses and strains, commonly found among professional sports people, are also common causes of fractures.

The fracture healing is an extremely complicated process of skeletal reconstruction. Many growth factors could promote osteoblast differentiation, proliferation, development and accelerate new bone formation in the process of fracture healing and remodeling (Pogoda et al., 2005). Bone morphogenetic proteins (BMPs) and neuropeptide Y (NPY) play important roles in bone fracture repair process (Oreffo RO., 2004). BMP-7 can induce cartilage and bone formation (Chen et al., 2002) and has been used to treat fracture models in rodents (Hak et al., 2006; Lu et al., 2010; den Boer et al., 2002). Some experimental and clinical reports illustrated the effect of BMP-7 on fracture healing (Blattert et al., 2002; White et al., 2007). NPY affects the activities of osteoblasts by inhibiting the synthesis of circle adenosine monophosphate (cAMP) during the fracture repair process (Linblad et al., 1994). As a skeletal maintenance regulation-related factor, NPY improves skeletal synthetic metabolism, controls bone remodeling, regulates bone balance, prevents bone loss, and maintains bone stability (Lee et al., 2009; Teixeira et al., 2009). NPY participates in fracture remodeling not only from the central nervous system, but also from the tissue surrounding fracture (Liu et al., 2009).

Current fracture care includes internal and external fixation with early mobilization to restore function earlier and more completely. But fracture fixation could cause serious trauma and mostly need the secondary operation. In addition, it increases the risk of infection and the rates of delayed union, and nonunion (Zhao et al., 2011). Traditional Chinese medicine formula Zhuangjin Xugu decoction (ZJXG decoction) has been clinically used for promoting fracture healing for many years (Li K et al., 2009). The exact therapeutic mechanism by which ZJXG decoction enhances healing in rodent model, however, still remains unclear. Here we aim to elucidate if the effects of ZJXG decoction in fracture repair were related to the expression of BMP-7 and NPY.

2   Materials and methods

2.1   Animal model and grouping

Fifty male adult Wistar rats [Experiment Animal Center of Qingdao Drug Inspection Institute, SCXK (LU) 20090010] weighting 190~210 g were used in this study. All experimental procedures were approved by the Ethics Committee of Qingdao University Medical College (No. QUMC 2011-09). The rats were anesthetized with injecting intraperitoneally 100 g/L chloral hydrate (300 mg/kg) and then restrained in a supine position for operation. The animal's hind limb was shaved and then a medial prepatellar incision was created. The femoral fracture model was established by cutting the femur transversely at the middle section (about 1.0 cm below the great trochanter) (Wang et al., 2005). After the manual reduction, the fractured femur was fixed with intramedullary Kirschner wires (diameter 1.0 mm, Shanghai Medical Apparatus Co. Ltd.). The sham group was subjected to the same procedure except without cutting femur. Animals were allowed to drink and eat freely after surgery. The survival rate is 100%.

The rats were divided randomly into five groups of 10 rats in each group. The low, medium and high dose group rats were treated with 1.25 g/kg, 2.50 g/kg and 5.00 g/kg respectively while the vehicle was given at the same volume to sham and control group rats. At the time points of 7 d or 14 d, rats were subjected to X-ray image taking after chloral hydrate anesthesia and then euthanized for blood and tissue collection.

2.2   Preparation of ZJXG decoction

ZJXG decoction was derived from the ZJXG pellet recorded in *Shangke Dacheng* written by Zhao Lian of the Qing Dynasty in China. It is composed of 10 constituents (Chinese herbal medicines) listed in Table 1-1.

Table 1-1　Chinese herbal medicines of ZJXG decoction

Sources	Chinese Name	English Name	Lating Name	Dose
Gansu	Danggui	Chinese Angelica	Radix Angelicae Sinensis	12 g
Sichuan	Chuanxiong	Rhizoma Chuanxiong	Rhizoma Chuanxiong	12 g
Henan	Shudi	Radix Rehmanniae Preparata	Radix Rehmanniae Preparata	10 g
Inner Mongolia	Huangqi	Milkvetch Root	Radix Astragali	12 g
Sichuan	Duzhong	Eucommia Bark	Eucommia ulmoides Oliv	12 g
Sichuan	Chuanxuduan	Himalayan Teasel Root	Radix Dipsaci Asperoides	12 g
Guangxi	Gusuibu	Fortune's Drynaria Rhizome	Rhizoma Drynariae	12 g
Yunnan	Sanqi	Sanchi	Radix Notoginseng	10 g
Inner Mongolia	Baishao	White Paeony Root	Radix Paeoniae Alba	10 g
Xinjiang	Honghua	Safflower	Flos Carthami	10 g
Total				112 g

The ZJXG decoction was decocted according to the *Standard of Decocting Herbal Medicine* promulgated by Chinese Administration Department of Traditional Chinese Medicine. The mixture of all herbal plants were immersed in distilled water for 20~30 min at 20~25 ℃ with relative humidity ≤ 85%, and then cooked to the boil, kept on simmer for 10~15 min to concentrate the extracts, protecting and maintaining all essential ingredients. The same procedure was repeated for twice. The two extractions yielded an amount of 224 mL liquid medicinal decoction containing 112 g of dry weight (concentration of 0.50 g/mL) which was packed with sterilized plastic bags and stored at −20 ℃ until use.

2.3　Radiological evaluation and gross observation

An initial X-ray examination was performed in all animals after the fracture. At day 7 and day 14 following surgery, all the rats were anesthetized for X-ray evaluation (GE Revolution RE/d, USA). The anesthetized rats were then sacrificed and the femurs were taken out, and washed in normal saline for general observation.

2.4　Histological analysis

For morphological analysis, the femur were cut and incubated in 40 g/L formaldehyde solution for 4 h and rinsed in distilled water for 4 h, and then decalcificated for 10 days in 20% ethylenediamine tetraacetic acid (EDTA). The samples were then dehydrated using graded ethanol, immersed in dimethylbenzene for 2 h, and embedded by paraffin. The 7 μm thickness slices were made by microtome (Leica RM 2015, Shanghai Leica Instruments, China) and attached to poly-L-lysine processed slides. Paraffin sections were deparaffinized in dimethylbenzene, hydrated in gradient ethanol and rinsed with distilled water. The sections were stained with hematoxylin-eosin and BMP-7 and NPY.

For immunostaining, antigen retrieval was made using a microwave oven. The sections were incubated with rabbit anti-rat BMP-7 (concentration) and NPY (concentration) polyclonal antibodies at 4 ℃ overnight. Negative control used PBS instead of primary antibodies. Immunohistochemical procedures were performed strictly according to the SABC kit manual. Four serial sections from each experimental rat were observed under a light microscope (manufacture). LEICA QWin micrograph analytical system was used to analyze the expression of immunosignals, illustrated by absorbance values (A).

2.5　Enzyme linked immunoabsorbent assay (ELISA)

About 4 mL blood was aseptically collected from abdominal aorta of each rat and centrifugalized for 10 min at 4000 r/min at 4 ℃ to separate the serum which was then kept at -20 ℃ until required for analysis. Anti-BMP-7 and anti-NPY were measured using commercially available ELISA kits (Blue Gene Co. Ltd.). The procedure was performed following manufacturer's instruction. The ODs were calculated with Bio-Rad 550 microplate reader (USA) set to 450 nm to reflect the level of BMP-7 and NPY.

2.6　Statistical analysis

The data was expressed by mean ± standard deviation (mean ± SD) and analyzed with SPSS 11.5 statistical software. Analysis of variance was used to compare whether there are obvious differences among groups. $P < 0.05$ was considered significantly.

3　Results

3.1　X-ray examination

X-rays revealed that the fracture-end of femur of the control group began forming fibrous callus at day 7 after surgery with the fracture line still clear; at day 14, the fracture line became unclear. In the treated groups, the fibrous callus was more than that in the control group and the fracture line became fuzzy at day 7 and tended to disappear at day 14 following treatment. There was no statistical significance between groups of low dose, medium dose and high dose.

3.2　Gross observation of fracture fragments

On day 7 in the control group, granulation tissue in the fracture breaking-end was observed and fibrous callus at day 14 following surgery. In the treated groups, fibrous callus formed at day 7 and the formation of cartilaginous and osseous callus was present on day 14 (Figure 1-1). There was no statistical difference among treatment groups.

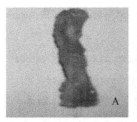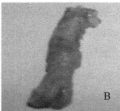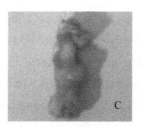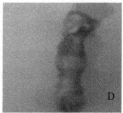

Figure 1-1   Gross observation of tissue samples on day 7 in control group (A) and low-dose treated group (B), day 14 in control group (C) and low-dose treated group (D)

3.3   HE staining

On day 7, in the control group, the inflammatory cell infiltration, the formation of granulation tissues occurred between fracture fragments and the proliferation of fibroblasts and osteoblasts under periosteum was localized in the fracture gap. On day 14 of control rats, the number of fibroblasts and osteoblasts increased and fibrous callus had formed with a small cartilaginous callus. In the treated groups, the inflammatory cells decreased and the fibroblasts and osteoblasts increased in the fractured bone end 7 days after treatment compared to the control group, while on day 14 a lot of fibrous, cartilaginous and osseous callus tissues had developed and newly formed bone trabeculae appeared (Figure 1-2).

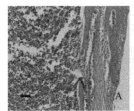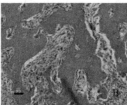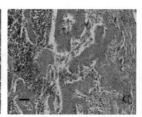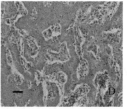

Figure 1-2   Hematoxylin and eosin staining on tissues collected on day 7 in control group (A) and treatment group (B), on day 14 in control group (C) and treatment group (D)
Scale bar =50 μm.

3.4   Immunohistochemistry

Minimal expression of BMP-7 and NPY was detected in the sham group ($F = 14.12$, $q = 2.39 \sim 7.69$, $P > 0.05$). BMP-7 and NPY positive cells were observed in callus tissues in the control group on day 7 and the absorbance values on day 14 was greater compared to 7 d control group ($F = 14.12$, $q = 2.39 \sim 7.69$, $P < 0.05$). In paired comparisons of groups, the grade of values of absorbance (A) of BMP-7 and NPY was significantly higher in the treatment groups compared to the control group ($F = 14.12$, $q = 2.39 \sim 7.69$, $P < 0.05$). It was not significantly different among the high-dose, medium-dose and low-dose treated groups ($F =$

14.12, $q = 2.39 \sim 7.69$, $P > 0.05$) (Table 1-2 and Figure 1-3, Figure 1-4).

Table 1-2 The expression values of absorbance (A) of BMP-7 and NPY

(mean ± SD, $n = 5$)

Groups	Dose	BMP-7 (A)		NPY (A)	
		7 d	14 d	7 d	14 d
Sham group	NS	0.24 ± 0.07	0.25 ± 0.06	0.27 ± 0.05	0.25 ± 0.07
Control group	NS	0.28 ± 0.06^a	$0.43 \pm 0.08^{a,c}$	0.38 ± 0.06^a	$0.46 \pm 0.11^{a,c}$
Low-dose group	1.25 g/kg	0.65 ± 0.12^b	$0.71 \pm 0.14^{b,c}$	0.56 ± 0.10^b	$0.70 \pm 0.10^{b,c}$
Medium-dose group	2.50 g/kg	0.62 ± 0.12^b	$0.81 \pm 0.12^{b,c}$	0.57 ± 0.12^b	$0.71 \pm 0.13^{b,c}$
High-dose group	5.00 g/kg	0.63 ± 0.13^b	$0.83 \pm 0.15^{b,c}$	0.57 ± 0.16^b	$0.68 \pm 0.13^{b,c}$

[a]$P < 0.05$ *vs* sham group, [b]$P < 0.05$ *vs* control group, [c]$P < 0.05$ *vs* treated 7 d.

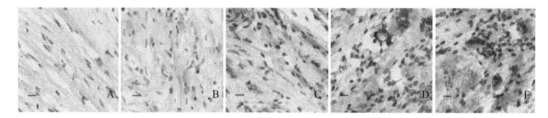

Figure 1-3 The expression of BMP-7

DAB × 200, Scale Bar = 25 μm. A: Sham group, B: 7 days in control group, C: 7 days in low-dose group, D: 14 days in control group, E: 14 days in low-dose group.

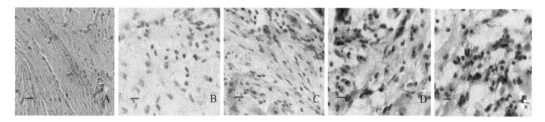

Figure 1-4 Immunohistochemistry of BMP-7

DAB × 200, Scale Bar = 25 μm. A: Sham group, B: 7 days in control group, C: 7 days in low-dose group; D: 14 days in control group, E: 14 days in low-dose group.

3.5 The serum levels of BMP-7 and NPY

There was no significant difference of serum levels of BMP-7 and NPY between day 7 and day 14 in the sham operation group ($P > 0.05$). It is significantly different between day 7 and day 14 within other each group, with higher levels on day 14 ($P < 0.05$). At the same time points, the serum levels of BMP-7 and NPY in the control group were significantly higher than those in the sham operation group and significantly lower than those in the treated groups ($P < 0.05$). No significant difference among the high-dose, medium-dose and low-dose groups was observed ($P > 0.05$) (Table 1-3).

Table 1-3   The serum levels of BMP-7 and NPY determined by ELISA (mean ± SD, $n = 5$)

Groups	Dose	BMP-7/(ng/L)		NPY/(ng/L)	
		7 d	14 d	7 d	14 d
Sham group	NS	112.24 ± 10.71	115.50 ± 12.20	121.27 ± 13.55	135.20 ± 23.20
Control group	NS	386.28 ± 41.04[a]	430.37 ± 45.00[a, c]	283.36 ± 20.06[a]	363.61 ± 28.05[a, c]
Low-dose group	1.25 g/kg	679.15 ± 64.62[b]	783.15 ± 73.41[b, c]	562.35 ± 46.78[b]	706.00 ± 65.10[b, c]
Medium-dose group	2.50 g/kg	722.15 ± 70.12[b]	861.56 ± 75.12[b, c]	573.32 ± 50.32[b]	710.00 ± 70.36[b, c]
High-dose group	5.00 g/kg	730.24 ± 75.00[b]	853.35 ± 81.05[b, c]	575.55 ± 53.16[b]	688.64 ± 63.73[b, c]

[a] $P < 0.05$ vs sham group, [b] $P < 0.05$ vs control group, [c] $P < 0.05$ vs treatment group 7 d.

4   Discussion

Bone healing is a natural process which, in most cases, will occur automatically. Fracture treatment is usually aimed at making sure there is a best possible function of the injured part after healing.Treatment also focuses on providing the injured bone with the best circumstances for optimum healing (immobilization). For the natural healing process to begin, the ends of the broken bone need to be lined up — this is known as reducing the fracture. The patient is usually asleep under a general anesthetic when fracture reduction is done. Fracture reduction may be done by manipulation, closed reduction (pulling the bone fragments), or surgery. If there was damage to the skin and soft tissue around the affected bone or joint, plastic surgery may be required.

If a broken bone has been aligned properly and kept immobile, the healing process is usually straightforward. Osteoclasts (bone cells) absorb old and damaged bone while osteoblasts (other bone cells) are used to create new bone. Callus is new bone that forms around a fracture. It forms on either side of the fracture and grows toward each end until the fracture gap is filled. Eventually, the excess bone smoothes off and the bone is as it was before. The patient's age, which bone is affected, the type of fracture, as well as the patient's general health are all factors which influence how rapidly the bone heals. If the patient smokes regularly, the healing process will take longer.

Immobilization: as soon as the bones are aligned they must stay aligned while they heal. This may include: (1) Plaster casts or plastic functional braces: these hold the bone in position until it has healed. (2) Metal plates and screws: current procedures may use minimally invasive techniques. (3) Intramedullary nails: internal metal rods are placed down the center of long bones. Flexible wires may be used in children. (4) External fixators: these may be made of metal or carbon fiber; they have steel pins that go into the bone directly through the skin. They are a type of scaffolding outside the body.

Usually, the fractured bone area is immobilized for 2 ~ 8 weeks. The duration depends on which bone is affected and whether there are any complications, such as a blood supply problem or an infection. After the bone has healed, it may be necessary to restore muscle strength as well as mobility to the affected area. If the fracture occurred near or through a joint, there is a risk of permanent stiffness or arthritis — the individual may not be able to bend that joint as well as before.

Complications include: (1) Heals in the wrong position: this is known as a malunion; either the fracture heals in the wrong position or it shifts (the fracture itself shifts). (2) Disruption of bone growth: if a childhood bone fracture affects the growth plate, there is a risk that the normal development of that bone may be affected, raising the risk of a subsequent deformity. (3) Persistent bone or bone marrow infection: if there is a break in the skin, as may happen with a compound fracture, bacteria can get in and infect the bone or bone marrow, which can become a persistent infection (chronic osteomyelitis). (4) Patients may need to be hospitalized and treated with antibiotics. Sometimes, surgical drainage and curettage is required. (5) Bone death (avascular necrosis): if the bone loses its essential supply of blood it may die.

RhBMP previous clinical studies have demonstrated that applications of ZJXG decoction enhanced healing of fractured humerus and femur (Zhang et al., 2006; Liang et al., 2005; Kuang et al., 2003; Li et al., 2010). Consistent with these empirical observations, here we presented the first robust evidence of the effectiveness of ZJXG decoction in the promotion of fracture healing in the experimental animal. Fracture healing is an extremely complex process which is reportedly influenced by multiple cytokines and growth factors (Westerhuis et al., 2005). In the present study, we hypothesized that the efficacy of ZJXG decoction can be mediated via the up-regulation of local and systematic BMP-7 and NPY. Bone morphogenetic proteins (BMPs) are known to play critical roles in the formation of cartilage and bone during embryonic development, and the loss of certain BMP molecules leads to a severe impairment of osteogenesis (Bandyopadhyay et al., 2006). The molecules of BMP-2, BMP-4, BMP-5, BMP-6, BMP-7, and BMP-9 have effects on osteogenic action (Xiao et al., 2007), though different members play specific roles in bone formation during different stages. BMP-7 induces osteogenic differentiation of mesenchymal stem cells by regulating the transcription factors Runx2 and Osterix.

In addition to the effects in skeletal development, BMP-7 has been well characterized for its involvement in the fracture healing. For example, Kloen et al. (2003) showed the presence of BMP molecules including BMP-7 in human fracture callus. In another study, clinical application of BMP-7 could induce the osteoblastic activity and repair bony defects (Geesink et al., 1999). Furthermore, BMP-7 accelerated the healing in distal tibial fractures treated by external fixation (Ristiniemi et al., 2007). The results of these studies suggest BMP-7 can be a positive modulator of fracture healing. This experiment showed that the BMP-7 expression in blood and in the femoral fracture callus tissue of rats significantly increased after treatment with ZJXG decoction at different stages; meanwhile, HE staining and X-ray evaluation demonstrated the efficacy of ZJXG decoction in enhancing the fracture healing. The current data suggested the involvement of BMP-7 be an important mediator in the accelerated healing by ZJXG decoction. Other Chinese herbal medicines such as the mixture of kidney-tonifying also increased BMPs concentration in the area of implant-synostosis and promoted fracture healing of rats. It is therefore possible that up-regulation of MBP-7 could be a common therapeutic mechanism employed by different treatments for enhancing fracture healing.

Immunohistochemical experiments revealed that neuropeptides including NPY widely distributed in bones (Elefterious, 2005; Nunes et al., 2010). Several lines of evidence suggest that NPY mediate the bone reconstruction. Nunes et al. (2010) demonstrated that NPY could promote the synthesis of osteoblasts, cartilage cells and bone cells, and increase the bone mass by increasing ceramide contents during embryonic and adult periods. The bone fracture remodeling was enhanced not only by the NPY from the central nervous system, but also by the peripheral NPY surrounding the fractures (Long et al., 2010). NPY also influenced the osteoblasts activity by inhibiting synthesis of cAMP in osteoblasts (Linblad et al., 1994). In this experiment, higher level of NPY was detected in the fibroblasts and osteoblasts in fracture callus following treatment with ZJXG decoction, and the concentration of NPY also exhibited an increase in blood serum of rats with ZJXG decoction by ELISA. At the same time points, X-ray showed the fracture line became dim and the fibrous and cartilaginous callus formed at fracture-site by HE staining after treatment with ZJXG decoction. In combination, our findings suggest that accelerated fracture healing induced by ZJXG decoction may also be mediated by an increase in NPY expression.

In conclusion, the current data demonstrated that ZJXG decoction significantly promotes the fracture healing in a fracture rat model. Moreover, the fracture healing effects by ZJXG decoction might partially be due to its influence on the expression of growth factors of BMP-7 and NPY. This study provided information useful for elucidating the mechanistic details underlying the therapeutic effects of ZJXG decoction on bone. Future studies will be needed to investigate which signaling pathways are affected by ZJXG decoction.

Acknowledgement

This study was supported by grant-in-aids for the Best Article Culture Fund for Graduate of Qingdao University (No. YSPY2011012). We also thank Dr. Li Yonggang from Department of Anatomy and Neurobiology, Morehouse School of Medicine (MSM), Atlanta for copyediting this paper.

References

[1]　Bandyopadhyay A, Tsuji K, Cox K, et al. Genetic analysis of the roles of BMP2, BMP4, and BMP7 in limb patterning and skeletogenesis. PLoS Genet, 2006, 2(12): e216.

[2]　Blattert T R, Delling G, Dalal P. Successful transpedicular lumbar interbody fusion by means of a composite of osteogenic protein-1(rhBMP-7) and hydroxyapatite carrier: a comparison with autograft and hydroxyapatite in the sheep spine. Spine, 2002, 27(10): 2697-2705.

[3]　Chen X, Kidder L S, Lew W D. Osteogenic protein-1 induced bone formation in an infected segmental defect in the rat femur. J Orthop Res, 2002, 20(2): 142-150.

[4]　den Boer F C, Bramer J A, Blokhuis T J. Effect of recombinant human osteogenic protein-1 on the healing of a freshly closed diaphyseal fracture. Bone, 2002, 31(2): 158-164.

[5]　Elefteriou F. Neuronal signaling and the regulation of bone remodeling. Cell Mol Life Sci, 2005, 62(10): 2339-2349.

[6]　Geesink R G, Hoefnagels N H, Bulstra S K. Osteogenic activity of OP-1 bone morphogenetic protein (BMP-7) in a human fibular defect. J Bone Joint Surg Br, 1999, 81(4): 710-718.

[7]　Hak D J, Makino T, Niikura T. Recombinant human BMP-7 effectively prevents nonunion in both young and old rats. J Orthop Res, 2006, 24(1): 11-20.

[8]　Kloen P, Di Paola M, Borens O, et al. BMP signaling components are expressed in human fracture callus. Bone, 2003, 33(3): 362-371.

[9]　Komakil M, Asakura A, Rudnicki M A, et al. MyoD enhances BMP7-induced osteogenic differentiation of myogenic cell cultures. J Cell Sci, 2004, 117(8): 1457-1468.

[10]　Kuang J H, Kuang J H, Luo X H, et al. Jie Gu Li Shang decoction promoting fracture healing of 50 cases. Hunan Journal of Traditional Chinese Medicine, 2003, 19(3): 19-20.

[11]　Lee N J, Herzog H . NPY regulation of bone remodelling. Neuropeptides, 2009, 43(6): 457-463.

[12]　Li J B, Zhang J H. Therapeutic effect of Jie Gu syrup on fracture of rib and its clinical research. Hubei J Tradit Chin Med, 2010, 32(3): 26-27.

[13]　Li K, Shi M, Li W H. Experimental study of Traditional Chinese Medicine on postoperative healing of

fracture. J Liaoning Univ Tradit Chin Med, 2009, 11(10): 69-71.

[14]　Liang S Y, Liu Z J. Senile fracture of femur inter-tuberosity of 42 cases treated by integrative Traditional Chinese and Western medicine. Forum on Tradit Chin Med, 2005, 20(5): 45-46.

[15]　Lindblad B E, Nielsen L B, Jespersen S M, et al. Vasoconstrictive action of neuropeptide Y in bone. The porcine tibia perfused in vivo. Acta Orthop Scand, 1994, 65(6): 629-634.

[16]　Liu W L, Wang K Q, Jiao X L, et al. Effects of bone morphogenetic protein 7 in articular cartilage on the pathology course of osteoarthritis. J Tradit Chin Orthop Traumatol, 2009, 21(12): 17-19.

[17]　Long H, Ahmed M, Ackermann P, et al. Neuropeptide Y innervation during fracture healing and remodeling. A study of angulated tibial fractures in the rat. Acta Orthop, 2010, 81(5): 639-646.

[18]　Lu C Y, Xing Z, Yu Y Y, et al. Marcucio recombinant human bone morphogenetic Protein-7 enhances fracture healing in an ischemic environment. J Orthop Res, 2010, 28(5): 687-696.

[19]　Nunes A F, Liz M A, Franquinho F, et al. Neuropeptide Y expression and function during osteoblast differentiation-insights from transthyretin knockout mice. FEBS J, 2010, 277(1): 263-275.

[20]　Oreffo R O. Growth factors for skeletal reconstruction and fracture repair. Curr Opin Investig Drugs, 2004, 5(4): 419-423.

[21]　Pogoda P, Priemel M, Rueger J M, et al. Bone remodeling: new aspects of a key process that controls skeletal maintenance and repair. Osteoporos Int, 2005, 16(Suppl 2): S18-24.

[22]　Ristiniemi J, Flinkkilä T, Hyvönen P, et al. RhBMP-7 accelerates the healing in distal tibial fractures treated by external fixation. J Bone Joint Surg Br, 2007, 89(2): 265-272.

[23]　Teixeira L, Sousa D M, Nunes A F, et al. NPY revealed as a critical modulator of osteoblast function in vitro: new insights into the role of Y1 and Y2 receptors. J Cell Biochem, 2009, 107(5): 908-916.

[24]　Wang X, Song Y M, Pei F X. The effects of central nervous system injury on femur fracture healing of rats. Chin J Orthop Surg, 2005, 13(20): 1570-1572.

[25]　Westerhuis R J, van Bezooijen R L, Kloen P. Use of bone morphogenetic proteins in traumatology. Injury, 2005, 36(12): 1405-1412.

[26]　White A P, Vaccaro A R, Hall J A. Clinical applications of BMP-7/OP-1 in fractures, nonunions and spinal fusion. Int Orthop, 2007, 31(5): 735-741.

[27]　Xiao Y T, Xiang L X, Shao J Z. Bone morphogenetic protein. Biochem Biophys Res Commun, 2007, 362(3): 550-553.

[28]　Zhang X H, Guo X Q, Zeng S C, et al. The humeral fracture nonunion of 43 cases treated by unilateral function external fixation combing Traditional Chinese herbal medicines. Jiangxi J Tradit Chin Med, 2006, 37(8): 37-38.

[29]　Zhao Z C, Cao Z Q, Li H, et al. Progress of Traditional Chinese Medicine on the fracture healing. Shaanxi J Tradit Chin Med, 2011, 32(5): 636-637.

Section 4   Words of TCM

1. 中医学 traditional Chinese medicine (TCM)

2. 中药 traditional Chinese drugs; traditional Chinese materia medica (TCMM)

3. 中草药 herbal medicine; traditional Chinese herbal medicine

4. 整体观念 concept of holism

5. 病与证 disease and syndrome

6. 症状与体征 symptom and physical sign

7. 辨病与辨证 disease diagnosing and syndrome differentiation

8. 辨证论治 syndrome differentiation and treatment variation

9. 黄帝内经（内经） huangdi neijing; huangdi's canon of medicine (neijing)

10. 素问 suwen; simple questions

11. 灵枢 lingshu; spiritual axis

12. 黄帝八十一难经（难经）classic of questioning (nanjing)

13. 伤寒杂病论 shanghan zabing lun; treatise on cold pathogenic and miscellaneous diseases

14. 金匮要略 jinkui yaolüe; synopsis of golden chamber

15. 神农本草经（本草经或本经） shennong bencao jing; shennong's classic of materia medica

16. 本草纲目 compendium of materia medica

17. 本草从新 new compilication materia medica

18. 新修本草 newly-revised meteria medica

19. 外科精义（外科精要）main points for surgery; essential points for surgery

20. 千金翼方 qianjin yifang; a supplement to recipes worth a thousand gold

21. 千金要方 qianjin yaofang; valuable prescriptions

22. 肘后备急方 zhouhou beiji fang; prescriptions for emergent reference

23. 诸病源候论 zhubing yuanhou lun; general treatise on causes and manifestations of all diseases

24. 太平圣惠方 taiping shenghui fang; taiping holy prescriptions for universal relief

25. 圣济总录 shengji zonglu; the complete record of holy benevolence

26. 济生方 jisheng fang; prescription for succouring the sick

27. 扁鹊心书 Bianque xinshu; Bianque heart book

28. 素问玄机原病式 exploration to pathogenesis in familiar conversation

29. 儒门事亲 rumen shiqin; confucians' duties to parents

30. 脾胃论 piwei lun; theory of spleen and stomach

31. 格致余论 gezhi yulun; theory of over due

32. 医学正传 yixue zhengzhuan; medical biography

33. 慎斋遗书 shenzhai yishu; shen zhai's suicide note

34. 景岳全书 Jingyue quanshu; Jingyue complete works

35. 瘟疫论 theory of the plague

36. 温热论 treatise on epidemic febrile diseases

37. 温病条辨 wenbing tiaobian; differentiation on febrile disease

38. 医林改错 correction of the errors of medical works

39. 血证论 a treatise on blood troubles

40. 医学衷中参西录 records of tradition Chinese and Western medicine in combination

(Guo Yunliang, Zhang Rui)

Chapter 2　Infection

Section 1　Antibiotics

What are antibiotics? Which infections do they treat?

Antibiotics are among the most frequently prescribed medications in modern medicine. Antibiotics cure disease by killing or injuring bacteria. The first antibiotic was penicillin, discovered accidentally from a mold culture. Today, over 100 different antibiotics are available to cure minor or life-threatening infections.

Although antibiotics are useful in a wide variety of infections, it is important to realize that antibiotics only treat bacterial infections. Antibiotics are useless against viral infections (for example, the common cold) and fungal infections (such as ringworm). Doctors can best determine if an antibiotic is right for your condition.

What are the side effects of antibiotics?

Antibiotics may have side effects. Some of the common side effects may include: (1) soft stools or diarrhea, (2) mild stomach upset. You should notify your doctor if you have any of the following side effects: (1) vomiting, (2) severe watery diarrhea and abdominal cramps, (3) allergic reaction (shortness of breath, hives, swelling of lips, face or tongue, fainting), (4) rash, (5) vaginal itching or discharge, and (6) white patches on the tongue.

What are symptoms of an allergic reaction to an antibiotic?

Some people are allergic to certain types of antibiotics, most commonly penicillin. If you have a question about a potential allergy, ask your doctor or pharmacist before taking the medicine. Allergic reactions commonly have the following symptoms: shortness of breath; rash; hives; itching; swelling of the lips, face or tongue; fainting.

Types of antibiotics

Although there are well over 100 antibiotics, the majority come from only a few types of drugs. These are the main classes of antibiotics: penicillins such as penicillin and amoxicillin; cephalosporins such as cephalexin (Keflex); macrolides such as erythromycin (E-Mycin), clarithromycin (Biaxin), and azithromycin (Zithromax); fluoroquinolones such as ciprofolxacin

(Cipro), levofloxacin (Levaquin), and ofloxacin (Floxin); sulfonamides such as co-trimoxazole (Bactrim) and trimethoprim (Proloprim); tetracyclines such as tetracycline (Sumycin, Panmycin) and doxycycline (Vibramycin); aminoglycosides such as gentamicin (Garamycin) and tobramycin (Tobrex).

Most antibiotics have two names — the trade or brand name, created by the drug company that manufactures the drug, and a generic name, based on the antibiotic's chemical structure or chemical class. Trade names such as Keflex and Zithromax are capitalized. Generics such as cephalexin and azithromycin are not capitalized.

Each antibiotic is effective only for certain types of infections, and your doctor is best able to compare your needs with the available medicines. Also, a person may have allergies that eliminate a class of antibiotic from consideration, such as a penicillin allergy preventing your doctor from prescribing amoxicillin.

In most cases of antibiotic use, a doctor must choose an antibiotic based on the most likely cause of the infection. For example, if you have an earache, the doctor knows what kinds of bacteria cause most ear infection. He or she will choose the antibiotic that best combats those kinds of bacteria. In another example, a few bacteria cause most kinds of pneumonia in previously healthy people. If you are diagnosed with pneumonia, the doctor will choose an antibiotic that will kill these bacteria.

In some cases, laboratory tests may be used to help a doctor make an antibiotic choice. Special strains of the bacteria such as Gram stains, can be used to identify bacteria under the microscope and may help narrow down which species of bacteria is causing infection. Certain bacterial species will take a stain, and others will not. Cultures may also be obtained. In this technique, a bacterial sample from your infection is allowed to grow in a laboratory. The way bacteria grow or what they look like when they grow can help to identify the bacterial species. Cultures may also be tested to determine antibiotic sensitivities. A sensitivity list is the roster of antibiotics that kill a particular bacterial type. This list can be used to double check that you are taking the right antibiotic.

How should I take antibiotics?

It is important to learn how to take antibiotics correctly. Read the label to see how many pills to take and how often to take your medicine. Also, ask your pharmacist if there is anything you should know about the medication.

An important question to ask is how the medication should be taken. Some medications need to be taken with something in your stomach such as a glass of milk or a few crackers, and others only with water. Taking your antibiotics incorrectly may affect their absorption, reducing or eliminating their effectiveness.

It is also important to store your medication correctly. Many children's antibiotics need to be refrigerated (Amoxicillin), while others are best left at room temperature (Biaxin).

Take your entire course of antibiotics. Even though you may feel better before your medicine is entirely gone, follow through and take the entire course. This is important for your healing. If an antibiotic is stopped in midcourse, the bacteria may be partially treated and not completely killed, causing the bacteria to be resistant to the antibiotic. This can cause a serious problem if those now-resistant bacteria grow enough to cause a reinfection.

What drugs interact with antibiotics?

Antibiotics may have interactions with other prescription and nonprescription medications. For example, clarithromycin (Biaxin, an antibiotic) should not be taken with metoclopramide (Reglan, a digestive system drug).

Be sure your doctor and pharmacist know about all the other medications you are taking while on antibiotics.

What is antibiotic resistance? Am I at risk?

One of the foremost concerns in modern medicine is antibiotic resistance. Simply put, if an antibiotic is used long enough, bacteria will emerge that cannot be killed by that antibiotic. This is known as antibiotic resistance. Infections that are caused by bacteria resistant to some antibiotics exist today. The existence of antibiotic-resistant bacteria creates the danger of life-threatening infections that don't respond to antibiotics.

There are several reasons for the development of antibiotic-resistant bacteria. One of the most important is antibiotic overuse. This includes the common practice of prescribing antibiotics for the common cold or flu. Even though antibiotics do not affect viruses, many people expect to get a prescription for antibiotics when they visit their doctor. Although the common cold is uncomfortable, antibiotics do not cure it, nor change its course. Each person can help reduce the development of resistant bacteria by not asking for antibiotics for a common cold or flu.

Recent studies published in the *New England Journal of Medicine* contend that most people with the raspy breathing problem called bronchitis shouldn't get an antibiotic. Two physicians at the Virginia Commonwealth University School of Medicine, who surveyed the world literature on bronchitis (research studies, clinical trials and anything related to bronchitis and its treatment), said that physicians should be encouraged to avoid antibiotics in most cases.

The primary reason for over-prescription of antibiotics is that most cases of bronchitis, which is inflammation of the tiny airways of the lungs, are caused by viruses for which we have no therapy yet. Only a small percentage of acute bronchitis cases are caused by bacteria that can be treated, such as whooping cough. Yet doctors keep prescribing antibiotics. It is estimated that 70% ~ 80% of bronchitis patients are given a course of antibiotics lasting 5 ~ 10 days.

In the United States, one of every 20 American adults will get bronchitis in a given year. The first reason for them not taking antibiotics is that the drugs cost money, in an era when the mounting cost of health care is a major concern. The second reason is that all antibiotics have side effects, such as rash, diarrhea and abdominal pain. Side effects are acceptable only when a medication helps the patient. The third reason for not prescribing antibiotics is impressive pressure it puts on organisms to select more resistant strains, so that the ones we use will no longer be effective. While economists worry about medical costs, physicians worry about antibiotic-resistant strains of bacteria.

With all those arguments against the practice, why do doctor still write those prescriptions? One reason is convenience. Think of all the patients we have to move through the office. Doctor could take 15 minutes to explain why an antibiotic is not needed or write a prescription in 30 seconds. Bronchitis tends to be overlooked as a subject of medical interest and isn't considered very jazzy. It doesn't get highlights in medical journals or educational conferences in the past 10 years.

The information on bronchitis is there for any doctor who cares to look. The American Academy of Family Physicians notes that because acute bronchitis is usually caused by viruses, antibiotics usually do not help. The academy recommends getting lots of rest, drinking lots of non-caffeinated fluids, keeping the indoor humidity high and waiting for the condition to go away after a few days or a week. If coughing and other symptoms persist, it could be a sign of a more serious condition, such an asthma or pneumonia.

One big reason for antibiotic prescriptions is patients' demand, but patients are getting much savvier. They understand that a lot of infections are viral and that giving them an antibiotic places them at risk. People with the bothersome symptoms of bronchitis shouldn't insist on a prescription. They should understand that it may be the best course of treatment not to give an antibiotic. The message is getting out, a little bit at a time. There is a better understanding than there was, say, 10 years ago, that sometimes an antibiotic is not the better treatment.

Section 2   Theory of Yin and Yang

The philosophical origins of Chinese medicine have grown out of the tenets of Daoism (also known as Taoism). Daoism bases much of its thinking on observing the natural world and manner in which it operates, so it is no surprise to find that the Chinese medical system draws extensively on natural metaphors. In Chinese medicine, the metaphoric views of the human body based on observations of nature are fully articulated in the theory of yin-yang and the system of five elements.

The direct meanings of yin and yang in Chinese are bright and dark sides of an object. Chinese philosophy uses yin and yang to represent a wider range of opposite properties in the universe: cold and hot, slow and fast, still and moving, masculine and feminine, lower and upper, etc.. In general, anything that is moving, ascending, bright, progressing, hyperactive, including functional disease of the body, pertains to yang. The characteristics of stillness, descending, darkness, degeneration, hypo-activity, including organic disease, pertain to yin.

The function of yin and yang is guided by the law of unity of the opposites. In other words, yin and yang are in conflict but at the same time mutually dependent. The nature of yin and yang is relative, with neither being able to exist in isolation. Without cold there would be no hot; without moving there would be no still; without dark, there would be no light. The most illustrative example of yin-yang interdependence is the interrelationship between substance and function. Only with ample substance can the human body function in a healthy way; and only when the functional processes are in good condition, can the essential substances be appropriately refreshed.

The concepts of yin and yang and the five agents provided the intellectual framework of much of Chinese scientific thinking especially in fields like biology and medicine. The organs of the body were seen to be interrelated in the same sort of way as other natural phenomena, and best understood by looking for correlations and correspondences. Illness was seen as a disturbance in the balance of yin and yang or the five agents caused by emotions, heat or cold, or other influences. Thus, therapy depended on accurate diagnosis of the source of the imbalance. The earliest surviving medical texts are fragments of manuscript from early Han tombs. Besides general theory, these texts cover drugs, gymnastics, minor surgery and magic spells. The text which was to become the main source of medical theory also apparently dates from the Han. It is the *Yellow Emperor's Classic of Medicine*, supposed to have been written during the third millennium BC by the mythical Yellow Emperor. A small portion of it is given below.

The Yellow Emperor said: The principle of yin and yang is the foundation of the entire universe. It underlies everything in creation. It brings about the development of parenthood; it is the root and source of life and death; it is found with the temples of the gods. In order to treat and cure diseases one must search for their origins. Heaven was created by the concentration of yang, the force of light; Earth was created by the concentration of yin, the forces of darkness. Yang stands for peace and serenity; yin stands for confusion and turmoil. Yang stands for destruction; yin stands for conservation. Yang brings about disintegration; yin gives shape to things … The pure and lucid element of light is manifested in the upper orifices and the turbid element of darkness is manifested in the lower orifices. Yang, the element of light, originates in the pores. Yin, the element of darkness, moves within the five viscera. Yang, the lucid force of light, truly is represented by the four extremities, and yin, the turbid force of darkness, stores the power of the six treasures of nature. Water is an embodiment of yin as fire is an embodiment of yang. Yang creates the air, while yin creates the senses, which belong to the physical body. When the physical body dies, the spirit is restored to the air, its natural environment. The spirit receives its nourishment through the air, and the body receives its nourishment through the senses. If yang is overly powerful, then yin may be too weak. If yin is particularly strong, then yang is apt to be defective. If the male force is overwhelming, then there will be excessive heat. If the female force is overwhelming, then there will be excessive cold. Exposure to repeated and severe heat will induce chills. Cold injures the body while heat injures the spirit. When the spirit is hurt, severe pain will ensue. When the body is hurt, there will be swelling. Thus, when severe pain occurs first and swelling comes on later, one may infer that a disharmony in the spirit has done harm to the body. Likewise, when swelling appears first and severe pain is felt later on, one can say that a dysfunction in the body has injured the spirit ... Nature has four seasons and five elements. To grant long life, these seasons and elements must store up the power of creation in cold, heat, dryness, moisture and wind. Man has five viscera in which these five climates are transformed into joy, anger, sympathy, grief and fear. The emotions of joy and anger are injurious to the spirit just as cold and heat are injurious to the body. Violent anger depletes yin; violent joy depletes yang. When rebellious emotions rise to Heaven, the pulse expires and leaves the body. When joy and anger are without moderation, then cold and heat exceed all measure, and life is no longer secure. Yin and yang should be respected to an equal extent.

The Yellow Emperor asked: Is there any alternative to the law of yin and yang?

Qi Bo answered: When yang is stronger, the body is hot, the pores are closed, and people begin to pant; they become boisterous and coarse and do not perspire. They become feverish, their mouths are dry and sore, their stomachs feel tight, and they die of constipation. When yang is stronger, people can endure winter but not summer. When yin is stronger, the body is cold and covered with perspiration. People realize they are ill; they tremble and feel chilly. When they feel chilled, their spirits become rebellious. Their stomachs can no long digest food and they die. When yin is stronger, people can endure summer but not winter. Thus yin and yang alternate. Their ebbs and surges vary, and so does the character of the diseases.

The Yellow Emperor asked: Can anything be done to harmonize and adjust these two principles of nature?

Qi Bo answered: If one has the ability to know the seven injuries and the eight advantages, one can bring the two principles into harmony. If one does not know how to use this knowledge, his life will be doomed to early decay. By the age of 40, the yin force in the body has been reduced to one-half of its natural vigor and an individual's youthful prowess has deteriorated. By the age of 50, the body has grown heavy. The ears no longer hear well. The eyes no longer see clearly. By the age of 60, the life producing power of yin has declined to a very low level. Impotence sets in. The nine orifices no longer benefit each other ... Those who seek wisdom beyond the natural limits will retain good hearing and clear vision. Their bodies will remain light and strong. Although they grow old in years, they will stay able-bodied and vigorous and be capable of governing to great advantage. For this reason, the ancient sages did not rush into the affairs of the world. In their pleasures and joys they were dignified and tranquil. They did what they thought best and did not bend their will or ambition to the achievement of empty ends. Thus their allotted span of life was without limit, like that of Heaven and Earth. This is the way the ancient sages controlled and conducted themselves. By observing myself, I learn about others, and their diseases become apparent to me. By observing the external symptoms, I gather knowledge about the internal diseases. One should watch for things out of the ordinary. One should observe minute and trifling things and treat them as if they were big and important. When they are treated, the danger they pose will be dissipated. Experts in examining patients judge their general appearance; they feel their pulse and determine whether it is yin or yang that causes the disease … To determine whether yin or yang predominates, one must be able to distinguish a light pulse of low tension from a hard pounding one. With a disease of yang, yin predominates. With a disease of yin, yang predominates. When one is filled with vigor and strength, yin and yang are in proper harmony.

Section 3   Research Article

The hypoglycemic effect of the kelp on diabetes mellitus model induced by alloxan in rats

[Abstract]Hypoglycemic effects and the use of kelp in diabetes mellitus (DM) model rats induced by alloxan were investigated. Sixty healthy male rats were used to establish DM models by injecting alloxan intraperitoneally. Kelp powder was added to the general forage for the rats. The levels of fasting blood glucose (FBG) were determined by an automatic blood glucose device. Electrochemiluminescence immunoassay was applied to determine the serum levels of insulin. The serum levels of malondialdehyde (MDA) were measured by thiobarbituric acid assay and nitric oxide (NO) by nitrate reductase assay. The activities of superoxide dismutase (SOD) were determined by xanthinoxidase assay and glutathione peroxidase (GSH-Px) by chemical colorimetry. The shape and structure of islet cells were observed with Hematine-Eosin staining, and the expressions of SOD and inducible nitric oxide synthase (iNOS) in islet cells were detected by immunohistochemical assay. The results showed that the serum levels of insulin after treatment with kelp powder increased significantly compared to those in the DM-model group, while the FBG in the medium-high dose treated groups decreased significantly compared to those in the DM-model group ($P < 0.05$). The levels of MDA and NO in the kelp powder groups were lower than those in the DM-model group, while the activities of SOD and GSH-Px were higher than those in the DM-model group, of which a significant difference existed between the medium-high dose treated groups and the DM-model group ($P < 0.05$). The shape and structure of islet cells improved with the SOD up-expressing and iNOS down-expressing in the medium-high dose treated groups compared to those in the DM-model group ($P < 0.05$). There were no significant differences between the medium and high dose treated groups, all above indexes ($P > 0.05$). It is suggested that kelp might aid recovery of the islet cells' secreting function and reduce the level of FBG by an antioxidant effect.

Keywords: kelp; diabetes mellitus; alloxan; oxidative stress; rats

1　Introduction

Diabetes mellitus (DM) is a common disease in the world and type 2 DM accounts for about 90% ~ 95% of cases. Although the etiology of type 2 DM is complex and its pathogenesis is not completely understood, the disease is associated with the level of free radicals and the antioxidant system dysfunction. It has been well established that oxidative stress is a commonly used approach to DM and its complications [1]. Malondialdehyde (MDA) can reflect oxygen free radicals (OFR) that are produced in the body when OFR oxidizes polyunsaturated fatty acids in biomembranes [2]. The gas free radical, nitric oxide (NO), is important in initiating type 2 DM, insulin resistance and secondary effects as well as the islet beta cell function obstacle [3-4]. The natural enzyme superoxide dismutase (SOD) can capture free radicals in the body and the catalytic oxidation enzyme glutathione peroxidase (GSH-Px) is widespread in the body. These enzymes work to eliminate OFR in the body when decline in activity leads to OFR accumulation [5-6]. *Laminaria japonica* (*L. japonica*) is widely cultivated kelp, with China being the largest producer [7]. In China, the kelp is used for food in daily life and also used in traditional medicine. According to the *Compendium of Materia Medica* [8], kelp is cold, salty, and has efficacy in clearing water, softening solid, dissipating node and dissolving phlegm [9], as well as alleviate edema, and eliminate carbuncle. Kelp belongs to the Phaeophyta Laminariaceae *Laminaria*, containing laminarin, ammonium alginate, mannitol, vitamins, amino acids and various normal and trace elements, with a variety of 40 active components [10]. The variety of physiological functions of the kelp relate to the biological activity of polysaccharides which can improve the immunity function, anti-aging, anti-tumor [11], antiatheroscloresis, anti-diabetics [12-13] and other such biological activities. Until now, there has been only limited research and reports on *L. japonica*'s anti-diabetic functions and mechanism [14]. Therefore, the experiment described in this study expands the exploration of the hypoglycemic effect along with a possible mechanism of the effect of kelp on alloxan-induced diabetic rats.

2　Results and discussion

2.1　General situation

Before alloxan was injected, all rats reacted nimbly, had hair that was bright and smooth and there was no significant variation in body weights ($F = 0.05$, $q = 0.03 \sim 0.55$, $P > 0.05$). After alloxan was injected and before kelp powder, forage was administered, and the animals showed typical signs of diabetes mellitus(DM): clumsiness, slow actions, dull colored fur and marasmus. Average body weights reduced significantly before alloxan was injected ($F = 1643.22$, $q = 21.77 \sim 104.53$, $P < 0.05$) and there was no significant difference between the weights of kelp-treated rats and DM-model rats ($P > 0.05$).

After kelp powder forage was administered, the action and hair color of animals in kelp treated and DM-model groups recovered gradually, with body weight becoming significantly higher than before treatment, lower than that of the control group ($F = 149.29$, $q = 22.82 \sim 29.00$, $P < 0.05$). Average body weight of animals in the DM-model and kelp-treated groups was significant lower than that in the control group ($F = 149.29$, $q = 22.82 \sim 30.06$, $P < 0.05$). There was no significant difference between the low-dose group and DM-model rats ($P > 0.05$). Average body weight of animals in the medium-dose and high-dose groups was significantly higher than in the DM-model rats ($P < 0.05$), but there was no significant difference between the medium-dose and high-dose groups ($P > 0.05$) (Table 2-1).

Table 2-1   The average body weight of animals in the experiment (mean ± SD)

Groups	n	Kelp dose	Before modeled/g	Before treated/g	After treated/g
Control group	10	General forage	151.76 ± 3.45	168.50 ± 4.22	189.69 ± 4.55
Model group	10	General forage	151.85 ± 3.67	133.62 ± 5.35[a]	139.46 ± 5.36
Low group	10	1.25 g/kg	151.68 ± 3.38	134.46 ± 5.23[a]	141.24 ± 5.32[b, c]
Medium group	10	5.00 g/kg	152.26 ± 3.51	135.27 ± 5.18[a]	150.24 ± 5.45[b, c, d]
High group	10	12.50 g/kg	151.65 ± 3.43	133.55 ± 5.27[a]	151.56 ± 5.67[b, c, d]

[a] $P < 0.05$ *vs* before modeled; [b] $P < 0.05$ *vs* before treated; [c] $P < 0.05$ *vs* model group; [d] $P < 0.05$ *vs* low group.

2.2   The level of fasting blood glucose (FBG)

Before injecting alloxan, there were no obvious differences in FBG levels among the control group, DM-model rats and kelp-treated groups ($F = 0.05$, $q = 0.03 \sim 0.55$, $P > 0.05$). After injecting alloxan and before administering kelp powder forage, FBG levels increased significantly compared to those of DM-model rats and the control group ($F = 79.52$, $q = 19.68 \sim 20.19$, $P < 0.05$). There was no significant difference between kelp-treated groups and DM-model rats ($P > 0.05$).

After administering kelp powder forage, FBG levels in kelp-treated groups were significantly lower than those in the DM-model rats and higher than those in the control group ($F = 189.19$, $q = 9.24 \sim 36.44$, $P < 0.05$). After the experiment, FBG levels in the DM-model rats and kelp-treated groups were significantly higher than those in the control group ($F = 188.99$, $q = 9.20 \sim 36.41$, $P < 0.05$). There was no significant difference between the low-dose group and DM-model rats ($P > 0.05$). FBG levels in the medium-dose and high-dose groups were significantly lower than those in the DM-model rats ($P < 0.05$), but there was no significant difference between the medium-dose group and the high-dose group ($P > 0.05$). Results indicated that medium-dose kelp could achieve an ideal hypoglycemic effect.

2.3 The serum level of insulin

The serum levels of insulin in the DM-model group (11.23 ± 3.45, pmol/L) were significantly lower than those in the control group (71.38 ± 15.26, pmol/L), while those in kelp-treated groups were significantly higher than those in the DM-model group ($F = 13.25$, $q = 5.12 \sim 9.73$, $P < 0.05$), but there was no significant difference between the high-dose (26.22 ± 4.85, pmol/L), medium-dose (24.17 ± 5.09, pmol/L) and low-dose (18.78 ± 4.56, pmol/L) groups ($P > 0.05$)(Table 2-2).

Table 2-2   The levels of fasting blood glucose (FBG) in the experiment (mean ± SD)

Groups	n	Kelp dose	FBG/(mmol/L)			Insulin/(pmol/L)
			Before modeled	Before treated	After treated	
Control group	10	General forage	4.78 ± 0.39	4.95 ± 0.34	4.97 ± 0.33	71.38 ± 15.26
Model group	10	General forage	4.82 ± 0.33	17.86 ± 2.26^a	13.32 ± 1.40^b	11.23 ± 3.45
Low group	10	1.25 g/kg	4.55 ± 0.35	18.12 ± 2.28^a	12.63 ± 1.67^b	18.78 ± 4.56^c
Medium group	10	5.00 g/kg	4.81 ± 0.37	17.79 ± 2.31^a	$9.37 \pm 1.70^{b, c, d}$	24.17 ± 5.09^c
High group	10	12.50 g/kg	4.65 ± 0.34	18.05 ± 2.35^a	$9.18 \pm 1.65^{b, c, d}$	26.22 ± 4.85^c

[a] $P < 0.05$ *vs* before modeled; [b] $P < 0.05$ *vs* before treated; [c] $P < 0.05$ *vs* model group; [d] $P < 0.05$ *vs* low group.

2.4 The levels of MDA and NO and the activities of SOD and GSH-Px

Serum levels of MDA and NO were significantly higher and actions of SOD and GSH-Px were sharply lower in the DM-model rats and kelp-treaded groups than those in the control group ($F = 12.60$, $q = 3.72 \sim 7.17$, $P < 0.05$). MDA and NO serum levels were significantly lower and actions of SOD and GSH-Px were higher in medium-dose and high-dose groups than those in DM-model groups ($P < 0.05$). There was no significant difference between the medium-dose and high-dose groups ($P > 0.05$). Results indicated that medium-dose kelp could achieve on ideal anti-oxidant effect (Table 2-3).

Table 2-3 The levels of MDA and NO and the activities of SOD and GSH-Px in the experiment (mean ± SD)

Groups	n	Kelp dose	MDA/ (mmol/L)	NO/ (μmol/L)	SOD/ (U/mL)	GSH-Px/ (U/mL)
Control group	10	General forage	7.15 ± 0.68	14.96 ± 1.56	156 ± 14.02	922 ± 22.16
Model group	10	General forage	9.38 ± 1.24[a]	23.86 ± 2.17[a]	122 ± 11.26[a]	828 ± 15.46[a]
Low group	10	1.25 g/kg	8.93 ± 1.02	21.50 ± 2.24	127 ± 18.35	837 ± 24.82
Medium group	10	5.00 g/kg	8.02 ± 0.45[b,c]	17.13 ± 1.41[b,c]	143 ± 22.26[b,c]	890 ± 24.58[b,c]
High group	10	12.50 g/kg	7.83 ± 0.51[b,c]	16.32 ± 1.73[b,c]	145 ± 19.38[b,c]	886 ± 25.72[b,c]

[a]$P < 0.05$ vs control group; [b]$P < 0.05$ vs model group; [c]$P < 0.05$ vs low group.

2.5 Pancreatic islets tissue pathology

The cells of pancreatic islets in the control group are oval in shape, uniform in size and evenly dispersed in the pancreatic gland bubble. DM-model rats have shrunken islets, a reduced number of islet cells that are unevenly dispersed, vacuolar degeneration and karyolysis, etc., but this improved significantly in the medium-dose and high-dose kelp-treated groups. The index of pancreatic B cells in the medium-dose and high-doses kelp-treated groups is higher than those in the DM-model rats (Table 2-4).

Table 2-4 The B cell index and the expressions of SOD and iNOS in the pancreatic tissue (mean ± SD)

Groups	n	Kelp dose	B cell index/%	SOD (A)	iNOS (A)
Control group	10	General forage	61.48 ± 9.13	0.48 ± 0.15	0.16 ± 0.05
Model group	10	General forage	28.16 ± 5.64[a]	0.18 ± 0.06[a]	0.41 ± 0.12[a]
Low group	10	1.25 g/kg	31.49 ± 6.28	0.22 ± 0.08	0.35 ± 0.10
Medium group	10	5.00 g/kg	45.37 ± 6.82[b]	0.31 ± 0.10[b]	0.24 ± 0.09[b]
High group	10	12.50 g/kg	46.71 ± 7.36[b]	0.33 ± 0.12[b]	0.23 ± 0.08[b]

[a]$P < 0.05$ vs control group; [b]$P < 0.05$ vs model group.

2.6 Immunohistochemistry of SOD and iNOS

SOD expression in pancreatic islet cells of the control group rats was strong and scattered focally with deep-yellow color. SOD expression was reduced in the DM-model rats ($t = 7.89$, $P < 0.05$). In medium-dose and high-dose kelp-treated group rats, SOD expression in islet cells was stronger than that in DM-model rats ($t = 4.73 \sim 4.76$, $P < 0.05$). There was no significant difference between the low-dose kelp-treated group and the DM-model rats ($t = 1.69$, $P > 0.05$). (Table 2-4 and Figure 2-1).

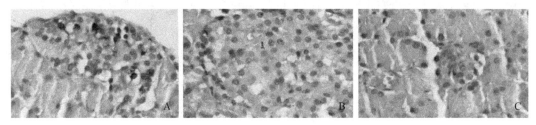

Figure 2-1   The expression of inducible nitric oxide synthase (iNOS) in the pancreatic islet cells

SABC × 400, bar 25 μm. A: Control group, B: DM-model group, C: Medium-dose kelp-treated group.

iNOS expression in pancreatic islet cells of the control group rats was weak and scattered focally with light-yellow color and was significantly stronger in DM-model rats ($t = 8.16$, $P < 0.05$). In medium-dose and high-dose kelp treated group rats, iNOS expression in islet cells was weaker than that in the DM-model rats ($t = 4.81 \sim 5.30$, $P < 0.05$). There was no significant difference between the low-dose kelp treated group and the DM-model rats ($t = 1.90$, $P > 0.05$) (Table 2-4 and Figure 2-2).

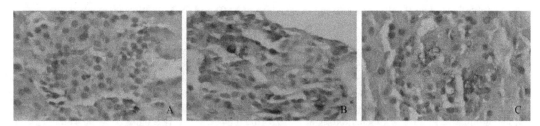

Figure 2-2   The expression of superoxide dismutase (SOD) in the pancreatic islet cells

SABC × 400, bar 25 μm. A: Control group, B: DM-model group, C: Medium-dose kelp-treated group.

2.7 Discussion

Hyperglycemia and oxidative stress are closely related to diabetes mellitus and its complications. The common soil theory of Ceriello et al. [15-16] holds that oxidative stress is a common feature of insulin resistance, diabetes mellitus and cerebrovascular diseases [17]. In a body suffering from various harmful stimuli, there is an increase in free radicals, and decreased elimination of those radicals can upset the balance of the oxidation system and antioxidant system, and damage tissues and function [18-19]. At the same time, an overflow of oxygen free radicals (OFR) causes lipid peroxidation (LPO), which increases the damage of the oxidative stress through a chain reaction [20-21]. Diabetes mellitus patients with long-term hyperglycemia produce more OFR due to increased glucose autoxidation and protein saccharification, which weakens oxidation resistance and initiates oxidation stress [22]. Increased OFR plays an important role in initiating type 2 diabetes mellitus, insulin resistance and secondary effects, and the islet beta cell function obstacle. It becomes an important media for various factors that cause type 2 diabetes mellitus [23].

Alloxan has a specific toxic effect on islet beta cells that can cause damage by producing a superoxide radical, damage the DNA of the cell and activate polyphosphate ADP ribosomes synthase. This can reduce the coenzyme I, impair mRNA function and cause proinsulin decrease and insulin shortage [24]. In the process of diabetes mellitus development, the anti-oxidant defense level drops and the ability to eliminate free radicals weakens [25-26]. Bottino et al. [27] separated and purified islet cells by using an anti-oxidant to disrupt islet cells at an early stage and found that if blocking oxidative stress reduces damage to the islet cells and promotes their proliferation, it provides a new way of thinking about early diagnosis and intervention for diabetes mellitus. Our previous researches confirmed that kelp has antioxidant effects on the organism and can improve the oxidative stress [12,13].

In this experiment, the serum MDA and NO content in DM-model rats were significantly higher than those in the control group. The action of serum SOD and GSH-Px in DM-model rats was significantly less than that in the control group. At the same time, SOD expression in pancreatic islet cells in the DM-model rats was significantly lower and iNOS expression was higher than that in the control group. The number of islet cells and beta cells reduced significantly and became partly pyknotic and there was necrosis related to a decrease in serum insulin levels as well as increases in fasting blood glucose levels. Such features indicate that diabetes mellitus models, induced by alloxan, caused much lipid peroxidation in the rat body, injured the structure and secretion function of the islet cells and increased fasting blood glucose levels.

After kelp powder was added to interfere with the diabetes mellitus models induced by alloxan, serum levels of MDA and NO decreased significantly, and the actions of serum SOD and GSH-Px increased in comparison with the DM-model group. Immunochemical stain showed that SOD expression in pancreatic islet cells was significantly higher and iNOS expression was lower than that in the DM-model group. The structure of the pancreatic islet cells in kelp powder treated groups clearly improved in comparison with the DM-model group. Apparently, kelp enhances anti-oxidant enzyme activity, reduces lipid peroxidation (LPO), products induced by diabetes mellitus and shows an antioxidant effect in the organism. Changes in fasting blood glucose (FBG) levels, serum insulin levels and animal weights show that FBG levels in kelp powder treated groups were significantly lower than those in the DM-model group, while serum insulin levels and animal weights were higher than those in the DM-model group. Results indicate that kelp could play a hypoglycemic role by enhancing anti-oxidation and enabling recovery of the pancreatic islet cell secreting function.

3 Experimental section

3.1 The creation of diabetic models

Sixty SPF grade healthy male Wistar rats weighing 140 ~ 160 g were purchased from the Experiment Animal Center of Qingdao Drug Inspection Institute [SCXK (LU) 20090100]. Local regulations related to ethical experimentation on animals and guidelines for the care and use of laboratory animals were followed in all animal procedures in this experiment. This experiment was approved by the Ethics Committee of Qingdao University Medical College (No. QUMC 2011-09). Animals were acclimatized for seven days and allowed free access to food and water at room temperature [(23 ± 2)°C] and humidity-controlled housing with natural illumination. Initially, an extracted blood sample (0.5 mL) from the tail vein was used for the serum separation and determination of fasting blood glucose (FBG) levels. Subsequently, ten (n = 10) experimental animals were randomized as a control group and injected with equivalent normal saline and the remaining fifty rats were injected intraperitoneally (i.p.) with 1.5% alloxan (100 mg/kg body weight), once every three days and three times continuously [28-29]. Three days after the final injection, the FBG level was determined and FBG > 15.00 mmol/L served as the standard in successful diabetes mellitus (DM) models. Ten of the fifty experimental rats were excluded because they did not satisfy the standard. The remaining forty DM-model rats were subjected to experiment and randomly divided into a DM-model group (n = 10), and three kelp treated groups: a low-dose group (1.25 g/kg, n = 10), a medium-dose group (5.0 g/kg, n = 10) and a high-dose group (12.5 g/kg, n = 10).

3.2 The general forage and kelp powder forage

The main components of the general forage: soybean meal 20.4%, corn flour 31.7%, wheat bran 7.2%, wheat flour 28.8%, fish meal 7.2%, yeast 2.4%, salt 0.2%, bone meal 1.4%, cod liver oil 0.04%, Vitamin E powder 0.04%, milk powder 0.18%, and trace elements 0.04%.

"Zhongke No. 1" kelp powder forage is derived from kelp products manufactured at the Institute of Oceanology, Chinese Academy of Sciences. Chemical analysis shows the main components to be dietary fiber 26.1%, protein 8.5%, lipid 0.39%, total amino acid 10.49

mg/100g, Vitamin A 273 μg/100g, and Vitamin C 3 μg/100g.

The kelp powder forage used as an ingredient in the feed for the rats was pressed into a block, air dried and reserved. The low-dose forage contains general forage 97.5% and kelp powder 2.5%, the medium-dose forage contains general forage 90% and kelp powder 10%, and the high-dose forage contains general forage 75% and kelp powder 25%.

3.3 Inference of tests

Rats in the control group and the DM-model group were fed with general forage for two weeks. Rats in the kelp-treated groups were fed with kelp powder forage for two weeks.

The low-dose kelp powder (2.5%) equals 1.25 g/kg body weight per day, the medium-does kelp powder (10%) equals 5.0 g/kg body weight per day and the high-dose kelp powder (25%) equals 12.5 g/kg body weight per day.

3.4 Preparation of samples

3.4.1 Serum preparation

At the end of this experiment, all rats were denied food for 12 h, then FBG was determined and 4 mL blood was collected from the eye artery using heparinized capillary tubes. Blood samples were centrifuged for 10 minutes at 4000 r/min to separate serum and then stored at −20 °C.

3.4.2 Pancreatic tissue

At the end of this experiment, animals were sacrificed by cervical dislocation and pancreatic tissues were immediately collected. Rudimental blood was fully washed with normal saline at −4 °C, and placed in 4% formaldehyde for fixing.

3.5 Index of determinations

3.5.1 FBG level

An automatic blood glucose meter (Johnson & Johnson Medical Equipment Co., Ltd., Germany) and blood glucose test strips (Onetouch, Ultra) were used to detect FBG level (mmol/ L).

3.5.2 The serum level of insulin

Serum samples were thawed at room temperature and centrifuged again. Electrochemiluminescence immunoassay (ECLIA) was applied to determine the serum level of insulin with Elecsys 2010 and Cobase 411 analyzers and Roche diagnostics reagent kits (12017547). All standards were prepared before starting the assay procedure. The first incubation: insulin from 20 μL serum sample, a biotinylated monoclonal insulin-specific antibody, and a monoclonal insulin-specific antibody labeled with a ruthenium complex form a sandwich complex. The second incubation: after addition of streptavidin-coated microparticles, the complex becomes bound to the solid phase via interaction of biotin and strepavidin. Then the reaction mixture is aspirated into the measuring cell where the microparticles are magnetically captured onto the surface of the electrode. Unbound substances are then removed with ProCell. A voltage is applied to the electrode to induce chemiluminescent emission which is measured by a photomultiplier. The results are determined via a calibration curve which is instrument-specifically generated by 2-point calibration and a master curve provided via the reagent barcode. Finally, the analyzer automatically calculates the analyte concentration of each sample. The measuring range of the assay is 1.39 ~ 6945 pmol/L.

3.5.3　MDA and NO values

MDA values were detected by thiobarbituric acid and NO values were detected by nitratase reductase using kits purchased from Jiancheng Institute of Biomedical Technology, Nanjing, China. Standardization was conducted on an ultraviolet spectrophotometer (Bechmann DU640, USA) and the selected wavelengths were 532 nm for MDA and 550 nm for NO. Assay sensitivity is 0.1 mmol/L (MDA) and 0.1 μmol/L (NO).

3.5.4　SOD and GSH-Px activities

SOD action was detected by xanthinoxidase and GSH-Px action was detected by chemical colorimetry with kits supplied by Jiancheng Institute of Biomedical Technology, Nanjing, China. Standardization was conducted on an ultraviolet spectrophotometer and the selected wavelengths were 550 nm for SOD and 412 nm for GSH-Px. Assay sensitivity is 0.1 U/mL (SOD and GSH-Px).

3.5.5　Histopathological assay

Pancreatic tissue samples fixed in 4% formaldehyde were gradually dehydrated in alcohol, hyalinized by dimethylbenzene, embedded in paraffin, sectioned at a thickness of 5 μm, adhered to sections prepared with poly-L-Lysine and stored at 4 °C. Paraffin sections were deparaffinized by dimethylbenzene, hydrated in gradient ethanol washed with distilled water and stained by Hematoxylin-Eosin (HE) staining that showed nuclei with a blue color and cytoplasm with a red color under light microscopy. Under a 400-fold light microscope, the average index of pancreatic B cells was calculated in five views selected randomly in each section from each animal. Index of pancreatic B cell in each view = (the number of pancreatic islets B cells/total number of cells) × 100.

3.5.6　Immunohistochemical assay

Rabbit anti-rat SOD and iNOS multiclonal antibody, and strept actividin-biotin peroxidase complex (SABC) kit, diaminobenzidine (DAB) kit were supplied by Wuhan Boster Biological Technology Co. Ltd., China. Paraffin-embedded sections were deparaffinated in dimethylbenzene, hydrated successively in gradient ethanol and antigen was restored twice in a microwave oven. All procedures were strictly performed in accordance with the manufacturers' directions. Under a microscope, cells with brown granulation in cytoplasm or nucleus were considered to be positive. Negative control slides added 0.01 mol/L PBS (containing 1 : 200

blocking serum of non-immunized animals) instead of a primary antibody that has no immunological reaction. Under a 400× light microscope, five sections were randomly chosen from each experimental rat and observed in five views detected in islets. Absorbance values (*A*) of each view were detected by a LEICA QWin microgramme analytical system (Leica Company, Shanghai, China).

3.6　Statistical analysis

SPSS17.0 software was used for statistical analysis. Data were expressed as mean ± standard deviation (mean ± SD). Multi-group comparison was made by the analysis of variance (ANOVA) and students' test, and two-group comparison was by *t*-test. Values were considered to be significant when $P < 0.05$.

4　Conclusions

This study suggested that kelp might enable the recovery of islet cell secretion function and reduce the FBG level by an antioxidant effect. Future researches should focus on the hypoglycemic effect and the mechanism of kelp.

Acknowledgement

This study was supported by the National Natural Science Foundation of China (No. 40976085) and Key Projects in the National Science & Technology Pillar Program during the Twelve Five-Year Plan Period.

Conflict of Interest

This article does not compromise our adherence to *Int. J. Mol. Sci.* policies on sharing data and materials.

References

[1]　Shih C C, Wu Y W, Lin W C. Antihyperglycaemic and anti-oxidant properties of Anoectochilus formosanus in diabetic rats. Clinical & Experimental Pharmacology & Physiology, 2002, 29(8): 684-688.

[2]　Surapaneni K M, Venkataramana G. Status of lipid peroxidation, glutathione, ascorbic acid, vitamin E and antioxidant enzymes in patients with osteoarthritis. Indian Journal of Medical Sciences, 2007, 61(1): 284.

[3]　Bian K, Ke Y, Kamisaki Y, et al. Proteomic modification by nitric oxide. Japanese Journal of

Pharmacology, 2006, 101(4): 271.

[4]　Challa S R, Akula A, Metla S, et al. Partial role of nitric oxide in infarct size limiting effect of quercetin and rutin against ischemia-reperfusion injury in normal and diabetic rats. Indian Journal of Experimental Biology, 2011, 49(3): 207-210.

[5]　Aguilar A, Alvarez-Vijande R, Capdevila S, et al. Antioxidant patterns (superoxide dismutase, glutathione reductase, and glutathione peroxidase) in kidneys from non-heart-beating-donors: experimental study. Transplantation Proceedings, 2007, 39(1): 249-252.

[6]　Chung S S, Min K, Youn B S, et al. Glutathione peroxidase mediates the antioxidant effect of peroxisome proliferator-activated receptor in human skeletal muscle cells. Molecular & Cellular Biology, 2008, 29(1): 20-30.

[7]　Tseng C K. Algal biotechnology industries and research activities in China. Journal of Applied Phycology, 2001, 13(4): 375-380.

[8]　Huang L, Guo H W, Huang Z Y, et al. The association of Lipoprotein lipase gene polymorphism with hyperlipidemia and dietary predisposition of obesity. Acta Nutrimenta Sinica, 2007, 29(3): 228-231.

[9]　Chinese Pharmcopoeia Commission. Chinese Pharmacopoeia: Part I. Beijing: Chemical Industry Press, 2000.

[10]　Zhu L, Zhang Q, Wang Y F, et al. Determination of polysaccharide from Ecklonia kurome. Chinese Journal of Marine Drugs, 2005, 24: 47-48.

[11]　Zhou Q F, Li M Y, Na G S, et al. Progress in research of antitumor mechanisms of marine polysaccharides. Chinese Pharmacological Bulletin, 2009, 25(8): 995-997.

[12]　Ying X X, Li S, Liang G Y, et al. Regulating effects and mechanism of Laminaria japonica on serum lipid of hyperlipidemia rats. Chinese Journal of Marine Drugs, 2009, 28: 1-4.

[13]　Li S, Ying X X, Liang G Y, et al. Study on the antioxidant effects of Laminaria japonica in hyperlipemia rats. Chinese Journal of Marine Drugs, 2010, 29: 1-4.

[14]　Wang T X, Pang J.H. Study on the hypoglycemic and hypolipidemic effect of Laminarina japonica polysaccharides. Acta Nutr. Sin., 2007, 29: 99-100.

[15]　Ceriello A, Motz E. Is oxidative stress the pathogenic mechanism underlying insulin resistance, diabetes, and cardiovascular disease? The common soil hypothesis revisited. Arteriosclerosis Thrombosis & Vascular Biology, 2004, 24(5): 816.

[16]　Capellini V K, Baldo C F, Celotto A C, et al. Oxidative stress is not associated with vascular dysfunction in a model of alloxan-induced diabetic rats. Arquivos Brasileiros De Endocrinologia E Metabologia, 2010, 54(6): 530.

[17]　Vanguilder H D, Bixler G V, Kutzler L, et al. Multi-modal proteomic analysis of retinal protein expression alterations in a rat model of diabetic retinopathy. Plos One, 2011, 6(1): e16271.

[18]　Mircescu G. Oxidative stress: an accomplice to uremic toxicity. Journal of Renal Nutrition, 2006, 16(3): 194-198.

[19]　Lushchak V I. Free radical oxidation of proteins and its relationship with functional state of organisms.

Biochemistry, 2007, 72(8): 809-827.

[20]　Zhou T, Zhou K K, Lee K, et al. The role of lipid peroxidation products and oxidative stress in activation of the canonical wingless-type MMTV integration site (WNT) pathway in a rat model of diabetic retinopathy. Diabetologia, 2011, 54(2): 459-468.

[21]　Chaiyasut C, Kusirisin W, Lailerd N, et al. Effects of phenolic compounds of fermented indigenous plants on oxidative stress in streptozotocin-induced diabetic rats. Evidence-Based Complementray and Alternative Medicine, 2011, 11(9): 74-77.

[22]　Kröncke K D, Fehsel K, Suschek C, et al. Inducible nitric oxide synthase-derived nitric oxide in gene regulation, cell death and cell survival. International Immunopharmacology, 2001, 1(8): 1407-1420.

[23]　Chapman J, Miles P D, Ofrecio J M, et al. Osteopontin is required for the early onset of high fat diet-induced insulin resistance in mice. Plos One, 2010, 5(11): e13959.

[24]　Soto C, Pérez J, García V, et al. Effect of silymarin on kidneys of rats suffering from alloxan-induced diabetes mellitus. Phytomedicine, 2010, 17(14): 1090-1094.

[25]　Silva K C, Rosales M A, Biswas S K, et al. Diabetic retinal neurodegeneration is associated with mitochondrial oxidative stress and is improved by an angiotensin receptor blocker in a model combining hypertension and diabetes. Diabetes, 2009, 58: 1382-1390.

[26]　Ouslimani N, Peynet J, Bonnefont-Rousselot D, et al. Metformin decreases intracellular production of reactive oxygen species in aortic endothelial cells. Metabolism-clinical & Experimental, 2005, 54(6): 829-834.

[27]　Bottino R, Balamurugan A N, Tse H, et al. Response of human islets to isolation stress and the effect of antioxidant treatment. Diabetes, 2004, 53(10): 2559.

[28]　Liu L P, Huang J, Chen B L, et al. Research on the hypoglycemic effection of marine alga Porphyridium cruentum in experimental diabetic mice. Chinese Journal of Marine Drugs, 2005, 24: 18-20.

[29]　Owu D U, Antai A B, Udofia K H, et al. Vitamin C improves basal metabolic rate and lipid profile in alloxan-induced diabetes mellitus in rats. Journal of Biosciences, 2006, 31(5): 575-579.

Section 4　Words of TCM

1. 百家学说 schools of various medical thoughts
2. 阴阳学说 theory of yin-yang
3. 五行学说 theory of five elements
4. 藏象学说 theory of visceral manifestation
5. 经络学说 theory of meridian and collateral; meridian doctrine
6. 精 jing (as the world origin in ancient philosophy); essence
7. 气 qi (as the world origin in ancient philosophy); energy

8. 气化学说 theory of qi transformation

9. 精气学说 theory of jing and qi (in ancient philosophy)

10. 病因病机学说 theory of etiology and pathology

11. 水地说 hypothesis of jing originating from water and earth

12. 云气说 hypothesis of qi originating from cloud and air

13. 气一元论 / 元气一元论 monism of qi

14. 同病异治 different treatments for the same disease

15. 异病同治 the same treatment for different diseases

16. 因地制宜 environment-concerned treatment

17. 因时制宜 climate-concerned treatment

18. 因人制宜 individuality-concerned treatment

19. 五脏六腑 five zang-organs and six fu-organs

20. 奇恒之腑 extraordinary fu-organs

21. 温养脏腑 warming and nourishing zang-organs and fu-organs

22. 先天禀赋，精微物质 inheritance, essential substance

23. 形神合一 harmonization between soma and spirit

24. 形神统一 unity of body and spirit

25. 形与神俱 inseparability of body and spirit

26. 神色形态 spirit, complexion and physical build

27. 元神之府 mentality house

28. 脑为髓海 brain being marrow sea

29. 髓海不足 insufficiency of marrow sea

30. 精神萎靡 dispiritedness; listlessness; lower spirit

31. 醒脑开窍 consciousness restore resuscitate

32. 神明，失神 mental activities, depletion of spirit

33. 心藏神 heart storing spirit

34. 调摄精神 regulating mental states

35. 安神醒脑法 mind-tranquilizing and brain-refreshing manipulation

36. 健脑益智法 mind-invigorating manipulation for improving intelligence

37. 养心益神法 heart-nourishing and mind-benefiting manipulation

38. 延年益寿 prolonging life; promising longevity

39. 调心调身法 mind-regulating and body-regulating methods

40. 调息法 respiration-regulating methods

(Guo Yunliang, Zhang Rui)

Chapter 3   Renal Diseases

Section 1   Kidney Stones

The existence of kidney stones was first recorded thousands of years ago, and lithotomy for the removal of stones is one of the earliest known surgical procedures. In 1901, a stone discovered in the pelvis of an ancient Egyptian mummy was dated to 4800 BC. Medical texts from ancient Mesopotamia, India, China, Persia, Greece and Rome all mentioned calculous disease. Part of the *Hippocratic Oath* suggests there were practicing surgeons in ancient Greece to whom physicians were to defer for lithotomies. The Roman medical treatise *De Medicina* by Aulus Cornelius Celsus contained a description of lithotomy, and this work served as the basis for this procedure until the 18th century.

New techniques in lithotomy began to emerge in 1520, but the operation remained risky. After Henry Jacob Bigelow popularized the technique of litholapaxy in 1878, the mortality rate dropped from about 24% to 2.4%. However, other treatment techniques continued to produce a high level of mortality, especially among inexperienced urologists. In 1980, Dornier MedTech introduced extracorporeal shock wave lithotripsy for breaking up stones via acoustical pulses, and this technique has since come into widespread use.

Kidney stones affect all geographical, cultural and racial groups.The lifetime risk is about 10% ~ 15% in the developed world, but can be as high as 20% ~ 25% in the Middle East. The increased risk of dehydration in hot climates, coupled with a diet 50% lower in calcium and 250% higher in oxalates compared to western diets, accounts for the higher net risk in the Middle East. In the Middle East, uric acid stones are more common than calcium-containing stones. The number of deaths due to kidney stones is estimated at 19 000 per year being fairly consistent between 1990 and 2010.

In North America and Europe, the annual number of new cases per year of kidney stones is roughly 0.5%. In the United States, the frequency in the population of urolithiasis has increased from 3.2% to 5.2% from the mid-1970s to the mid-1990s. In the United States, about 9% of the population has had a kidney stone.

The total cost for treating urolithiasis was 2 billion US$ in 2003. About 65% to 80% of those with kidney stones are men; most stones in women are due to either metabolic defects (such as cystinuria) or infection. Men most commonly experience their first episode between

30 and 40 years of age, whereas for women, the age at first presentation is somewhat later. The age of onset shows a bimodal distribution in women, with episodes peaking at 35 and 55 years. Recurrence rates are estimated at 50% over a 10-year and 75% over a 20-year period, with some people experiencing ten or more episodes over the course of a lifetime.

Kidney stones are often present with acute renal colic and diagnosed basically on symptomatology and diagnostic tests, which include urinalysis, abdominal radiology and excretory urography. Urinalysis provides information related to hematuria, infection, the presence of stone-forming crystals and urine pH. At least 90% of stones are radiopaque and are readily visible on a plain film of the abdomen. Excretory urography uses a contrast medium that is filtered in the glomeruli to visualize the collecting system of the kidneys and the ureters. Retrograde urography, ultrasonography, computer tomography (CT) scanning and magnetic resonance imaging may also be used.

Treatment of acute renal colic usually is supportive. Pain relief may be needed during acute phases of obstruction, and antibiotic therapy may be necessary to treat urinary infections. Most stones that are less than 5 mm in diameter pass spontaneously. All urine should be strained during an attack in the hope of retrieving the stone for chemical analysis and determination of type. This information, along with a careful history and laboratory tests, affords the basis for long-term preventive measures.

A major goal of treatment in people who have passed kidney stones or have had them removed is to prevent their recurrence. Prevention requires investigation into the cause of stone formation by using urine tests, blood chemistries and stone analysis. Underlying disease conditions, such as hyper-parathyroidism, are treated. Adequate fluid intake reduces the saturation of stone-forming crystals and needs to be encouraged. Depending on the type of stone formed, dietary changes or medications or both may be used to alter the concentration of stone-forming elements in the urine. For example, people who form calcium oxalate stones may need to decrease their intake of foods that are high in oxalate. Thiazide diuretics lower urinary calcium excretion by increasing the fractional absorption of calcium and reducing intestinal calcium absorption. Measures to change the pH of urine can also influence kidney stone formation. In people who lose the ability to lower the pH of their urine or acidify their urine, there is an increase in the divalent and trivalent forms of urine phosphate that combines with calcium to form calcium phosphate stones. The formation of uric acid stones, on the other hand, is increased in acid urine; stone formation can be reduced by raising the pH of urine to $6.0 \sim 6.5$ with potassium alkali salts.

It is necessary to remove the kidney stone in some cases. There are several methods available for removal of kidney stones: ureteroscopic removal, percutaneous removal and extracorporeal lithotripsy. All these procedures eliminate the need for an open surgical procedure, which is another form of treatment. Struvite stones cannot be passed and require removal; extracorporeal lithotripsy and percutaneous removal can be used to reduce the damage incurred by these stones.

Ureteroscopic removal involves the passage of an instrument through the urethra into the bladder and then into the ureter. The development of high quality optics has improved both the ease with which this procedure is performed and its outcome. The procedure, which is performed under fluoroscopic guidance, involves the use of various instruments for dilating the ureter and for grasping and removing the stone. Preprocedure radiologic studies using a contrast medium (excretory urography) are done to determine the position of the stone and direct the placement of the ureteroscope.

Percutaneous nephrostomy involves the insertion through the flank of a small-gauge needle into the collecting system of the kidney; the needle tract is then dilated, and an instrument called a nephroscope is inserted into the renal pelvis. The procedure is performed under fluoroscopic guidance. Preprocedure radiologic and ultrasound examinations of the kidney and ureter are used in determining the placement of the nephroscope. Stones up to 1.0 cm can be removed through this method. Larger stones must be broken up with an electrohydraulic or ultrasonic lithotripter (stone-breaker).

A nonsurgical treatment called extracorporeal shock wave lithotripsy has been applied for treatment of stones primarily in the renal calix and pelvis and the upper third of the ureter. The procedure uses acoustic shock waves to fragment calculi into sand-like particles that are passed in the urine over the next few days. Because of the large amount of stone particles that are generated during the procedure, a ureteral catheter may be inserted to ensure adequate urine drainage. The catheter may be left in place for several weeks, depending on the stone burden and likelihood of ureteral obstruction.

Section 2   Interstitial Nephritis

Interstitial nephritis or tubulo-interstitial nephritis is a form of nephritis affecting the interstitium of the kidneys surrounding the tubules, i.e., is inflammation of the spaces between renal tubules. This disease can be either acute, meaning it occurs suddenly, or chronic, meaning it is ongoing and eventually ends in kidney failure.

1   Causes of Interstitial Nephritis

Common causes include infection, or reaction to medication such as an analgesic or antibiotics such as methicillin (meticillin). Reaction to medications causes 71% to 92% of cases. This disease is also caused by other diseases and toxins that damage the kidney. Both acute and chronic tubulo-interstitial nephritis can be caused by a bacterial infection in the kidneys known as pyelonephritis, but the most common cause is by an adverse reaction to a medication. The medications that are known to cause this sort of reaction are β-lactam antibiotics such as penicillin and cephalexin, and nonsteroidal anti-inflammatory drugs (aspirin less frequently than others), as well as proton-pump inhibitors, rifampicin, sulfa medications, fluoroquinolones, diuretics, allopurinol, mesalamine, and phenytoin. The time between exposure to the drug and the development of acute tubulo-interstitial nephritis can be anywhere from 5 days to 5 months (fenoprofen-induced).

2　Diagnosis of Interstitial Nephritis

At times, there are no symptoms of this disease, but when they do occur they are widely varied and can occur rapidly or gradually. When caused by an allergic reaction, the symptoms of acute tubulo-interstitial nephritis are fever (27% of patients), rash (15% of patients), and enlarged kidneys. Some people experience dysuria, and lower back pain. In chronic tubulo-interstitial nephritis the patient can experience symptoms such as nausea, vomiting, fatigue, and weight loss. Other conditions that may develop include a high concentration of potassium in the blood, metabolic acidosis, and kidney failure.

Blood tests: About 23% of patients have a high level of eosinophils in the blood.

Urinary findings: Urinary findings include: (1) eosinophiluria: original studies with methicillin-induced AIN showed sensitivity of 67% and specificity of 83%. The sensitivity is higher in patients with interstitial nephritis induced by methicillin or when the Hansel's stain is used. However, a 2013 study showed that the sensitivity and specificity of urine eosinophil testing are 35.6% and 68% respectively; (2) isosthenuria; (3) blood in the urine and occasional RBC casts; (4) sterile pyuria: white blood cells and no bacteria. Nephrotic-range amount of protein in the urine may be seen with NSAID-associated AIN.

Gallium scan: The sensitivity of an abnormal gallium scan has been reported to range from 60% to 100%.

3　Treatment of Interstitial Nephritis

Treatment consists of addressing the cause, such as by removing an offending drug. There is no clear evidence that corticosteroids help. Nutrition therapy consists of adequate fluid intake, which can require several liters of extra fluid.

4　Prognosis of Interstitial Nephritis

The kidneys are the only body system that is directly affected by tubulo-interstitial nephritis. Kidney function is usually reduced; the kidneys can be just slightly dysfunctional, or fail completely.

In chronic tubulo-interstitial nephritis, the most serious long-term effect is kidney failure. When the proximal tubule is injured, sodium, potassium, bicarbonate, uric acid, and phosphate reabsorption may be reduced or changed, resulting in low bicarbonate, known as metabolic acidosis, low potassium, low uric acid known as hypouricemia, and low phosphate known as hypophosphatemia. Damage to the distal tubule may cause loss of urine-concentrating ability and polyuria.

In most cases of acute tubulo-interstitial nephritis, the function of the kidneys will return after the harmful drug is not taken anymore, or when the underlying disease is cured by treatment. If the illness is caused by an allergic reaction, a corticosteroid may speed the recovery kidney function; however, this is often not the case.

Chronic tubulo-interstitial nephritis has no cure. Some patients may require dialysis. Eventually, a kidney transplant may be needed.

Section 3   Research Article

The risk factors and pathological mechanism and the treatment of kidney stone disease

Kidney stone disease, also known as urolithiasis, is when a solid piece of material (kidney stone) occurs in the urinary tract. Kidney stones typically form in the kidney and leave the body in the urine stream. A small stone may pass without causing symptoms. If a stone grows to more than 5 mm (0.2 in) it can cause blockage of the ureter resulting in severe pain in the lower back or abdomen. A stone may also result in blood in the urine, vomiting, or painful urination. About half of people will have another stone within ten years.

Most stones form due to a combination of genetics and environmental factors. Risk factors include high urine calcium levels, obesity, certain foods, some medications, calcium supplements, hyperparathyroidism, gout and not drinking enough fluids. Stones form in the kidney when minerals in urine are at high concentration. The diagnosis is usually based on symptoms, urine testing, and medical imaging. Blood tests may also be useful. Stones are typically classified by their location (nephrolithiasis in the kidney, ureterolithiasis in the ureter, cystolithiasis in the bladder), or by what they are made of (calcium oxalate, uric acid, struvite, cystine).

In those who have had stones, prevention is by drinking fluids so that more than two liters of urine are produced per day. If this is not effective enough, thiazide diuretic, citrate, or allopurinol may be taken. It is recommended that soft drinks containing phosphoric acid (typically colas) be avoided. When a stone causes no symptoms, no treatment is needed. Otherwise pain control is usually the first measure, using medications such as nonsteroidal anti-inflammatory drugs or opioids. Larger stones may be helped to pass with the medication tamsulosin or may require procedures such as extracorporeal shock wave lithotripsy, ureteroscopy or percutaneous nephrolithotomy.

Between 1% and 15% of people globally are affected by kidney stones at some point in their life. In 2015, 22.1 million cases occurred, resulting in about 16 100 deaths. They have become more common in the western world since the 1970s. Generally, more men are affected than women. Kidney stones have affected humans throughout history with descriptions of surgery to remove them dating from as early as 600 BC.

1   Signs and symptoms

The hallmark of a stone that obstructs the ureter or renal pelvis is excruciating, intermittent pain that radiates from the flank to the groin or to the inner thigh. This pain, known as renal colic, is often described as one of the strongest pain sensations known. Renal colic caused by kidney stones is commonly accompanied by urinary urgency, restlessness, hematuria, sweating, nausea and vomiting. It typically comes in waves lasting 20 to 60 minutes caused by peristaltic contractions of the ureter as it attempts to expel the stone.

The embryological link between the urinary tract, the genital system, and the gastrointestinal tract is the basis of the radiation of pain to the gonads, as well as the nausea and vomiting that are also common in urolithiasis. Postrenal azotemia and hydronephrosis can be observed following the obstruction of urine flow through one ureter or both ureters.

Pain in the lower-left quadrant can sometimes be confused with diverticulitis because the sigmoid colon overlaps the ureter, and the exact location of the pain may be difficult to isolate due to the close proximity of these two structures.

2   Risk factors

Dehydration from low fluid intake is a major factor in stone formation. Obesity is a leading risk factor as well.

High dietary intake of animal protein, sodium, sugars including honey, refined sugars, fructose and high fructose corn syrup, oxalate, grapefruit juice, and apple juice may increase the risk of kidney stone formation.

Kidney stones can result from an underlying metabolic condition, such as distal renal tubular acidosis, Dent's disease, hyperparathyroidism, primary hyperoxaluria, or medullary sponge kidney. 3% ~ 20% of people who form kidney stones have medullary sponge kidney.

Kidney stones are more common in people with Crohn's disease; Crohn's disease is associated with hyperoxaluria and malabsorption of magnesium.

A person with recurrent kidney stones may be screened for such disorders. This is typically done with a 24-hour urine collection. The urine is analyzed for features that promote stone formation.

Calcium oxalate: Calcium is one component of the most common type of human kidney stones, calcium oxalate. Some studies suggest that people who take calcium or vitamin D as a dietary supplement have a higher risk of developing kidney stones. In the United States, kidney stone formation was used as an indicator of excess calcium intake by the Reference Daily Intake Committee for calcium in adults.

In the early 1990s, a study conducted for the Women's Health Initiative in the US found that postmenopausal women who consumed 1000 mg of supplemental calcium and 400 international units of vitamin D per day for seven years had a 17% higher risk of developing kidney stones than subjects taking a placebo. The Nurses' Health Study also showed an association between supplemental calcium intake and kidney stone formation.

Unlike supplemental calcium, high intakes of dietary calcium do not appear to cause kidney stones and may actually protect against their development. This is perhaps related to the role of calcium in binding ingested oxalate in the gastrointestinal tract. As the amount of calcium intake decreases, the amount of oxalate available for absorption into the bloodstream increases; this oxalate is then excreted in greater amounts into the urine by the kidneys. In the urine, oxalate is a very strong promoter of calcium oxalate precipitation—about 15 times stronger than calcium.

A 2004 study found that diets low in calcium are associated with a higher overall risk for kidney stone formation. For most individuals, other risk factors for kidney stones, such as high intakes of dietary oxalates and low fluid intake, play a greater role than calcium intake.

Other electrolytes: Calcium is not the only electrolyte that influences the formation of kidney stones. For example, by increasing urinary calcium excretion, high dietary sodium may increase the risk of stone formation.

Drinking fluoridated tap water may increase the risk of kidney stone formation by a similar mechanism, though further epidemiological studies are warranted to determine whether fluoride in drinking water is associated with an increased incidence of kidney stones. High dietary intake of potassium appears to reduce the risk of stone formation because potassium promotes the urinary excretion of citrate, an inhibitor of calcium crystal formation.

Kidney stones are more likely to develop and to grow larger, if a person has low dietary magnesium. Magnesium inhibits stone formation.

Animal protein: Diets in western nations typically contain a large proportion of animal protein. Consumption of animal protein creates an acid load that increases urinary excretion of calcium and uric acid and reduced citrate. Urinary excretion of excess sulfurous amino acids (e.g., cysteine and methionine), uric acid, and other acidic metabolites from animal protein acidifies the urine, which promotes the formation of kidney stones. Low urinary-citrate excretion is also commonly found in those with a high dietary intake of animal protein, whereas vegetarians tend to have higher levels of citrate excretion. Low urinary citrate, too, promotes stone formation.

Vitamins: The evidence linking vitamin C supplements with an increased rate of kidney stones is inconclusive. The excess dietary intake of vitamin C might increase the risk of calcium-oxalate stone formation; in practice, this is rarely encountered. The link between vitamin D intake and kidney stones is also tenuous. Excessive vitamin D supplementation may increase the risk of stone formation by increasing the intestinal absorption of calcium, while correction of a deficiency does not.

Other: There are no conclusive data demonstrating a cause-and-effect relationship between alcoholic beverage consumption and kidney stones. However, some people have theorized that certain behaviors associated with frequent and binge drinking can lead to dehydration, which can, in turn, lead to the development of kidney stones.

3　Pathophysiology

Hypocitraturia: Hypocitraturia or low urinary-citrate excretion (defined as less than 320 mg/d) can cause kidney stones in up to 2/3 of cases. The protective role of citrate is linked to several mechanisms; in fact, citrate reduces urinary supersaturation of calcium salts by forming soluble complexes with calcium ions and by inhibiting crystal growth and aggregation. The therapy with potassium citrate, or magnesium potassium citrate, is commonly prescribed in clinical practice in order to increase urinary citrate and to reduce stone formation rates.

Supersaturation of urine: When the urine becomes supersaturated (when the urine solvent contains more solutes than it can hold in solution) with one or more calculogenic (crystal-forming) substances, a seed crystal may form through the process of nucleation. Heterogeneous nucleation (where there is a solid surface present on which a crystal can grow) proceeds more rapidly than homogeneous nucleation (where a crystal must grow in a liquid medium with no such surface), because it requires less energy. Adhering to cells on the surface of a renal papilla, a seed crystal can grow and aggregate into an organized mass. Depending on the chemical composition of the crystal, the stone-forming process may proceed more rapidly when the urine pH is unusually high or low.

Supersaturation of the urine with respect to a calculogenic compound is pH-dependent. For example, at a pH of 7.0, the solubility of uric acid in urine is 158 mg/100 mL. Reducing the pH to 5.0 decreases the solubility of uric acid to less than 8 mg/100 mL. The formation of uric-acid stones requires a combination of hyperuricosuria (high urine uric-acid levels) and low urine pH; hyperuricosuria alone is not associated with uric-acid stone formation if the urine pH is alkaline. Supersaturation of the urine is a necessary, but not a sufficient, condition for the development of any urinary calculus. Supersaturation is likely the underlying cause of uric acid and cystine stones, but calcium-based stones (especially calcium oxalate stones) may have a more complex cause.

Inhibitors of stone formation: Normal urine contains chelating agents, such as citrate, which inhibit the nucleation, growth, and aggregation of calcium-containing crystals. Other endogenous inhibitors include calgranulin (an S100 calcium-binding protein), Tamm-Horsfall protein, glycosaminoglycans, uropontin (a form of osteopontin), nephrocalcin (an acidic glycoprotein), prothrombin F1 peptide, and bikunin (uronic acid-rich protein). The biochemical mechanisms of action of these substances have not yet been thoroughly elucidated. However, when these substances fall below their normal proportions, stones can form from an aggregation of crystals.

Sufficient dietary intake of magnesium and citrate inhibits the formation of calcium oxalate and calcium phosphate stones; in addition, magnesium and citrate operate synergistically to inhibit kidney stones. Magnesium's efficacy in subduing stone formation and growth is dose-dependent.

4　Diagnosis

Diagnosis of kidney stones is made on the basis of information obtained from the history, physical examination, urinalysis, and radiographic studies. Clinical diagnosis is usually made on the basis of the location and severity of the pain, which is typically colicky in nature (comes and goes in spasmodic waves). Pain in the back occurs when calculi produce an obstruction in the kidney. Physical examination may reveal fever and tenderness at the costovertebral angle on the affected side.

Imaging studies: In people with a history of stones, those who are less than 50 years of age and are presenting with the symptoms of stones without any concerning signs do not require helical CT scan imaging. A CT scan is also not typically recommended in children.

Otherwise a noncontrast helical CT scan with 5 mm (0.2 in) sections is the diagnostic modality of choice in the radiographic evaluation of suspected nephrolithiasis. All stones are detectable on CT scans except very rare stones composed of certain drug residues in the urine, such as from indinavir. Calcium-containing stones are relatively radiodense, and they can often be detected by a traditional radiograph of the abdomen that includes the kidneys, ureters, and bladder (KUB film). About 60% of all renal stones are radiopaque. In general, calcium phosphate stones have the greatest density, followed by calcium oxalate and magnesium ammonium phosphate stones. Cystine calculi are only faintly radiodense, while uric acid stones are usually entirely radiolucent.

Renal ultrasonography can sometimes be useful, because it gives details about the presence of hydronephrosis, suggesting that the stone is blocking the outflow of urine. Radiolucent stones, which do not appear on KUB, may show up on ultrasound imaging studies. Other advantages of renal ultrasonography include its low cost and absence of radiation exposure. Ultrasound imaging is useful for detecting stones in situations where X-rays or CT scans are discouraged, such as in children or pregnant women. Despite these advantages, renal ultrasonography in 2009 was not considered a substitute for noncontrast helical CT scan in the initial diagnostic evaluation of urolithiasis. The main reason for this is that, compared with CT, renal ultrasonography more often fails to detect small stones (especially ureteral stones) and other serious disorders that could be causing the symptoms. A 2014 study confirmed that ultrasonography rather than CT as an initial diagnostic test results in less radiation exposure and did not find any significant complications.

Laboratory examination: Laboratory investigations typically carried out include: (1) microscopic examination of the urine, which may show red blood cells, bacteria, leukocytes, urinary casts and crystals; (2) urine culture to identify any infecting organisms present in the urinary tract and sensitivity to determine the susceptibility of these organisms to specific antibiotics; (3) complete blood count, looking for neutrophilia (increased neutroph il granulocyte count) suggestive of bacterial infection, as seen in the setting of struvite stones; (4) renal function tests to look for abnormally high blood calcium blood levels (hypercalcemia); (5) 24-hour urine collection to measure total daily urinary volume, magnesium, sodium, uric acid, calcium, citrate, oxalate and phosphate; (6) collection of stones (by urinating through a StoneScreen kidney stone collection cup or a simple tea strainer) is useful. Chemical analysis of collected stones can establish their composition, which in turn can help to guide future preventive and therapeutic management.

Composition: Where a CT scan is unavailable, an intravenous pyelogram may be performed to help confirm the diagnosis of urolithiasis. This involves intravenous injection of a contrast agent followed by a KUB film. Uroliths present in the kidneys, ureters or bladder may be better defined by the use of this contrast agent. Stones can also be detected by a retrograde pyelogram, where a similar contrast agent is injected directly into the distal ostium of the ureter (where the ureter terminates as it enters the bladder).

Calcium-containing stones: By far, the most common type of kidney stones worldwide contains calcium. For example, calcium-containing stones represent about 80% of all cases in the United States; these typically contain calcium oxalate either alone or in combination with calcium phosphate in the form of apatite or brushite. Factors that promote the precipitation of oxalate crystals in the urine, such as primary hyperoxaluria, are associated with the development of calcium oxalate stones. The formation of calcium phosphate stones is associated with conditions such as hyperparathyroidism and renal tubular acidosis.

Oxaluria is increased in patients with certain gastrointestinal disorders including inflammatory bowel disease such as Crohn's disease or in patients who have undergone resection of the small bowel or small-bowel bypass procedures. Oxaluria is also increased in patients who consume increased amounts of oxalate (found in vegetables and nuts). Primary hyperoxaluria is a rare autosomal recessive condition that usually presents in childhood.

Calcium oxalate crystals in urine appear as "envelopes" microscopically. They may also form dumbbells.

Struvite stones: About 10% ~ 15% of urinary calculi are composed of struvite (ammonium magnesium phosphate, $NH_4MgPO_4\cdot6H_2O$). Struvite stones (also known as infection stones, urease, or triple-phosphate stones) form most often in the presence of infection by urea-splitting bacteria. Using the enzyme urease, these organisms metabolize urea into ammonia and carbon dioxide. This alkalinizes the urine, resulting in favorable conditions for the formation of struvite stones. *Proteus mirabilis*, *Proteus vulgaris* and *Morganella morganii* are the most common organisms isolated; less common organisms include *Ureaplasma urealyticum* and some species of *Providencia*, *Klebsiella*, *Serratia* and *Enterobacter*. These infection stones are commonly observed in people who have factors that predispose them to urinary tract infections, such as those with spinal cord injury and other forms of neurogenic bladder, ileal conduit urinary diversion, vesicoureteral reflux, and obstructive uropathies. They are also commonly seen in people with underlying metabolic disorders, such as idiopathic hypercalciuria, hyperparathyroidism and gout. Infection stones can grow rapidly, forming large calyceal staghorn (antler-shaped) calculi requiring invasive surgery such as percutaneous nephrolithotomy for definitive treatment.

Struvite stones (triple-phosphate/magnesium ammonium phosphate) have a coffin lid morphology by microscopy.

Uric acid stones: About 5% ~ 10% of all stones are formed from uric acid. People with certain metabolic abnormalities, including obesity, may produce uric acid stones. They also may form in association with conditions that cause hyperuricosuria (an excessive amount of uric acid in the urine) with or without hyperuricemia (an excessive amount of uric acid in the serum). They may also form in association with disorders of acid/base metabolism where the urine is excessively acidic (low pH), resulting in precipitation of uric acid crystals. A diagnosis of uric acid urolithiasis is supported by the presence of a radiolucent stone in the face of persistent urine acidity, in conjunction with the finding of uric acid crystals in fresh urine samples.

As noted above (section on calcium oxalate stones), people with inflammatory bowel disease (Crohn's disease, ulcerative colitis) tend to have hyperoxaluria and form oxalate stones. They also have a tendency to form urate stones. Urate stones are especially common after colon resection.

Uric acid stones appear as pleomorphic crystals, usually diamond-shaped. They may also look like squares or rods which are polarizable.

Patients with hyperuricosuria can be treated with allopurinol, which will reduce urate formation. Urine alkalinization may also be helpful in this setting.

Other types: People with certain rare inborn errors of metabolism have a propensity to accumulate crystal-forming substances in their urine. For example, those with cystinuria, cystinosis and Fanconi syndrome may form stones composed of cystine. Cystine stone formation can be treated with urine alkalinization and dietary protein restriction. People afflicted with xanthinuria often produce stones composed of xanthine. People afflicted with adenine phosphoribosyl transferase deficiency may produce 2,8-dihydroxy adenine stones, alkaptonurics produce homogentisic acid stones, and iminoglycinurics produce stones of glycine, proline and hydroxyproline. Urolithiasis has also been noted to occur in the setting of therapeutic drug use, with crystals of drug forming within the renal tract in some people currently being treated with agents such as indinavir, sulfadiazine and triamterene.

Location: Urolithiasis refers to stones originating anywhere in the urinary system, including the kidneys and bladder. Nephrolithiasis refers to the presence of such stones in the kidneys. Calyceal calculi are aggregations in either the minor or major calyx, parts of the kidney that pass urine into the ureter (the tube connecting the kidneys to the urinary bladder). The condition is called ureterolithiasis when a calculus is located in the ureter. Stones may also form or pass into the bladder, a condition referred to as bladder stones.

Size: Stones less than 5 mm (0.2 in) in diameter pass spontaneously in up to 98% of cases, while those measuring 5 ~ 10 mm (0.2 ~ 0.4 in) in diameter pass spontaneously in less than 53% of cases.

Stones that are large enough to fill out the renal calyces are called staghorn stones, and are composed of struvite in a vast majority of cases, which forms only in the presence of urease-forming bacteria. Other forms that can possibly grow to become staghorn stones are those composed of cystine, calcium oxalate monohydrate and uric acid.

5   Prevention

Preventative measures depend on the type of stones. In those with calcium stones, drinking lots of fluids, thiazide diuretics and citrate are effective as is allopurinol in those with high uric acid levels in the blood or urine.

Dietary measures: Specific therapy should be tailored to the type of stones involved. Diet can have a profound influence on the development of kidney stones. Preventive strategies include some combination of dietary modifications and medications with the goal of reducing the excretory load of calculogenic compounds on the kidneys. Current dietary recommendations to minimize the formation of kidney stones include:

(1) Increasing total fluid intake to more than two liters per day of urine output.

(2) Increasing citric acid intake; lemon/lime juice is the richest natural source.

(3) Moderate calcium intake.

(4) Limiting sodium intake.

(5) Avoidance of large doses of supplemental vitamin C.

(6) Limiting animal protein intake to no more than two meals daily (an association between animal protein consumption and recurrence of kidney stones has been shown in men).

(7) Limiting consumption of cola soft drinks, which contain phosphoric acid, to less than one liter of soft drink per week.

Maintenance of dilute urine by means of vigorous fluid therapy is beneficial in all forms of nephrolithiasis, so increasing urine volume is a key principle for the prevention of kidney stones. Fluid intake should be sufficient to maintain a urine output of at least 2 litres (68 USfloz) per day. A high fluid intake has been associated with a 40% reduction in recurrence risk. The quality of the evidence for this, however, is not very good.

Calcium binds with available oxalate in the gastrointestinal tract, thereby preventing its absorption into the bloodstream, and reducing oxalate absorption decreases kidney stone risk in susceptible people. Because of this, some nephrologists and urologists recommend chewing calcium tablets during meals containing oxalate foods. Calcium citrate supplements can be taken with meals if dietary calcium cannot be increased by other means. The preferred calcium supplement for people at risk of stone formation is calcium citrate because it helps to increase urinary citrate excretion.

Aside from vigorous oral hydration and consumption of more dietary calcium, other prevention strategies include avoidance of large doses of supplemental vitamin C and restriction of oxalate-rich foods such as leaf vegetables, rhubarb, soy products and chocolate. However, no randomized, controlled trial of oxalate restriction has yet been performed to test the hypothesis that oxalate restriction reduces the incidence of stone formation. Some evidence indicates magnesium intake decreases the risk of symptomatic nephrolithiasis.

Urine alkalinization: The mainstay for medical management of uric acid stones is alkalinization (increasing the pH) of the urine. Uric acid stones are among the few types amenable to dissolution therapy, referred to as chemolysis. Chemolysis is usually achieved through the use of oral medications, although in some cases, intravenous agents or even instillation of certain irrigating agents directly onto the stone can be performed, using antegrade nephrostomy or retrograde ureteral catheters. Acetazolamide (Diamox) is a medication that alkalinizes the urine. In addition to acetazolamide or as an alternative, certain dietary supplements are available that produce a similar alkalinization of the urine. These include sodium bicarbonate, potassium citrate, magnesium citrate and Bicitra (a combination of citric acid monohydrate and sodium citrate dihydrate). Aside from alkalinization of the urine, these supplements have the added advantage of increasing the urinary citrate level, which helps to reduce the aggregation of calcium oxalate stones.

Increasing the urine pH to around 6.5 provides optimal conditions for dissolution of uric acid stones. Increasing the urine pH to a value higher than 7.0 increases the risk of calcium phosphate stone formation. Testing the urine periodically with nitrazine paper can help to ensure the urine pH remains in this optimal range. Using this approach, stone dissolution rate can be expected to be around 10 mm (0.4 in) of stone radius per month.

Diuretics: One of the recognized medical therapies for prevention of stones is the thiazide and thiazide-like diuretics, such as chlorthalidone or indapamide. These drugs inhibit the formation of calcium-containing stones by reducing urinary calcium excretion. Sodium restriction is necessary for clinical effect of thiazides, as sodium excess promotes calcium excretion. Thiazides work best for renal leak hypercalciuria (high urine calcium levels), a condition in which high urinary calcium levels are caused by a primary kidney defect. Thiazides are useful for treating absorptive hypercalciuria, a condition in which high urinary calcium is a result of excess absorption from the gastrointestinal tract.

Allopurinol: For people with hyperuricosuria and calcium stones, allopurinol is one of the few treatments that have been shown to reduce kidney stone recurrences. Allopurinol interferes with the production of uric acid in the liver. The drug is also used in people with gout or hyperuricemia (high serum uric acid levels). Dosage is adjusted to maintain a reduced urinary excretion of uric acid. Serum uric acid level at or below 6 mg/100 mL) is often a therapeutic goal. Hyperuricemia is not necessary for the formation of uric acid stones; hyperuricosuria can occur in the presence of normal or even low serum uric acid. Some practitioners advocate adding allopurinol only in people in whom hyperuricosuria and hyperuricemia persist, despite the use of a urine-alkalinizing agent such as sodium bicarbonate or potassium citrate.

6　Treatment

Stone size influences the rate of spontaneous stone passage. For example, up to 98% of small stones [less than 5 mm (0.2 in) in diameter] may pass spontaneously through urination within four weeks of the onset of symptoms, but for larger stones [5 ~ 10 mm (0.2 ~ 0.4 in) in diameter], the rate of spontaneous passage decreases to less than 53%. Initial stone location also influences the likelihood of spontaneous stone passage. Rates increase from 48% for stones located in the proximal ureter to 79% for stones located at the vesicoureteric junction, regardless of stone size. Assuming no high-grade obstruction or associated infection is found in the urinary tract, and symptoms are relatively mild, various nonsurgical measures can be used to encourage the passage of a stone. Repeat stone formers benefit from more intense management, including proper fluid intake and the use of certain medications. In addition, careful surveillance is clearly required to maximize the clinical course for people who are stone formers.

Pain management: Management of pain often requires intravenous administration of NSAIDs or opioids. NSAIDs appear somewhat better than opioids or paracetamol in those with normal kidney function. Medications by mouth are often effective for less severe discomfort. The use of antispasmodics does not have further benefit.

Medical expulsive therapy: The use of medications to speed the spontaneous passage of stones in the ureter is referred to as medical expulsive therapy. Several agents, including alpha adrenergic blockers (such as tamsulosin) and calcium channel blockers (such as nifedipine), have been found to be effective. Alpha blockers appear to lead to both higher and faster stone clearance rates. Alpha blockers, however, only appear to be effective for stones over 4 mm but less than 10 mm in size. A combination of tamsulosin and a corticosteroid may be better than tamsulosin alone. These treatments also appear to be useful in addition to lithotripsy.

Lithotripsy: Extracorporeal shock wave lithotripsy (ESWL) is a noninvasive technique for the removal of kidney stones. Most ESWL is carried out when the stone is present near the renal pelvis. ESWL involves the use of a lithotriptor machine to deliver externally applied, focused, high-intensity pulses of ultrasonic energy to cause fragmentation of a stone over a period of around 30 ~ 60 min. Following its introduction in the United States in February 1984, ESWL was rapidly and widely accepted as a treatment alternative for renal and ureteral stones. It is currently used in the treatment of uncomplicated stones located in the kidney and upper ureter, provided the aggregate stone burden (stone size and number) is less than 20 mm (0.8 in) and the anatomy of the involved kidney is normal.

For a stone greater than 10 mm (0.4 in), ESWL may not help break the stone in one treatment; instead, two or three treatments may be needed. Some 80% ~ 85% of simple renal calculi can be effectively treated with ESWL. A number of factors can influence its efficacy, including chemical composition of the stone, presence of anomalous renal anatomy and the specific location of the stone within the kidney, presence of hydronephrosis, body mass index, and distance of the stone from the surface of the skin. Common adverse effects of ESWL include acute trauma, such as bruising at the site of shock administration, and damage to blood vessels of the kidney. In fact, the vast majority of people who are treated with a typical dose of shock waves using currently accepted treatment settings are likely to experience some degree of acute kidney injury.

ESWL-induced acute kidney injury is dose-dependent (increases with the total number of shock waves administered and with the power setting of the lithotriptor) and can be severe, including internal bleeding and subcapsular hematomas. On rare occasions, such cases may require blood transfusion and even lead to acute renal failure. Hematoma rates may be related to the type of lithotriptor used; hematoma rates of less than 1% and up to 13% have been reported for different lithotriptor machines. Recent studies show reduced acute tissue injury when the treatment protocol includes a brief pause following the initiation of treatment, and both improved stone breakage and a reduction in injury when ESWL is carried out at slow shock wave rate.

In addition to the aforementioned potential for acute kidney injury, animal studies suggest these acute injuries may progress to scar formation, resulting in loss of functional renal volume. Recent prospective studies also indicate elderly people are at increased risk of developing new-onset hypertension following ESWL. In addition, a retrospective case-control study published by researchers from the Mayo Clinic in 2006 has found an increased risk of developing diabetes mellitus and hypertension in people who had undergone ESWL, compared with age and gender-matched people who had undergone nonsurgical treatment. Whether or not acute trauma progresses to long-term effects probably depends on multiple factors that include the shock wave dose (i.e., the number of shock waves delivered, rate of delivery, power setting, acoustic characteristics of the particular lithotriptor, and frequency of retreatment), as well as certain intrinsic predisposing pathophysiologic risk factors.

To address these concerns, the American Urological Association established the Shock Wave Lithotripsy Task Force to provide an expert opinion on the safety and risk-benefit ratio of ESWL. The task force published a white paper outlining their conclusions in 2009. They concluded the risk-benefit ratio remains favorable for many people. The advantages of ESWL include its noninvasive nature, the fact that it is technically easy to treat most upper urinary tract calculi, and that, at least acutely, it is a well-tolerated, low-morbidity treatment for the vast majority of people. However, they recommended slowing the shock wave firing rate from 120 pulses per minute to 60 pulses per minute to reduce the risk of renal injury and increase the degree of stone fragmentation.

Surgery: Most stones under 5 mm (0.2 in) pass spontaneously. Prompt surgery may, nonetheless, be required in persons with only one working kidney, bilateral obstructing stones, a urinary tract infection and thus, it is presumed, an infected kidney, or intractable pain. Beginning in the mid-1980s, less invasive treatments such as extracorporeal shock wave lithotripsy, ureteroscopy and percutaneous nephrolithotomy began to replace open surgery as the modalities of choice for the surgical management of urolithiasis. More recently, flexible ureteroscopy has been adapted to facilitate retrograde nephrostomy creation for percutaneous nephrolithotomy. This approach is still under investigation, though early results are favorable. Percutaneous nephrolithotomy or, rarely, anatrophic nephrolithotomy, is the treatment of choice for large or complicated stones (such as calyceal staghorn calculi) or stones that cannot be extracted using less invasive procedures.

Ureteroscopic surgery: Ureteroscopy has become increasingly popular as flexible and rigid fiberoptic ureteroscopes have become smaller. One ureteroscopic technique involves the placement of a ureteral stent (a small tube extending from the bladder, up the ureter and into the kidney) to provide immediate relief of an obstructed kidney. Stent placement can be useful for saving a kidney at risk for postrenal acute renal failure due to the increased hydrostatic pressure, swelling and infection (pyelonephritis and pyonephrosis) caused by an obstructing stone. Ureteral stents vary in length from 24 cm to 30 cm (9.4 ~ 11.8 in) and most have a shape commonly referred to as a double-J or double pigtail, because of the curl at both ends. They are designed to allow urine to flow past an obstruction in the ureter. They may be retained in the ureter for days to weeks as infections resolve and as stones are dissolved or fragmented by ESWL or by some other treatment. The stents dilate the ureters, which can facilitate instrumentation, and they also provide a clear landmark to aid in the visualization of the ureters and any associated stones on radiographic examinations. The presence of indwelling ureteral stents may cause minimal to moderate discomfort, frequency or urgency incontinence and infection, which in general resolves on removal.

More definitive ureteroscopic techniques for stone extraction (rather than simply by passing the obstruction) include basket extraction and ultrasound ureterolithotripsy. Laser lithotripsy is another technique, which involves the use of a holmium: yttrium aluminium garnet (Ho: YAG) laser to fragment stones in the bladder, ureters and kidneys.

Ureteroscopic techniques are generally more effective than ESWL for treating stones located in the lower ureter, with success rates of 93% ~ 100% using Ho: YAG laser lithotripsy. Although ESWL has been traditionally preferred by many practitioners for treating stones located in the upper ureter, more recent experience suggests ureteroscopic techniques offer distinct advantages in the treatment of upper ureteral stones. Specifically, the overall success rate is higher, fewer repeat interventions and postoperative visits are needed, and treatment costs are lower after ureteroscopic treatment when compared with ESWL. These advantages are especially apparent with stones greater than 10 mm (0.4 in) in diameter. However, because ureteroscopy of the upper ureter is much more challenging than ESWL, many urologists still prefer to use ESWL as a first-line treatment for stones of less than 10 mm, and ureteroscopy for those greater than 10 mm in diameter. Ureteroscopy is the preferred treatment in pregnant and morbidly obese people, as well as those with bleeding disorders.

Section 4   Words of TCM

1. 先天之本 congenital basis
2. 先天之精 congenital/genetic/ innate essence
3. 后天之精 acquired essence
4. 精气 essence; essential qi; essence and qi
5. 元气 / 原气 primordial/original qi
6. 真气 original/primordial qi

7. 营 / 卫 / 宗气 nutrient/defensive/thoracic qi

8. 人体之气 body qi; vital energy

9. 气主响之，血主濡之 qi promoting, blood nourishing

10. 气能生血 / 行血 qi promoting blood production and circulation

11. 气能生津 / 行津 qi promoting body fluid production and circulation

12. 气能摄血 / 摄津 qi governing blood and body fluid

13. 血 / 津能载气 blood/body fluid conveying qi

14. 精能化气 essence transforming into qi

15. 气能生精 qi promoting essence production

16. 津血同源 body fluid and blood sharing the same source

17. 血汗同源 blood and sweat sharing the same source

18. 精血同源 essence and blood sharing the same origin

19. 津停气滞 body fluid retention causing qi stagnation

20. 膻中，虚里 danzhong, heat apex

21. 六气 / 淫 / 邪 six climates/excesses/exopathogens or evils

22. 伤寒，中寒 exogenous febrile disease, cold stroke

23. 瘟疫，疠气 prestilence, epidemic pathogens

24. 正邪相争 struggle between healthy qi and pathogenic factors

25. 表里关系 exterior-interior relationship

26. 发热恶寒 fever with aversion to cold

27. 清热泻火 clearing away heat and purging fire; clearing way heat to remove fire

28. 风性主动 / 轻扬 wind tending to migrate/drift

29. 寒性凝滞 / 收引 cold tending to coagulate and stagnate/contract

30. 暑性升散 summer heat tending to ascend and disperse

31. 暑多夹湿 summer heat usually accompanied with dampness

32. 湿性重浊 dampness being heavy and turbid

33. 湿性黏滞 dampness being viscous and lingering

34. 燥性干涩 dryness tending to desiccate

35. 火性趋上 fire tending to flare up

36. 火易生风动血 fire causing wind and bleeding

37. 风热眩晕 vertigo due to wind-heat

38. 寒证化热 cold syndrome transforming into heat syndrome

39. 寒热错杂 simultaneous occurrence of cold and heat

40. 表邪入里 invasion of exterior pathogen into interior

(Ni Tongshang, Wang Tingting)

Chapter 4　Tuberculosis

Section 1　Fight Against Tuberculosis

Tuberculosis (TB) is one of the leading infectious diseases and a serous health problem around the world. The World Health Organization (WHO) reports that two billion people, about 1/3 of the world's total population, are infected with the TB bacteria. One in ten (10%) people infected with the TB bacteria will become sick with tuberculosis at some time during their life. Almost nine million people become sick with the disease each year and about 1 600 000 people will die of the disease this year.

Tuberculosis is an infectious disease usually caused by the bacterium Mycobacterium tuberculosis (MTB).Tuberculosis generally affects the lungs, but can also affect other parts of the body. Most infections do not have symptoms, in which case it is known as latent tuberculosis. About 10% of latent infections progress to active disease which, if left untreated, kills about half of those infected. The classic symptoms of active TB are a chronic cough with blood-containing sputum, fever, night sweats, and weight loss. The historical term consumption came about due to the weight loss. Infection of other organs can cause a wide range of symptoms. Tuberculosis is spread through the air when people who have active TB in their lungs cough, spit, speak, or sneeze. People with latent TB do not spread the disease. Active infection occurs more often in people with HIV/AIDS and in those who smoke. Diagnosis of active TB is based on chest X-rays, as well as microscopic examination and culture of body fluids. Diagnosis of latent TB relies on the tuberculin skin test (TST) or blood tests.

Prevention of TB involves screening those at high risk, early detection and treatment of cases, and vaccination with the bacillus Calmette-Guérin (BCG) vaccine. Those at high risk include household, workplace, and social contacts of people with active TB. Treatment requires the use of multiple antibiotics over a long period of time. Antibiotic resistance is a growing problem with increasing rates of multiple drug-resistant tuberculosis (MDR-TB) and extensively drug-resistant tuberculosis (XDR-TB).

Presently, one-third of the world's population is thought to be infected with TB. New infections occur in about 1% of the population each year. In 2016, there were more than 10 million cases of active TB which resulted in 1.3 million deaths. This makes it the number one cause of death from an infectious disease. More than 95% of deaths occurred in developing countries, and more than 50% in India, China, Indonesia, Pakistan, and the Philippines. The number of new cases each year has decreased since 2000. About 80% of people in many Asian and African countries test positive while 5% ~ 10% of people in the United States population test positive by the tuberculin test. Tuberculosis has been present in humans since ancient times.

Tuberculosis is a disease of poverty and affects mostly young adults in their most productive years. The large majority of deaths from the disease are in developing countries and more than half of all deaths happen in Asia. The WHO declared TB a public health emergency in 1993. A new report shows tuberculosis rates around the world are falling or unchanged. The report says the rates were unchanged in 2005 after reaching record high levels one year earlier. If this continues for the next three or four years, WHO officials believe their Millennium Development Goal could be reached. The goal is to discover at least 75% of TB cases and successfully treat 85% of those cases by the year 2015.

Tuberculosis is a bacterial infection that usually attacks the lungs. Most people infected with the bacteria never develop active TB. However, people with weak body defense systems often develop the disease. TB can damage a person's lungs or other parts of the body and cause serious health problems. The disease is spread by people who have active, untreated TB bacteria in their throat or lungs. The bacteria are spread into the air when people with the disease talk or expel air suddenly. People who breathe infected air from a TB victim can become infected with the tuberculosis bacteria. However, most people with active tuberculosis don't expel very many TB bacteria. So, the spread of the disease usually does not happen unless a person spends large amount of time with a TB patient. Those most at risk are family members, friends and people who live or work closely with a patient.

If a person becomes infected with the TB bacteria, it does not mean he or she has the disease. Having the infection means that the bacteria are in the body, but they may be neutral, or inactive. When TB bacteria are inactive, they cannot damage the body or spread to other people. People with the inactive bacteria are infected, but they are not sick. They probably do not know they are infected. For most of them, the bacteria will always be inactive and they will never suffer signs of tuberculosis.

If the natural immune system against disease is weak, however, a person can get tuberculosis soon after the TB bacteria enter the body. Also, inactive TB bacteria may become active if the immune system becomes weak. When this happens, the bacteria begin reproducing and damaging the lungs or other organs and causing serious sickness. The inactive TB bacteria can become active under several conditions. When a person becomes old, the immune system may become too weak to protect against the bacteria. The virus diseases can cause TB bacteria to become active. Also, people who drink too much alcohol or use drugs have a higher risk of becoming sick from the TB bacteria.

Tuberculosis can attack any part of the body. However, the lungs are the most common targets of the bacteria. People with the disease show several signs. They may expel air from the lungs suddenly with an explosive noise. This kind of cough continues for a long period of time. People with a more severe case of tuberculosis also may have hemoptysis. People with the disease often have high body temperatures. They suffer what are called night sweats, during which their bodies release large amounts of water through the skin. TB victims also are tired all the time and not interested in eating. So their bodies lose weight.

It is especially dangerous about TB that people with moderate signs of the disease may not know they have it. They may spread the disease to others without even knowing it, so it is very important for people to get tested for tuberculosis. There are several ways to test for TB. The first is the TB skin test known as the Mantoux skin test. The test can identify most people infected with tuberculosis 6 ~ 8 weeks after the bacteria entered their bodies. A purified protein derivative is injected under the skin of the arm. The place of the injection is examined 2 ~ 3 days later. If a raised red area or swelling forms, the person may have been infected with the tuberculosis bacteria. However, this does not always mean the disease is active. If the skin test shows that TB bacteria have entered the body, doctors can use other methods to discover if the person has active TB. However, this sometimes can be difficult because tuberculosis may appear similar to other diseases. Doctors must consider other physical signs. Also, they must decide if a person's history shows that he or she has been in situations where tuberculosis was present. Doctors also use an X-ray examination to show if there is evidence of TB infection, such as damage to the lungs. Another way to test for the presence of active tuberculosis is to examine the fluids from a person's mouth. It is very important to identify which kind of TB bacteria are present so the doctors can decide which drugs to use to treat the disease. Most TB cases can be successfully treated with medicines. However, the death rate for untreated patients is reported to be about 50%. Successful treatment of TB requires close cooperation among patients, doctors and other health care workers.

The WHO has a five-step program to guarantee that TB patients take their medicine correctly. The program is called Directly Observed Treatment, Short-course, or DOTS which means local health care workers watch to make sure patients take their medicine every day. Full treatment usually lasts for 6 ~ 9 months to destroy all signs of the bacteria.

It is very important for patients to be educated about the disease and its treatment. Sometimes patients fail to finish taking the medicine because of feeling better after only 2 ~ 4 weeks of treatment and stop taking their medicine. This can lead to the TB bacteria becoming resistant to drugs and growing stronger, more dangerous and more difficult to treat.

Tuberculosis is a preventable disease. The goal of health organizations is to quickly identify infected persons, especially those who have the highest risk of developing the disease. There are several drugs to prevent TB in these people. TB can be cured if it is discovered early and if patients take their medicine correctly. And, like other diseases, education and understanding are extremely important in preventing and treating TB.

Progression from TB infection to overt TB disease occurs when the bacilli overcome the immune system defenses and begin to multiply. In primary TB disease (some 1% ~ 5% of cases), this occurs soon after the initial infection. However, in the majority of cases, a latent infection occurs with no obvious symptoms. These dormant bacilli produce active tuberculosis in 5% ~ 10% of these latent cases, often many years after infection.

Section 2　Buzhong Yiqi Tang

Within the Chinese medical journal literature there are several different genres of articles, of which is the new uses genre. In this type of essay, the author takes an ancient or classical formula and present several case histories exemplifying new uses of this formula. From a western medical perspective, these would be called off-label uses. This is the use of a formula for a disease or disorder for which this formula is not standardly indicated. This is an example of the basic dictum of professional Chinese medicine — Treatment is based on pattern discrimination (Bianzheng Lunzhi). In other words, although a formula may not be normally indicated for the treatment of this or that disease, if the patient's pattern fits the formula's pattern discrimination, then the formula may be used. This genre of article underscores the fundamental, over-riding importance of basing a patient's treatment primarily on their pattern discrimination and not simply or even primarily on their disease diagnosis.

Buzhong Yiqi Tang: Buzhong Yiqi Tang (supplement the center and boost the qi decoction) is one of the famous doctor in Jin-Yuan Dynasty, Li Dongyuan's most famous formulas. It is comprised of Radix Astragali Membranacei (Huangqi), Radix Panacis Ginseng (Renshen), Rhizoma Atractylodis Macrocephalae (Baizhu), Radix Angelicae Sinensis (Danggui), Rhizoma Cimicifugae (Shengma), Pericarpium Citri Reticulatae (Chenpi), Radix Bupleuri (Chaihu), and mix-fried Radix Glycyrrhizae (Gancao). This formula banks and supplements the spleen and stomach, supplements the center and boosts the qi, up-bears yang and lifts the fallen. It treats all conditions of spleen-stomach qi vacuity with clear yang falling down. However, as originally conceived by Li Dongyuan, it also sweetly and warmly clears qi vacuity heat or yin fire via up-bearing and out-thrusting. In addition, based on an analysis of its individual ingredients, it supplements the spleen and boosts the qi, courses the liver and rectifies the qi. Therefore, for those who truly understand this formula, its scope of application is much greater than qi vacuity downward falling conditions. The following is a summary of three case histories taken from an article published in *Sichuan Zhongyi* (Sichuan Journal of Traditional Chinese Medicine) by Qiu Liming.

Case 1: The patient was 34 years old, male, firstly examined on Oct. 25, 1998. He had had recurrent oral ulcers for five years. For the last two months, the number of these oral sores had increased and both burning hot and peppery painful, so the man was not able to eat. He had already taken various Chinese medicinal to clear heat and drain fire as well as vitamin B complex and several Western medicines, all without effect. Accompanying the oral sores were ventral and abdominal glomus and fullness, torpid intake, loose stools, lassitude of the spirit, lack of strength, a dry throat, somnolence, a pale, fat tongue with teeth-marks on its edges and thin, white fur, and a deep, fine, rapid pulse. On examination, there were ulcers on the man's upper and lower lips and the mucus membrane on both sides of his cheeks. The tip of his tongue also had many ulcerated sores whose bases were concave and depressed. The color of these sores was ashen white, and pressure pain was pronounced.

Based on the above signs and symptoms, the man's pattern was categorized as spleen-stomach vacuity weakness with clear yang not being up-borne and yin fire ascending and flaming, steaming and burning the mouth and tongue. Thus treatment should supplement the center and boost the qi, subdue and downbear yin fire. The formula used was Buzhong Yiqi Tang with additions and subtractions: Rasix Astragali Membranacei (Huangqi) 30 g, Radix Codonopsitis Pilosulae (Dangshen) and Rhizoma Atractylodis Macrocephalae (Baizhu) 15 g each, Rhizoma Cimicifugae (Shengma), Radix Bupleuri (Chaihu), Herba Lophatheri Gracilis (Danzhuye) and Fructus Evodiae Rutecarpae (Wuzhuyu) 10 g each, Pericarpium Citri Reticulatae (Chenpi) and mix-fried Radix Glycyrrhizae (Gancao) 6 g each, and Cortex Cinnamomi Cassiae (Rougui) 3 g. After administering seven doses (ji) of this formula, the ulcers had shrunk and become smaller and eating was no longer painful. All the man's symptoms were greatly reduced. Ten more doses (ji) were administered continuously and the ulcers were cured as well as all other symptoms. On follow-up in 2000, there had been no recurrence.

Comment: According to Chinese medical theory, the spleen opens into the orifice of the mouth, and oral cavity ulcers and sores are mostly due to heart-spleen brewing heat or yin vacuity fire effulgence. In this case, there was spleen-stomach qi vacuity with clear yang not being up-borne. Thus yin fire was taking advantage of spleen-stomach vacuity and flaming upward. This was then steaming and burning the mouth and tongue, hence producing the sores and ulcers. This is as Li Dongyuan's *Piwei Lun* (treatise on the spleen and stomach). In terms of the spleen and stomach's production of yin fire, the grain qi becomes blocked and obstructed and pours downward. The clear qi is not up-borne and the results in the nine orifices become inhibited.

Normally, one uses either bitter cold medicinal to drain fire or sweet cold medicinal to downbear fire. However, in this case, either of these would further harm the central qi, thus further aggravating yin fire. This is why the previous treatments had not been effective. Instead, the author of this case used Buzhong Yiqi Tang to supplement the center and boost the qi and, therefore, regulated the mechanisms of upbearing and downbearing. Once the spleen recovered its fortification and movement, clear yang ascended and was upborne, yin fire was hidden and stored, and all the symptoms were automatically cured.

Case 2: The patient was female, 29 years old, examined firstly on Dec. 2, 1997. She had caught cold two years earlier after having given birth and had lost her regular nourishment. This resulted in the emission of chill in both her lower extremities. Initially this was not serious. However, during the last year, this condition had gradually worsened to the point that all four limbs emitted chill. This was especially bad during the cold and chilly seasons. The woman had already seen several doctors and had been diagnosed with cold lodged in her blood vessels resulting in uneasy flow of the qi and blood. For this, she had been given yang-warming, cold-scattering, blood-quickening, and network vessel freeing Chinese medicines, after which there was slight improvement. The coldness and chilling were most severe below her elbows and knees. Her facial complexion was lusterless, and her stools were loose. Intake was torpid; there was bodily fatigue, and she lacked strength. The use of her body and limbs was normal, and there was no numbness, pain, or itching. Her tongue was pale with thin, white fur, and her pulse was deep and fine.

Based on the above signs and symptoms, the patient's Chinese medical pattern was categorized as middle burner vacuity cold with spleen qi unable to upbear, emit and spread clear yang to the four extremities. The treatment principles were to supplement the center and boost the qi, upbear and emit clear yang. The formula used was Buzhong Yiqi Tang with added flavors: Radox Astragali Membranacei (Huangqi) 50 g, Radix Codonopsitis Pilosulae (Dangshen) 30 g, Radix Angelicae Sinensis (Danggui), Rhizoma Atractylodis Macrocephalae (Baizhu) and Ramulus Cinnamomi Cassiae (Guizhi) 15 g each, and Rhizoma Cimicifugae (Shengma), Rsdix Bupleuri (Chaihu), Pericarpium Citri Reticulatae (Chenpi), dry Rhizoma Zingiberis (Ganjiang) and mix-fried Radix Glycyrrhizae (Gancao) 6 g each. Ten doses (ji) of these medicinal were administered orally, after which her four limbs were already warm, her intake of food had improved, and her loose stools had disappeared. Therefore, these same medicinal were administered for another half month when all her symptoms were eliminated. On follow-up after one year, there had been no recurrence.

Comment: According to Chinese medical theory, the four limbs are governed by tai yin spleen earth. This case was one of middle burner vacuity cold with spleen qi falling downward. Hence the spleen was unable to upbear and emit clear yang and spread it to the four extremities. This resulted in emission of chill in the four limbs. Therefore, Buzhong Yiqi Tang was used in order to supplement the center and boost the qi, thus promoting fullness and sufficiency of the spleen qi. The yang qi became effulgent and exuberant, the light of yang was able to shine in all directions, and yin chill was automatically scattered. This effect was increased by the addition of dry Ginger (Shengjiang) and Cinnamon Twigs (Guizhi) which warm the center and invigorate yang, and warm and free the flow of the blood vessels. Hence cold qi was eliminated and the treatment effect was good.

In actual fact, the symptoms of spleen qi downward fall were, in this case, minimal — really only the loose stools. This shows that this formula has a greater scope of application than spleen qi downward fall conditions. It can be used for simple spleen qi vacuity weakness, even though modern Chinese authors typically feel compelled to talk about upbearing the clear and lifting the fallen whenever discussing this formula.

Case 3: The patient was female, 30 years old, and examined firstly on Mar. 5, 1998. One year previously she had caught cold after giving birth which resulted in leaking urine as coughing. Initially this was not severe, and she did not seek treatment for it. However, two months ago, this condition had become more pronounced and her urination had become incontinent. Whenever the patient was fatigued, this incontinence was worse. Other symptoms included low back soreness, weak lower limbs, lassitude of the spirit, shortness of breath, dizziness, blurred vision, occasional venter and stomach distention and fullness, a fat body, a pale red tongue which was also slightly fat with thin, white fur, and a vacuous, fine, forceless pulse.

Based on these signs and symptoms, the woman's Chinese medical pattern was categorized as spleen-kidney qi vacuity with the bladder not doing its duty. The treatment principles were to supplement the center, boost the qi and regulate the qi. The formula used was modified Buzhong Yiqi Tang: Radix Astragali Membranacei (Huangqi) 30 g, Radix Codonopsitis Pilosulae (Dangshen), Rhizoma Atractylodis Macrocephalae (Baizhu) and Radix Angelicae Sinensis (Danggui) 20 g each. Pericarpium Citri Reticulatae (Chenpi), Rhizoma Cimicifugae (Shengma), Radix Bupleuri (Chaihu) and Cortex Eucommiae Ulmoidis (Duzhong) 10 g each, Fructus Corni Officinalis (Shanzhuyu) 15 g, Ramulus Cinnamomi Cassiae (Guizhi) and mix-fried Radix Glycyrrhizae (Gancao) 6 g each. After taking 10 doses (ji) of this formula, the urinary incontinence disappeared. This prescription was then administered for another month, after which all her symptoms disappeared. On follow-up after two years, there had been no recurrence.

Comment: According to the *Suwen* (simple questions), the bladder holds the office of the river island which stores fluids and humors. When its qi transforms, fluids are able to exit. The basic disease mechanism of urinary incontinence is inhibition of the bladder qi's transformation. In this case, it was due to spleen-kidney qi vacuity lacking strength to gather the fluids. Hence, the bladder qi was not able to control the urinary tract and urine easily exited. As said in the *Lingshu* (spiritual axis), when the central qi is insufficient, urination and defecation change (i.e., become abnormal). When the spleen qi is full and sufficient, the bladder's qi transformation function is normal. This is based on the fact that the latter heaven spleen and former heaven kidneys mutually promote and reinforce each other. Disease of the one typically eventually reaches the other. Therefore, Buzhong Yiqi Tang is a commonly used formula for treatment of spleen-kidney dual vacuity where spleen vacuity is more pronounced than kidney vacuity. In that case, kidney-supplementing medicinal are added to this formula as in the above case.

Due to the prevalence of spleen vacuity, or more accurately liver-spleen disharmony, among Western patients seeking treatment with Chinese medicine, Buzhong Yiqi Tang is one of the five most common guiding formulas. As the above cases illustrate, this formula treats more than just downward fall of the central qi resulting in prolapse of the stomach, intestines, uterus, and bladder. With the proper modifications, it can be used to treat a wide variety of conditions where spleen qi vacuity is the most prominent pattern present.

Section 3　Research Article

Primary study for the therapeutic dose and time window of picroside Ⅱ in treating cerebral ischemic injury in rats

[Abstract] This study aims to explore the optimal therapeutic dose and time window of picroside Ⅱ for treating cerebral ischemic injury in rats according to the orthogonal test. The middle cerebral artery occlusion (MCAO) models were established by inserting intraluminally a thread into middle cerebral artery (MCA) from left external carotid artery (ECA). The successful rat models were randomly divided into sixteen groups according to the orthogonal layout of $[L_{16}(4^5)]$ and treated by injecting picroside Ⅱ intraperitoneally with different dose at different time. The neurological behavioral function was evaluated by Bederson's test and the cerebral infarction volume was measured by tetrazolium chloride (TTC) staining. The expressions of neuron specific enolase (NSE) and neuroglial mark-protein S-100 were determined by immunohistochemisty assay. The results indicated that the optimal compositions of the therapeutic dose and time window of picroside Ⅱ in treating cerebral ischemic injury were ischemia 1.5 h with 20 mg/kg body weight according to Bederson's test, 1.0 h with 20 mg/kg body weight according to cerebral infarction volume, and 1.5 h with 20 mg/kg body weight according to the expressions of NSE and S-100 respectively. Based on the principle of the minimization of medication dose and maximization of therapeutic time window, the optimal composition of the therapeutic dose and time window of picroside Ⅱ in treating cerebral ischemic injury should be injecting picroside Ⅱ intraperitoneally with 20 mg/kg body weight at ischemia 1.5 h.

Keywords: picroside Ⅱ; cerebral ischemia; therapeutic dose; time window; NSE; S-100; rats

1　Introduction

Cerebral ischemic reperfusion injury is a pathological process relating to many factors, such as excitatory amino acids releasing, oxidative stress, calcium ion overloading, inflammatory reaction, apoptosis and so on[1-3]. Neuron-specific enolase and neuroglial mark-protein S-100 are closely related to the degree of cerebral injury and recovery[4-6]. The former study of cell culture proved that picroside Ⅱ could lessen the injury to PC12 induced by H_2O_2 and raise the cell survival rate[7-12]. Some animal experiments proved that picroside Ⅱ could inhibit apoptosis and the expression of related inflammatory factors in ischemic penumbra after ischemic reperfusion injury[13-15]. The authors' former experiments indicated that picroside Ⅱ could grow downwards degradation of the substrate, poly ADP-ribose polymerase (PARP) with catalytic activity, by inhibiting the expression toll-like receptor 4 (TLR4), nuclear transcription factor κB (NFκB), tumor necrotic factor α (TNFα) and Capase-3, and make PARP to utilize the remanent energy in the cells of ischemic penumbra to repair the nerve cells which have the reversibility of refreshing, so that to inhibit the ischemic injury leading to the apoptosis[16-23]. But in these experiments, the rats were treated by injecting picroside Ⅱ with a simple dose (20 mg/kg) at a simple time after ischemia 2 h from tail vein, and it is very inconvenient via tail vein injection. In this study, the authors aimed to explore the optimal therapeutic dose and time window of picroside Ⅱ by injecting intraperitoneally in cerebral ischemic injury in rats according to the design principle of orthogonal test.

2　Results and discussion

2.1　Neurobehavioral deficit score

After treated by picroside Ⅱ, all rats showed defect functionally at different degree. By the analysis of software of SPSS (set α=0.05), the probability of significant interaction of independent variable was 0.46 > 0.05 (Table 4-1), and namely there wasn't interaction between administering drug time and administering drug dose. From the result of analysis of variance, the significant probability of each independent variable was $P < 0.05$, namely medication time and dose had significant influence on the recovery of neurological function. All data were analysed by the statistical mean of two-way ANOVA (analysis of variance) and LSD (least significant difference) value, and the analytic results showed that there was no significant differences between administering drug at ischemia 1 h (A1) and 1.5 h (A2), and between administering drug at ischemia 2 h (A3) and 2.5 h (A4), $P > 0.05$. While there was no significant deviation between administering drug doses of 5 mg/kg (B1) and 10 mg/kg (B2) and between administering drug doses of 20 mg/kg (B3) and 40 mg/kg (B4), $P > 0.05$. There was a significant difference between each other for the rest groups, $P < 0.05$, so that the better composition of the therapeutic dose and time window of picroside Ⅱ were A1B3, A1B4, A2B3, A2B4. Considering the principles of medication dose minimization and therapeutic time maximization, it is presumed that A2B3 is the best composition, namely the best therapeutic time window and the best therapeutic dose of picroside Ⅱ is ischemia 1.5 h with 20 mg/ kg body weight.

Table 4-1   Analysis of variance about neurological function defect

Variation source	SS	df	MS	F	P
Time	3.19	3	1.06	17	0.02
Dose	3.19	3	1.06	17	0.02
Time×Dose	0.19	3	0.63	1	0.46
Error	0.38	6	0.63		

2.2   Volume of cerebral infarction

After treated by picroside Ⅱ, all rats showed an infarction volume at different degree in the area supplied by middle cerebral artery with TTC staining. According to the analysis with software of SPSS (set α = 0.05), the significant probability of the interaction of independent variables is 0.23 > 0.05, so there is no interaction between medication time and therapeutic dose (Table 4-2). The result of ANOVA showed that the significance probability of every independent variable was $P < 0.01$, which indicated the medication time and therapeutics dose of picroside Ⅱ influenced the cerebral infarction volume significantly. All data are analysed by the statistical mean of two-way ANOVA and LSD value, it is concluded that there was significant deviation between each other of medication time ($P < 0.05$), while no significant deviation between therapeutic dose 20 mg/kg (B3) and 40 mg/kg (B4) ($P > 0.05$), and there was a significant deviation between the rest combination, $P < 0.05$. So the better combination of medication time and therapeutic dose were A1B3 or A1B4. According to the principles of the minimization of medication dose and maximization of therapeutic time, it is presumed that A1B3 is the best composition group, i.e. the best therapeutic time window and the best therapeutic dose of picroside Ⅱ is ischemia 1 h with 20 mg/kg body weight.

Table 4-2　ANOVA of cerebral infraction volume

Variation source	SS	df	MS	F	P
Time	130.46	3	43.49	150.30	0.00
Dose	30.32	3	10.11	34.93	0.00
Time×Dose	1.67	3	0.56	1.92	0.23
Error	1.74	6	0.29		

2.3　Expression of NSE protein

The immunohistochemisty staining shows that NSE in brain tissue expressed at different degree, and mainly in cytoplasm with yellow or brown colors. The significance probability of the interaction of independent variables (the number of positive cells) is 0.78 > 0.05, so there is no interaction between medication time and therapeutics dose (Table 4-3). The result of ANOVA showed that the significance probability of every independent variable is less than 0.01, which proved the medication time and therapeutic dose of picroside Ⅱ could have significant influence on the expression of NSE. All data are analysed by the statistical mean of two-way ANOVA and LSD value, it is concluded that there was a significant deviation of NSE expression between each medication time ($P < 0.05$), while no significant deviation between 20 mg/kg (B3) and 40 mg/kg (B4) ($P > 0.05$), but there was significant deviation between the rest therapeutic dose combination ($P < 0.05$). So the better combination of medication time and therapeutics dose is A1B3 or A1B4. Considering the minimization of medication dose and maximization of therapeutic time, it is presumed that A1B3 is the best combination, namely the best therapeutic time window and the best therapeutic dose of picroside Ⅱ is ischemia 1.0 h with 20 mg/kg.

Table 4-3　ANOVA of positive cells of NSE

Variation source	SS	df	MS	F	P
Time	27.50	3	9.17	39.39	0.00
Dose	22.93	3	7.64	32.85	0.00
Time×Dose	0.25	3	0.08	0.36	0.78
Error	1.65	6	0.23		

2.4　Expression of S-100 protein

The staining of immunohistochemisty shows that the expression of S-100 in brain tissue was at different degree and mainly in cytoplasm. The significance probability of the interaction of independent variables (the number of positive cells) is 0.35 > 0.05, so there is no interaction between medication time and therapeutic dose (Table 4-4). The result of ANOVA showed that the significance probability of every independent variable is smaller than 0.01, which suggested the medication time and therapeutic dose of picroside II could significantly influence S-100 expression. All data were analysed by the statistical mean of two-way ANOVA and LSD value, and it is concluded that there was no significant deviation of S-100 expression between ischemia 1 h (A1) and ischemia 1.5 h (A2), also between ischemia 1.5 h (A2) and 2 h (A3) ($P > 0.05$), while there was a significant deviation between the rest combination ($P < 0.05$). Although no significant deviation between therapeutic dose 5 mg/kg (B1) and 10 mg/kg (B2), also between 20 mg/kg (B3) and 40 mg/kg (B4) ($P > 0.05$), there was a significant deviation between the rest combination ($P < 0.05$). So the better combination of medication time and therapeutic dose is A1B3 or A1B4 or A2B3 or A2B4. Considering the minimization of medication dose and maximization of therapeutic time, it is presumed that A2B3 is the best combination, namely the best therapeutic time window and the best therapeutic dose of picroside II is ischemia 1.5 h with 20 mg/kg body weight.

Table 4-4 ANOVA of positive cells of S-100

Variation source	SS	df	MS	F	P
Time	66.09	3	22.03	11.36	0.01
Dose	106.18	3	35.39	18.26	0.01
Time×Dose	7.69	3	2.56	1.32	0.35
Error	19.00	6	1.94		

2.5 Discussion

Orthogonal layout can balance sampling in the changing range of variable factors, and can enhance the representation of each test with minimum animal number and test times. Orthogonal layout owns characteristics of balanced scattering which satisfies some request of comprehensive test, shorten test cycle and elevated test efficiency to achieve better test aim. In this study, the authors applied orthogonal layout to design roundly, and compared synthetically with statistical analysis to obtain a better therapeutic schedule to get the best treatment effectiveness by a few number of tests.

In this experiment, the neurological behavioral function was evaluated by Bendeson's test to judge the therapeutic effect of picroside II on cerebral ischemic injury, TTC staining was observed and the cerebral infarction volume was calculated to indicate the severity of cerebral ischemic injury. The neuroglial mark-protein S-100[24-26] and the neuron-specific enolase (NSE) are sensitive indexes to evaluate cerebral ischemic injury [27-28]. NSE is a kind of acidic soluble protein only existing in nervous tissue. According to their three subunits with different immunity, enolases are divided into five kinds of isozymes as follows type αα, ββ, γγ, αβ and αγ, of which type γγ exists specially in nerve cells and being named as NSE. Enolases participate in the metabolism of glucolysis, catalysis α-phosphoglyceric acid into enolphospho-pyruvate. S-100 protein is an acidity calcium-binding protein, not simple protein but boodle of micromolecule protein with α and β subunits, of which the S-100 with β-subunit exist in nerve tissue specially, and mainly in gliocyte. S-100 is a kind of intercellular calcium-receptor protein and regulates energy metabolism, promotes axon growth and gliocyte proliferation, stabilizes internal environment of calcium ion, etc.. In the physiological circumstances, the contents of NSE and S-100 in brain tissue and serum are seldom and increase after brain ischemic injury to release in to the blood circulation because of cerebral ischemia injuring the blood-brain barrier. NSE and S-100 are neurochemistry markers reflecting the severity of brain tissue damage[25], so it could reflect the neuroprotective effects of picroside II on cerebral ischemia by detecting the contents of NSE and S-100 in brain tissue and serum.

In this experiment, the authors design four time point at 1 h, 1.5 h, 2 h and 2.5 h after brain ischemic injury, and inject intraperitoneally picroside II with four therapeutic doses of 5 mg/kg, 10 mg/kg, 20 mg/kg and 40 mg/kg. The experiment was carried out according to orthogonal table of $[L_{16}(4^5)]$ to explore the best therapeutic dose and best time window of picroside II in treating cerebral ischemic injury by neurological faction scale, TTC staining to measure cerebral infarction volume and the expressions of NSE and S-100, etc.. The results indicated that there is a significant difference between administering drug time and therapeutic drug dose of picroside II in influencing the multiple comparison of statistical analysis showed that the best combination isn't with accordant by different indexes. Considering minimization of medication dose and maximization of therapeutic time window, it is suggested the best choose of A1B3 composition, or the best therapeutic time window is at 1.5 h after ischemia and the best therapeutic dose of picroside II is 20 mg/kg. Because the mechanism of cerebral ischemic injury is very complicatedly and only four indexes was observed in this experiment, the results could not possible to be all right. So the effect and mechanism of picroside II and the golden evaluating indexes need to be further study in the next experiment.

3   Experimental section

3.1   Animal model of MCAO

Adult healthy male Wistar rat, SPF grade, weight 240 ~ 260 g, supplied by the Experiment Animal Center of Qingdao Drug Inspection Institute [SCXK (LU) 20090100]. The local legislation for ethics of experiment on animals and guidelines for the care and use of laboratory animals were followed in all animal procedures. This experiment was approved by the Ethics Committee of Qingdao University Medical College (No. QUMC 2011-09). All animals were acclimatized for 7 days and allowed free access to food and water in a room temperature [(23 ± 2)℃] and humidity-controlled housing with natural illumination and absolute diet at preoperative 12 h before operation. The rats were anesthetized by injecting intraperitoneally 100 g/L chloral hydrate (300 mg/kg) and fixed in supine position to conduct aseptic operation. The middle cerebral artery occlusion (MCAO) model were established by inserting intraluminally a monofilament suture from the left external-internal carotid artery (ECA-ICA) into middle cerebral artery (MCA) for cerebral ischemia[29]. Core body temperature was keeping with a rectal probe and maintained at 36 ~ 37 °C using a homeothermic blanket control unit (Qingdao Apparatus, China) during and after the surgery operation. The successful model rats showed left Horner's sign, right forelimb flexing and circling rightward as running.

3.2　Orthogonal experimental design

Sixteen successful MCAO rat models were internalized into the experiment and divided randomly according to the principle of orthogonal experimental design of $[L_{16}(4^5)]$ consisting of two impact factors with four impact levels (Table 4-5). The impact factor A is the therapeutic time widow designed four levels as ischemia 1.0 h, 1.5 h, 2.0 h, and 2.5 h. The impact factor B is the therapeutic drug dose which has four levels as following 5 mg/kg, 10 mg/kg, 20 mg/kg and 40 mg/kg body weight.

Table 4-5　Orthogonal experimental design of $[L_{16}(4^5)]$

Therapeutic dose	Ischemia 1.0 h (A1)	Ischemia 1.5 h (A2)	Ischemia 2.0 h (A3)	Ischemia 2.5 h (A4)
5 mg/kg (B1)	1.0×5	1.5×5	2.0×5	2.5×5
10 mg/kg (B2)	1.0×10	1.5×10	2.0×10	2.5×10
20 mg/kg (B3)	1.0×20	1.5×20	2.0×20	2.5×20
40 mg/kg (B4)	1.0×40	1.5×40	2.0×40	2.5×40

3.3　Treatment methods

Picroside Ⅱ (Tianjin Kuiqing Med. Tech. Co., Ltd., CAS No: 39012-20-9, purity > 98%) was diluted into 1% solution with 0.1 mol/L PBS and injected intraperitoneally according to the corresponding designed doses in the orthogonal layout $[L_{16}(4^5)]$. After 24 h of treatment, the rats were killed to detect the corresponding indexes.

3.4 Observation indexes

3.4.1 Neurological defect test

After treated with picroside Ⅱ, the neurological behavioral function scales was performed by Bederson's test [30] in each rats. The higher score, the severe neurological function defect. Score 0: no behavioral deficiency; Score 1: forelimb buckling (the tail lifting-suspension test positive); Score 2: lateral thrust resistance decreased (lateral thrust test positive) and forelimb buckling, no circling; Score 3: the same as midrange behavior and circling spontaneously.

3.4.2 The cerebral infarction volume

After treated with picroside Ⅱ, all rats were anesthetized with 100 g/L chloral hydrate (300 mg/kg) and then the brain was take out completely to be cut five coronal sections of 2 mm thickness backward from optic chiasma. Five coronal sections were put into 20 g/L TTC phosphate buffer at 37 ℃ and then fix in 40 g/L poly-formaldehyde. The normal brain tissues showed red and infarct tissue white. The infarct volume is determined by Adobe PhotoShop CS after taking a photograph, and expressed as the percentage of the brain infarct size and homonymy brain hemisphere (%).

3.4.3 Immunohistochemisty

After treated with picroside Ⅱ, all rats were anesthetized with 100 g/L chloral hydrate (300 mg/kg) and fixed with 40 g/L poly-formaldehyde from cardiac perfusion to take out the brain completely. The brain was dehydrated by gradient ethanol, cleared by xylene, embedded in paraffin and sliced backward from optic chiasma into pieces of thickness 5 μm. Then the slices were adhered to the sections prepared with poly-L-lysine, and finally stored at 4 ℃. Rabbit anti-rat NSE and S-100 monoclonal antibodies, SABC immunohistochemisty kit and DAB chromogenic liquor were provided by Boster Biological Company, Wuhan, China. The paraffin section were deparaffinized according to directions, then colored by DAB and observed under light microscope to count the positive cells with brown granules in cytoplasm. And the slides with the addition of 0.01 mmol/L PBS (containing 1∶200 non-immunity animal serum), instead of primary antibody, showed no response. Five serial section of each rat were randomly chosen and observed five visual fields of cortical area under light microscope (400 times) to count the number of positive cells of every visual fields and expressed as mean ± standard error (mean ± SD).

3.5 Statistical analysis

SPSS 17.0 software was used for data statistical analysis. According to the result, multi-group comparison was made by analysis of orthogonal test whether different level of administrating time and therapeutic dose had significant deviation or not, and whether their interaction on each detected index had significant deviation or not, meanwhile to explore the best therapeutic drug dose and the therapeutic time window. Values were considered to be significant when P was less than 0.05.

4   Conclusions

This study suggested the optimal composition of the therapeutic dose and time window of picroside Ⅱ in treating cerebral ischemic injury should be injecting picroside Ⅱ intraperitoneally with 20 mg/kg body weight at ischemia 1.5 h.

Acknowledgement

This study was supported by grant-in-aids for the Natural Science Foundation of China (grant No. 30873391 and No. 81041092) and the Natural Science Foundation of Shandong Province (ZR2011HM050).

Reference

[1]   Manneville S E, Manneville J B, Adamson P. et al. ICAM-1 coupled cytoskeletal tearrangements and transcendothelial lymphocyte migration involve intracellular calcium signaling in brain endothelial cell lines. Immunol, 2000, 165: 3375-3383.

[2]   Caso J R, Pradillo J M, Hurtado O, et al. Toll-like receptor 4 is involved in subacute stress-induced neuroinflammation and in the worsening of experimental stroke. Stroke. 2008, 39: 1314-1320.

[3]   Bi X, Yan B, Fang S, et al. Quetiapine regulates neurogenesis in ischemic mice by inhibiting NF-kappaB p65/p50 expression. Neurological Research, 2009, 31(2): 159-166.

[4]   Kruijk J R D, Leffers P, Menheere P P C A, et al. S-100B and neuron-specific enolase in serum of mild traumatic brain injury patients A comparison with healthy controls. Acta Neurologica Scandinavica, 2001, 103(3): 175-179.

[5]   Basile A M, Fusi C, Conti A A, et al. S-100 protein and neuron-specific enolase as markers of subclinical cerebral damage after cardiac surgery: preliminary observation of a 6-month follow-up study. European Neurology, 2001, 45(3): 151-159.

[6]   Kessler F H, Woody G, Portela L V, et al. Brain injury markers (S100B and NSE) in chronic cocaine dependents. Revista Brasileira De Psiquiatria, 2007, 29(2): 134-139.

[7]   Li P, Matsunaga K, Yamakuni T, et al. Potentiation of nerve growth factor-action by picrosides I and Ⅱ, natural iridoids, in PC12D cells. European Journal of Pharmacology, 2000, 406(2): 203-208.

[8]   Li P, Matsunaga K, Yamakuni T, et al. Picrosides I and Ⅱ, selective enhancers of the mitogen-activated protein kinase-dependent signaling pathway in the action of neuritogenic substances on PC12D cells.

Life Sciences, 2002, 71(15): 1821-1835.

[9]   Tao Y W, Liu J W, Wei D Z, et al. Protective effect of picroside-II on the damage of cultured PC12 cells in vitro. Chinese Journal of Clinical Pharmacology & Therapeutics, 2003, 8: 27-30.

[10]   Guo M C, Cao Y. Protective effects of picroside II on glutamate injury of PC12 cells. Chinese Journal of Clinical Pharmacology & Therapeutics, 2007, 12: 440-443.

[11]   Li T, Liu J W, Zhang X D, et al. The neuroprotective effect of picroside II from hu-huang-lian against oxidative stress. American Journal of Chinese Medicine, 2007, 35(4): 681-691.

[12]   Cao Y, Liu J W, Yu Y J, et al. Synergistic protective effect of picroside II and NGF on PC12 cells against oxidative stress induced by H_2O_2. Chinese Journal of Clinical Pharmacology & Therapeutics, 2007, 59(5): 573.

[13]   Yan W J, Zhen L I, Wang H P, et al. Picroside II inhibited apoptosis and expression of iNOS following cerebral ischemic reperfusion injury in rats. Chinese Pharmacological Bulletin, 2009, 25: 1677-1678.

[14]   Yang X W, Xu-Ming J I, Guo Y L. Effects of rhizoma picrorhizae on nerve growth factor in rat brain following cerebral ischemia. Acta Academiae Medicinae Qingdao Universitatis, 2008, 44: 69-71.

[15]   Zhen L I, Qin L I, Guo Y L, et al. Interference effect of picroside II on cerebral ischemia reperfusion injury in rats. Acta Anatomica Sinica, 2010, 41: 9-12.

[16]   Guo Y, Xu X, Li Q, et al. Anti-inflammation effects of picroside 2 in cerebral ischemic injury rats. Behavioral & Brain Functions, 2010, 6(1): 43.

[17]   Li Q, Li Z, Xu X Y, et al. Neuroprotective properties of picroside II in a rat model of focal cerebral ischemia. International Journal of Molecular Sciences, 2010, 11(11): 4580-4590.

[18]   Li Z, Xu X Y, Li Q, et al. Protective mechanisms of picroside II on aquaporin-4 expression in a rat model of cerebral ischemia/reperfusion injury. Neural Regeneration Research, 2010, 5(6): 411-417.

[19]   Li X, Xu X, Li Z, et al. Picroside II down-regulates matrix metalloproteinase-9 expression following cerebral ischemia/reperfusion injury in rats. Brain Injury, 2010, 5(18): 1403-1407.

[20]   Li Z, Xu X Y, Shen W, et al. The interferring effects of picroside II on the expressions of NF-κB and I-κB following cerebral ischemia reperfusion injury in rats. Chinese Pharmacological Bulletin, 2010, 26(1): 52-55.

[21]   Guo Y L, Shen W, Li Z, et al. The influence of picroside II on TLR4 and NFκB express after cerebral ischemia-reperfusion injury. Chin J Int Med, 2011, 31: 58-61.

[22]   Li Q, Guo Y L, Li Z, et al. The interference of picroside II on the expressions of Caspase-3 and PARP following cerebral ischemia reperfusion injury in rats. Chinese Pharmacological Bulletin, 2010, 26(3): 342-345.

[23]   Sun L, Li X D, Wang L, et al. The anti-oxidant effect and the possible mechanism of picroside II in cerebral ischemia reperfusion injury in rats. Neural Regen Res, 2011, 6: 1141-1146.

[24]   Butterworth R J, Wassif W S, Sherwood R A, et al. Serum neuron-specific enolase, carnosinase, and their ratio in acute stroke. Stroke, 1996, 27(11): 2064-2068.

[25]   Abraha H D, Butterworth R J, Bath P M, et al. Serum S-100 protein, relationship to clinical outcome in

acute stroke. Annals of Clinical Biochemistry, 1997, 34(5): 366-370.

[26] Naeimi Z S, Weinhofer A, Sarahrudi K, et al. Predictive value of S-100B protein and neuron specific-enolase as markers of traumatic brain damage in clinical use. Brain Inj, 2006, 20(5): 463-468.

[27] Jin L, Liu Z, Yang X. The expressions and serum levels of NSE and S-100 following cerebral ischemia and reperfusion in rabbits. Chinese Journal of Rehabilitation Medicine, 2007, 22(11): 964-967.

[28] Niu T X, Shi Z Y, Luo J J, et al. The change and clinical significance of NSE and S-100β protein in acute stroke in rats. Chin J Comp Med, 2009, 19: 34-37.

[29] Longa E Z, Weinstein P R, Carlson S, et al. Reversible middle cerebral artery occlusion without craniectomy in rats. Stroke, 1989, 20(1): 84.

[30] Bederson J B, Pitts L H, Tsuji M, et al. Rat middle cerebral artery occlusion: evaluation of the model and development of a neurologic examination. Stroke, 1986, 17(3): 472.

Section 4　Words of TCM

1. 心主神明 heart governing mental activities
2. 心主血脉 heart controlling blood and vessels or circulation
3. 心气下陷 heart qi descending
4. 心火亢盛 hyperactivity or exuberance of heart fire
5. 心肝血虚 asthenia or deficiency of heart and liver blood
6. 心肝火旺 exuberance of heart and liver fire
7. 心气充沛 abundance of heart qi
8. 肝主疏泄 liver governing distribution and excretion
9. 肝主藏血 liver storing blood
10. 肝为刚藏 liver being resolute zang-organ
11. 肝气升发 liver qi ascending and dispersing
12. 肝阳上亢 hyperactivity of liver yang
13. 肝气郁滞 stagnation of liver qi
14. 脾主运化 spleen governing transport and transformation
15. 脾主统血 spleen governing blood
16. 脾为孤脏 spleen being solitary zang-organ
17. 脾应四时 spleen corresponding to four seasons
18. 脾气升清 spleen qi lifting the clear
19. 脾喜燥恶湿 spleen preferring dryness to dampness
20. 肺主呼吸之气 lung governing respiratory air
21. 肺主一身之气 lung governing physical qi

22. 肺朝百脉 convergence of vessels of in the lungs

23. 肺主行水 lung governing water movement

24. 肺主治节 lung governing coordinative activities of viscera

25. 肺为华盖 lung being the canopy

26. 肺为娇脏 lung being the delicate organ

27. 宣发肃降 dispersion and descension

28. 升降出入 ascending, descending, outing and entering

29. 肾主纳气 kidney receiving respiratory qi

30. 肾气上升 kidney qi ascending

31. 肾主水 kidney governing water

32. 肾藏精 kidney storing essence

33. 命门，七冲门 vital gate, seven important portals

34. 胆主决断 gallbladder governing deciding

35. 胃为水谷之海 stomach being reservoir of water and grain

36. 上焦如雾 upper-jiao (energizer) resembling mist

37. 中焦如沤 middle-jiao resembling fermenter

38. 下焦如渎 lower-jiao resembling drainage

39. 疏肝和胃 smoothing the liver and mediating the stomach

40. 中气下陷 middle qi collapse or visceroptosis

(Ni Tongshang, Wang Tingting)

Chapter 5   Headache

Section 1   Vascular Headache

Vascular headache is a group of conditions that involve the dilation or swelling of blood vessels which cause headache pain. The blood vessels in the head become enlarged, distended and inflamed, which alters the normal pulsation of the vessels and leads to a throbbing pain that usually worsens with physical activity.

1   The types of vascular headache

Vascular headache is one of the four major types of headache, alongside muscle contraction (tension), traction and inflammatory headache. The definition of vascular headache is one from vascular disturbance. There are several types of vascular headaches, such as migraine, hypertension, cluster, miscellaneous, etc..

Migraine: The migraine is a periodic throbbing headache. It is the most common type of vascular headache and is more likely to affect women than men. The prodrome seems to be due to a vasoconstriction of the cerebral blood vessels (or the vessels leading into the brain), while the headache itself seems to be due to a vasodilation of the blood vessels with subsequent congestion of tissues. It is more often in women and is thought to affect up to 20% ~ 30% of the population. It usually begins at the ages of 10 ~ 30 and remissions commonly occur after age 50, which suggested a hormonal cause and a definitive familial component.

The symptoms and signs of migraine may be unilateral or bilateral that often located about or behind an eye spreading to one or both sides of the head. Frequently, there is nausea and vomiting, and a desire for darkness and quiet. The headache lasts from hours to 1 ~ 3 days. The classic type has a prodrome of various symptoms such as scintillating scotomas, mood swings, dizziness and tinnitus, dazzling zigzags, perhaps feeling of impending doom. Physical and neurological findings between attacks are unremarkable, and during attacks there may be transient neurological signs. The laboratory findings: rule out organic disease, skull X-ray, brain scan and EEG.

Hypertension headache: The hypertension headache is typically throbbing and located in the occiput or vertex. It is paroxysmal and has a history of renal or cardiovascular disease such as hypertension. Physical exam will reveal hypertension, with retinopathy, edema and cardiac findings. Generally, the hypertensive headache is associated with advanced hypertensive disease or attacks of potentially serious hypertension. The laboratory findings: blood chemistries and renal studies.

Cluster headache: The cluster (histamine headaches) is much more frequent in men and associated histaminic symptoms. It is paroxysmal, often wakes the patient at night, with abrupt severe pain and lasts $1 \sim 2$ hours. It occurs typically in clusters of days to weeks and then not experienced again for months or years. It is unilateral with associated histaminic symptoms include lacrimation, plugged nose, ptosis, cheek flushed and edemic. Remissions may occur lasting for years or permanently. Physical exam shows facial vasodilation, pupillary constriction, injected conjunctiva, tenderness to palpation of external and common carotid arteries.

Miscellaneous headache: The miscellaneous headache is moderate in intensity and caused by toxic states, infections, alcoholism, uremia, lead, arsenic, morphine, carbon monoxide, poisoning, encephalitides, etc.. There is a history of exposure to a toxin, or other signs and symptoms that would point to an associated microorganism. It has a history of exposure to a toxin, or other signs and symptoms that would point to an associated microorganism. The laboratory findings are specific to the causative agent, lumbar puncture, blood and urine studies, and course and prognosis.

2   Diagnosis of vascular headache

Types of vascular headache may be diagnosed based upon the presenting symptoms and a physical exam. It is useful if the patient records the nature of the condition in a headache diary for a period of time to help the health practitioner to obtain a more complete understanding of their condition.

Important information that will help in the diagnosis includes information about the headaches, such as time of attacks, location of the pain, description of the pain, duration of the pain, and frequency of the pain. Other factors that may help in the diagnosis of the condition include behavioral changes and other symptoms that present with attacks.

There are some diagnostic tests that can also help to confirm diagnosis of vascular headaches. This may include blood tests, X-rays, magnetic resonance imaging (MRI), computer tomography (CT) scan or a lumbar puncture.

3　Treatment of vascular headache

The treatment of vascular headaches depends on the specific characteristics of the condition and there are several factors that should be considered. These may include medical and family history, frequency and severity of symptoms, tolerance for medications and therapies, expected treatment outcomes and personal preferences.

Lifestyle alterations, particular in reducing activities with a high level of stress and prioritizing a healthy diet can make a significant difference in the frequency and severity of vascular headaches. Other treatment options for vascular headache may include: biofeedback training, stress reduction, nutritional modifications, physical therapy, pressure therapy and cold packs.

The first-line treatment options for vascular headaches in pharmacotherapy include analgesic medications, such as paracetamol, ibuprofen and aspirin. For severe pain that is not relieved by these medications, there are specific options that are indicated for the relief of pain associated with migraines. Additionally, preventative medications can help to reduce the frequency of vascular headaches for individuals that often suffer from severe attacks.

In general, migraine and cluster headaches are chronic conditions that recur and are not cured by conventional treatment. Although they are both benign, the pains can be debilitating and cause much morbidity. Conventional treatment usually involves ergotamine prophylaxis and narcotic analgesics. The hypertensive headache is correctable by controlling the patient's hypertension; if uncontrolled, then serious hypertensive sequelae may occur (e.g. stroke). The toxic headache is treated by dealing with the toxic exposure and ridding the body of the substance. Prognosis for migraine headache is favorable if thorough assessment and avoidance of triggers, along with biochemical/metabolic therapy are undertaken.

Section 2　Liuwei Dihuang Wan

Liuwei Dihuang Wan (LDW) is one of the most famous and frequently used formulas in traditional Chinese medicine. It is also known as Six Flavor Tea Pills, Liuwei Dihuang Pian, Six Ingredient Pill with Rehmannia, Six Flavor Rehmannia, and so on. It is so popular that nearly all Chinese have heard this name. Traditionally, it is used for vertigo, insomnia, tinnitus, weakness in the knees, poor hearing, poor eyesight, night sweats, heat in the five, weakness and soreness of the loins, and more. Today, it is also used to treat coronary heart disease, diabetes, Addison's disease, low adrenals, menopause, hypertension, infertility, impotence, and so on. For that reason, some people, especially middle-aged and older men and post-menopausal women, tend to use it for a long time to help boost libido and stay young. However, it is worth mentioning that this formula is not for everyone.

What is LDW?

This earliest version of this Chinese medicinal formula is Jinkui Shenqi Wan, which comes from *Shanghan Lun* or *Shanghan Zabing Lun* (Treatise on cold injury), a classic medicinal literature compiled by Zhang Zhongjing about 2000 years ago at the end of the Han Dynasty. Qian Yi, a royal physician in the Northern Song Dynasty, believed that kidney determines the growth and development of people, emphasizing the importance of reinforcing and reducing at the same time. So, in order to replenish yin due to the yin insufficiency of the kidney, according to his theory Qian Yi changed Jinkui Shenqi Wan slightly and created a 6-ingredient formula, which is later known as LDW. And it consists of Rehmanniae Radix (Shudihuang), Corni Fructus (Shanzhuyu), Dioscoreae Rhizoma (Shanyao), Alismatis Rhizoma (Zexie), Poria (Fuling), and Paeoniae Suffruticosa Cortex (Mudanpi).

Chinese medicine believes that the kidneys store congenital essence, which is the foundation of Zang-fu (yin-yang) organs and the source of life. So, the kidneys are associated with the gate of vitality or Mingmen in TCM. In this prescription, Shudihuang is the principal drug for enriching yin and nourishing kidney, Shanzhuyu for nourishing both liver and kidney, Shanyao for strengthening spleen and benefiting vital qi, Zexie for reducing dampness in the kidney, Mudanpi for clearing liver fire, and Fuling for resolving spleen dampness.

What is LDW good for?

First of all, it's important to note that it is not an elixir although it is a versatile Chinese patent medicine. According to incomplete statistics, this prescription involves 137 conditions in a variety of literature. The most common uses are to help suboptimal health status, boost immune system, and delay aging. This is why so many people take it as supplements for a long time in order to improve health. At the same time, as a therapeutic drug it is good for hypertension, diabetes, menopausal syndrome and other diseases too.

As a typical formula for insufficient liver and kidney yin in TCM, it is commonly used in various diseases due to liver and kidney yin deficiency. In recent years, it has been used for a variety of chronic diseases and difficult diseases and the result is quite positive.

1. Silicosis. According to reports, when it is combined with tetrandrine (100 mg 3 times/day) for 2 months, it significantly improves cough, expectoration, chest pain and dyspnea in patients with silicosis. Besides, by doing so it still decreases the risk of colds and bronchial infection by 52.94%.

2. Chronic rhinitis. It can be used to treat chronic rhinitis too. Usually the patients should take it twice a day and continue for at least 2 months to see a big improvement.

3. Allergic rhinitis. It can enhance cellular immune mechanisms, promote the synthesis of immune globulin, inhibit the formation of antibodies, inhibit allergic reactions, and play a two-way regulation. It works even better when combined with sodium cromoglycate.

4. Recurrent respiratory tract infections in pediatric patients. Some TCM practitioners ever used it to treat 60 cases of children with recurrent respiratory tract infection and the results were satisfactory. Besides, it has been observed that it significantly impacts the children's immune function and trace element levels.

5. Recurrent aphthous ulcers. Taking it 2 ~ 3 times a day for 3 ~ 5 days can help treat recurrent aphthous ulcers. And the patient won't relapse easily after treatment.

6. Xerostomia. It works for the elderly who are suffering from dry mouth, especially when there are no other primary diseases.

7. Mild to moderate hypertension. 38 cases of mild to moderate hypertension were randomly divided into two groups. While one group was treated with LDW along with Compound Danshen Tablet, the other group was given nifedipine and vitamin E. As a result, 90.9% participants saw a drop in blood pressure in the first group, compared to 87.5% in the second group.

8. Upper gastrointestinal bleeding. It has a certain therapeutic effect for patients with glucocorticoid-induced chronic gastrointestinal bleeding.

9. Nephrotic syndrome. It is good for nephrotic syndrome too. Usually a course of treatment (20 days) will significantly improve symptoms, signs and proteinuria.

10. Chronic nephritis. It treats both acute and chronic nephritis, but it has better effect for the latter, especially in patients with high blood pressure or edema too. Usually one course of treatment (1 month) can help eliminate proteinuria and edema, and promote the recovery of renal function.

11. Prostatitis. According to clinical reports, it is a highly effective treatment for patients with chronic prostatitis patients. Usually 10 days are a course of treatment.

12. Male infertility. It can act on the hypothalamus-pituitary-gonadal axis, improve sex hormone secretion, promote the normal sperm production, and thereby increase the success rate for getting pregnant.

13. Drug-induced leukopenia. It treats granulocytopenia caused by clozapine, anti-thyroid drugs and chemotherapy.

14. Toxic side effects of chemotherapy drugs. When used as adjuvant treatment, it can help achieve satisfactory result in enhancing the effect of chemotherapy drugs while reducing their toxic side effects. The method is to take it from the first day of chemotherapy, 9 grams each time, 3 times a day, and 20 days as one course of treatment.

15. Diabetes. Those who have pre-diabetes or even mild diabetes are very controllable with diet in some cases. Besides, LDW can help lower blood sugar and urine sugar and improve symptoms too.

16. Menopausal syndrome. Usually taking it for 3 months can help patients to improve flushing, hot flashes, sweating, palpitations, anxiety, insomnia and other symptoms.

17. Cerebral hemorrhage sequelae. It has good therapeutic efficacy for patients with sequelae from cerebral hemorrhage, such as trouble with speaking and understanding, paralysis or numbness of the face, arm or leg, blurred or blackened vision in one or both eyes, and so on.

18. Senile dementia. It has obvious antioxidant effect that is good for senile dementia. Related animal experiments show that it can improve learning and memory disorders and help to enhance memory. And clinical trials confirmed that it improves amnesia and senile dementia to some extent.

19. Fatigue syndrome. It helps mental fatigue, dizziness, loss of appetite, sleep loss and disturbed sleep, emotional instability, concentration difficulty, forgetfulness, memory problems, slow thinking, and the like.

20. Rheumatoid arthritis. It can replace glucocorticoid in the treatment of rheumatoid arthritis. In other words, it helps avoid the side effects of glucocorticoids.

21. Wrinkles. It has potent properties of strengthening kidney yin and helps the production of SOD (superoxide dismutase), one of the body's most powerful natural antioxidant enzymes. Since SOD can turn the superoxide ions that caused aging into harmless substances, it delays the aging of the human body to help people stay young.

22. Chronic pruritus in the elderly. The pathogenesis of this disease is mainly associated with dysfunction of sebaceous gland, lack of sebum and degradation of autonomic nervous system function. The good news is that LDW is good at nourishing kidney yin, enhancing androgen secretion, exciting gonadal axis, slowing down the sebaceous gland atrophy, relieving skin dryness and so on.

23. Premature aging. It helps blotchy hyperpigmentation, premature graying of hair, increased wrinkle formation, dry texture and other symptoms of premature aging.

24. Hair loss. As mentioned above, the kidney system is considered the foundation of the body's energy in TCM. And kidney governs the hair on the head. That's to say, hair loss is related to the state of the kidney and an outward sign of poor kidney health inside. So, kidney yin deficiency will fail to supply a regular supply of key nutrients to hair and cause thinning hair and hair loss.

25. Vitiligo. The disease is an acquired loss of skin color in blotches. LDW nourishes kidneys and liver, tonifies blood and essence, and moisturizes and lightens skin. Modern studies suggest that this formula activates tyrosine activity, accelerates the production of tyrosine-catalyzed melanin and promotes melanoma cell division and movement by improving the body's cellular immunity. By doing so, it restores color to the white patches of skin.

26. Systemic lupus erythematosus. This is an autoimmune disease characterized by the production of unusual antibodies in the blood. LDW can be a good option during stable stage and a reduction in the corticosteroid dose. This is mainly because it is able to strengthen healthy energy while fostering root, nourish kidney yin, improve immune system function, reduce steroid withdrawal syndrome or rebound effect and some other adverse reactions, help reduce the amount of hormones, and relieve negative feedback inhibition by adrenal glucocorticoids.

27. Low alpha-fetoprotein (AFP) levels. AFP is a tumor marker. Continuously elevated or decreased AFP blood levels can be found in certain tumors, especially hepatocellular carcinoma, or primary liver cancer, and some types of testicular and ovarian cancer. Long-term consumption of LDW can greatly reduce the incidence of liver cancer.

28. Eye diseases. It can help patients with senile cataracts to significantly improve vision, blurred vision, lens opacity and other symptoms. In addition, it also has a certain effect on treating traumatic corneal ulcer, Posner-Schlossman Syndrome (PSS), and so on.

29. Riehl's melanosis. As a photocontact dermatitis, Riehl melanosis is characterized by initial erythema, edema, pruritus, and followed hyperpigmentation. The pigmentation will gradually spread and then become stationary in the end. TCM believes that the pathogenesis of Riehl's melanosis is related to deficient kidney yin. So, this is where LDW comes in.

30. Chloasma. It is also known as melasma, facial pigmentation, and the mask of pregnancy. Chloasma is associated with endocrine disorders, autoimmune diseases, oral administration of certain drugs and pregnancy. There is no specific therapy so far. Luckily, LDW can be a good choice for the treatment of melasma.

Side effects of LDW

It is for those with obvious symptoms of kidney yin deficiency, which is manifested as weakness and soreness of the knees and the loins, hot palms of hands and soles of feet, dizziness, tinnitus, hot flashes, night sweats, dry mouth and throat, nocturnal emission, premature ejaculation, etc.. Although this formula tonifies kidney, long-term use may cause abdominal fullness or bloating, diarrhea, loss of appetite and so on in even healthy people who have not the above-mentioned symptoms.

It is not for those with obvious kidney and spleen yang deficiency, which is manifested as pale complexion, physical weakness, feeling of being cold without an apparent cause, and so on. For example, it will worsen erectile dysfunction due to kidney yang deficiency. In this case, another formula like Guifu Dihuang Wan would make more sense.

It is not for those with kidney yin deficiency having abnormal function in spleen and stomach. As mentioned previously, this formula mainly focuses on invigorating yin. Unfortunately, yin-natured ingredients tend to weaken the digestive function. So, caution should be taken for the elderly in long-term and continuous use of this prescription.

If LDW has been used for two weeks and the improvements are minimal, it may not be the right therapy. In this case, it is a good idea to visit a qualified TCM practitioner and let him or her assess the state of health and then carry out symptomatic treatment.

Section 3　Research Article

Anti-inflammation effects of Picroside Ⅱ in cerebral ischemic injury rats

[Abstract]Background: Excitatory amino acid toxicity, oxidative stress, intracellular calcium overload, as well as inflammation and apoptosis are involved in the pathological process after cerebral ischemic reperfusion injury. Picroside Ⅱ could inhibit neuronal apoptosis and play an anti-oxidant and anti-inflammation role in cerebral ischemia/reperfusion injuries, but the exact mechanism is not very clear. This study aims to explore the anti-inflammation mechanism of picroside Ⅱ in cerebral ischemic reperfusion injury in rats. Methods: The middle cerebral artery occlusion reperfusion models were established with intraluminal thread methods in 90 adult healthy female Wistar rats. Picroside Ⅱ and salvianic acid A sodium were respectively injected from tail vein at the dosage of 10 mg/kg for treatment. The neurobehavioral function was evaluated with Bederson's test and the cerebral infarction volume was observed with tetrazolium chloride (TTC) staining. The apoptotic cells were counted by in situ terminal deoxynucleotidyl transferase-mediated biotinylated deoxyuridine triphosphate nick end labeling (TUNEL) assay. The immunohistochemistry stain was used to determine the expressions of toll-like receptor 4 (TLR4), nuclear transcription factor κB (NFκB) and tumor necrosis factor α (TNFα). The concentrations of TLR4, NFκB and TNFα in brain tissue were determined by enzyme linked immunosorbent assay (ELISA). Results: After cerebral ischemic reperfusion, the rats showed neurobehavioral function deficit and cerebral infarction in the ischemic hemisphere. The number of apoptotic cells, the expressions and the concentrations in brain tissue of TLR4, NFκB and TNFα in ischemia control group increased significantly than those in the sham operative group ($P < 0.01$). Compared with the ischemia control group, the neurobehavioral scores, the infarction volumes, the apoptotic cells, the expressions and concentrations in brain tissue of TLR4, NFκB and TNFα were obviously decreased both in the picroside Ⅱ and salvianic acid A sodium groups ($P < 0.01$). There was no statistical difference between the two treatment groups in above indexes ($P > 0.05$). Conclusions: Picroside Ⅱ could down-regulate the expressions of TLR4, NFκB and TNFα to inhibit apoptosis and inflammation induced by cerebral ischemic reperfusion injury and improve the neurobehavioral function of rats.

Keywords: Picroside Ⅱ; anti-inflammation; cerebral ischemic injury; rats

1　Background

Excitatory amino acid toxicity, oxidative stress, intracellular calcium overload, as well as inflammation and apoptosis, are involved in the pathological process after cerebral ischemic reperfusion injury [1]. Among these, the inflammatory cytokines activate nuclear transcription factor κB (NFκB) through toll-like receptor 4 (TLR4)-NFκB signal transduction pathways, promote target gene activation, such as tumor necrosis factor α (TNFα), interleukin (IL), intercellular adhesion molecule (ICAM), and ultimately induce neuronal apoptosis[2-3]. Picrorhiza scrophulariflora belongs to the plant family composed of picroside I, II and III, of which picroside II is one of the most effective components extracted from the dried rhizome and roots of Picrorhiza kurrooa Royle ex Benth[4] and Picrorhiza scrophulariae flora Pennell [5]. It has been traditionally used to treat disorders of the liver, upper respiratory tract diseases, dyspepsia, chronic diarrhea and scorpion sting [5-6]. Current researches on picroside II are focused on its neuroprotective[7], antiapoptotic, anticholestatic, antioxidant, anti-inflammation, and immunemodulating activities[8-9]. It has been confirmed that picroside II could enhance nerve growth factor-induced PC12 cell axon growth, reduce H_2O_2 induced PC12 cell damage and improve cell survival in vitro[10-13]. Animal experiments showed that the extract of Picrorhizae could inhibit cell apoptosis in ischemic penumbra and improve neurobehavioral function in middle cerebral artery occlusion and reperfusion (MCAO/R) rats [14]. Our previous experiments [15-16] indicated that picroside II could inhibit the expressions of inducible nitric oxide synthase (iNOS), nuclear transcription factor κB (NFκB) and inhibitor of NFκB (IκB), and reduce the expressions of Caspase-3 and poly ADP-ribose polymerase (PARP) to inhibit the neuronal apoptosis and thus improve the neurobehavioral function of rats with cerebral ischemia reperfusion injury. However, it is poorly understood that how many ingredients there are in the extract Picrorhizae and which one can play the physiological role. In the study, we established the experimental MCAO/R model to investigate the effects of picroside II via tail vein injection on TLR4-NFκB signal transduction pathway and cell apoptosis, and to explore its anti-inflammatory mechanism in cerebral ischemic reperfusion injury.

2   Materials and methods

2.1   Establishment of animal models

The total of 90 adult female Wistar rats, weight 230 ~ 250 g, SPF grade, were granted by Qingdao Laboratory Animal Center [SCXK (LU) 20030010]. The guidance suggestions for care of laboratory animals was followed according to the *Guidelines for caring for experimental animals* released by the Ministry of Science and Technology of the People's Republic of China. All animals were reared in the laboratory environment, allowed free access to food and water in a temperature and humidity-controlled housing with natural illumination for a week, and fasted for 12 h before operation. 15 rats were randomly selected as a sham operated group (SO), and the rest 75 rats were subjected to the experimental middle cerebral artery occlusion 2 h and reperfusion 22 h (MCAO/R) models with intraluminal monofilament suture from left external-internal carotid artery [17-19]. Two hours after the operation, those with left Horner sign, right anterior limb flexible or circling towards right, were considered as symbols of successful models. Core body temperature was monitored with a rectal probe and maintained at $36 \sim 37$ ℃ using a homeothermic blanket control unit (Qingdao Apparatus, China) during and after the surgery operation. As a result, 45 successful models, as the candidate, were randomly divided into an ischemia control group (IC, $n = 15$), a salvianic acid A sodium group (SA, $n = 15$) and a picroside treated group (PT, $n = 15$) according to drug administration. Rats in the SO group were experimented with the same surgical procedure but the monofilament was advanced only about 10 mm and immediately withdrew. The 30 dead or unsuccessfully occluded rats were excluded from this experiment.

2.2   Intervention study

According to *the Pharmacopoeia of the People's Republic of China,* the molecular formula of picroside Ⅱ is $C_{23}H_{28}O_{13}$, molecular weight is 512.48; the molecular formula of salvianic acid A sodium is $C_9H_9O_5Na$, molecular weight is 221.17.

Picroside Ⅱ (Tianjin Kuiqing Med. Tech. Co. Ltd., CAS No: 39012-20-9, purity > 98%), as a treatment drug, was diluted into 1% injection with 0.1 mol/L PBS, and salvianic acid A sodium (Shanghai Huyun Medical Technology Co. Ltd., CAS No: 23028-17-3, purity > 98%) was also diluted into 1% solution as a positive control drug. According to Xiao's report [20], the rats in PT group were administrated picroside Ⅱ (10 mg/kg) 250 μL via tail vein at ischemia 2 h prior to reperfusion with a micro-syringe. Rats in SA group were given salvianic acid A sodium (10 mg/kg) 250 μL, while those in IC group and SO group were simultaneously suffered 0.1 mol / L PBS 250 μL.

2.3   Neurobehavioral function assessment

All animal neurobehavioral tests were performed at ischemia 2 h and reperfusion 22 h by an investigator who was blinded to the experiment according to the standard of Bederson's report [21]. 0 score: no neurological functional impairment; 1 score: any part of forepaw flexed (positive for tail suspension test) without other abnormal sign; 2 scores: lateral pushing resistance ability decreased (positive for lateral pushing experiment), accompanied with forepaw flexion without circling tendency; 3 scores: same behaviors as those for 2 scores, in addition to spontaneous rotation (circling around paralyzed limbs during free activity). The higher the score is got, the worse the neurobehavioral dysfunction is appeared, vice versa.

2.4   TTC staining

To determine the infarction volume, five rats in each group were deeply anesthetized by

10% chloral hydrate (300 mg/kg) and decapitated at given time after MCAO/R. The brain tissue was removed and successively sliced into 2.0 mm-thick coronal sections. The total of five brain slices were incubated in 2% TTC solution for 10 min at 37 ℃ and then transferred into 4% formaldehyde solution for fixation. The normal brain tissue appeared uniform red while the infarction region showed white. The infarction volumes were calculated in a blinded manner with Adobe PhotoShop CS analysis system. The data were expressed as the percentage of the infarction volume/the ipsilateral hemisphere volume (%) at the coronal section of optic chiasma.

2.5　Neuronal apoptosis assay

Five rats in each group were deeply anesthetized by 10% chloral hydrate (300 mg/kg), reperfused with sodium chloride and 4% formaldehyde 200 mL from the heart into the aorta, and then decapitated at given time. Brain samples were chosen from frontal fontanelle 2 mm to occipital fontanelle 4 mm by a stereotaxic point, post-fixed in 4% formaldehyde for 2 h, dehydrated in alcohol gradually, hyalinized by dimethylbenzene, embedded in paraffin, then sectioned at a thickness of 5 μm, adhered to the sections prepared with poly-L-Lysine, and finally stored at 4℃. To detect cell apoptosis, TUNEL staining was performed according to the protocol of DendEnd fluorometric TUNEL detection system (Santa Cruz Co. Ltd.). Coronal paraffin sections described as above were deparaffinized by dimethylbenzene, hydrated by gradient ethanol and washed by distilled water. Some sections added DNase I at a dose of 1 μg/mL were regarded as positive control samples, and those treated without TdT were the negative ones. Under a 400-fold immunofluorescent microscope (wavelength 488 nm), the apoptosis cells were appeared yellow-green fluorescence in nucleus, and averaged in four random views in cortex and striatum, respectively.

2.6　Immunohistochemical staining

Rabbit anti-rat TLR4, NFκB and TNFα monoclonal antibody (1:100) were purchased from Santa Cruz Co. Ltd. Strept-avidin-biotin complex (SABC) immunohisto-chemistry kit, and diaminobenzidine (DAB) dye were granted by Bostor biological company in Wuhan China. Paraffin-embedded sections were deparaffinized in dimethylbenzene, hydrated successively in gradient ethanol, restored antigen twice in a microwave oven. Immunohistochemical procedures were performed strictly according to the guidance of manufacture. Under a microscope, those with brown granules in cytoplasm or nucleus were considered as positive cells. And the slides added 0.1 mmol/L PBS (containing 1 : 200 non-immunity animal serum) instead of primary antibody had no response. Four serial sections were chosen from each experimental rat and observed randomly four views at cortex and striatum under a 400-fold microscope. Absorbance values (*A*) of each view was detected by a LEICA QWin microgramme analytical system (Leica Company).

2.7　Enzyme linked immunosorbent assay (ELISA)

Rat TLR4 (No. E02T0013), NFκBp65 (No. E02N0014) and TNFα (No. E02T0012) ELISA kits were purchased from Blue Gene Co. Ltd. Five rats in each group were deeply anesthetized and decapitated at given time after MCAO/R. The ischemic hemisphere tissue (0.5 g) was quickly removed and ground fully into brain tissue homogenate. Then added normal sodium 500 μL, mixed well and centrifugalized for 10 min at 12 000 r/min. The upper limpid liquid was collected and stored at –20 ℃ (Avoid repeated freeze-thawcycles). Prepare all standards before starting assay procedure. Secure the desired number of coated wells in the holder, and then add 50 μL of standards or samples to the appropriate well of the antibodypre-coated microtiter plate. Add 100 μL of conjugate to each well. Mix well, cover and incubate for 1 h at 37 °C. Wash the microtiter plate 5 times using distilled or deionized water. Add 50 μL substrate A&B to each well. Cover and incubate for 15minutes at 25°C. Add 50 μL of stop solution to each well. Mix well and calculate the mean absorbance value A_{450} for each set of reference standards and samples. The standard density is a X, and the B/B_0 is a Y, sitting to mark the study in the logit-log up draw a standard curve. According to the B/B_0 that needs to be measured the sample can from sit to mark the density value that the study looks up the sample up. The sensitivity by this assay is 1.0 pg/mL (TLR4 and TNFα) and 1.0 ng/mL (NFκB).

2.8　Statistical Analysis

SPSS11.5 software was used for statistical analysis. Data were expressed as mean ± standard error (mean ± SD). Multi-group comparison was made by analysis of variance (ANOVA) and students' test, and two-group comparison by t-test. Values were considered to be significant when P is less than 0.05.

3　Results

3.1　Neurobehavioral dysfunction score

There was no neurobehavioral dysfunction symptom in rats of the SO group, whose Bederson's score got 0 points. After cerebral ischemia-reperfusion injury, all animals showed neurobehavioral defects. The Bederson's scores both in the SA group and PT group were obviously lower than that in the IC group (F = 24.90, q = 8.38 ~ 8.88, P < 0.01). The scores in PT group is slightly lower than that in SA group, but no significant difference was found between these two groups (t = 0.50, P > 0.05). See Table 5-1.

3.2 The cerebral infarction volume

No cerebral ischemia infarction was shown in the brain slices of the SO group, while infarction lesion almost appeared in all the experimental rats after cerebral ischemic reperfusion injury. The volume of cerebral infarction in the SA group and PT group were significantly lower than that in the IC group ($F = 30.76$, $q = 8.66 \sim 10.33$, $P < 0.01$), but there is no statistical difference between the SA group and PT group ($t = 1.66$, $P > 0.05$). See table 5-1.

3.3 Neuronal apoptosis

A few apoptotic cells were scattered in the cortex and the striatum in SO group rats. Apoptotic cells were significantly increased in the IC group. As we expected, the number of apoptosis both in the SA group and PT group were obviously low compared with the IC group ($F = 29.05$, $q = 4.03 \sim 12.84$, $P < 0.01$), but no difference existed between the SA group and PT group ($t = 0.49$, $P > 0.05$). See Table 5-1.

Table 5-1 Bederson's score, infarction volume and apoptotic cells (mean ± SD)

Groups	Bederson's score ($n = 15$)	Infarction volume ($n = 5$)	Apoptotic cells ($n = 5$)
SO group	0.00 ± 0.00	0.00 ± 0.00	3.53 ± 1.13
IC group	$2.17 \pm 0.35^{\Delta}$	$77.32 \pm 3.06^{\Delta}$	$16.62 \pm 3.25^{\Delta}$
SA group	$1.33 \pm 0.43^{*}$	$70.11 \pm 3.13^{*}$	$8.13 \pm 2.15^{*}$
PT group	$1.28 \pm 0.38^{*\#}$	$68.73 \pm 3.46^{*\#}$	$7.64 \pm 2.08^{*\#}$

$^{\Delta}P < 0.01$ *vs* the SO group; $^{*}P < 0.01$ *vs* the IC group; $^{\#}P > 0.05$ *vs* the SA group.

3.4 The expressions of TLR4, NFκB and TNF α

With the help of immunohistochemistry, we found that there were no region differences between the cortex and the striatum. Thus we calculated the absorbance values (A) in four confirmed views instead of the random ones in each brain slice.

Few TLR4 positive cells with light yellow granules could be seen in the cortex and the striatum in SO group rats, and its expression was very weak. TLR4 expression in IC group was significantly elevated along with the increased A value as compared with the SO group rats. After the drug administration, the A values in the SA group and the PT group were obviously decreased in contrast to the IC group rats ($F = 4.33$, $q = 2.95 \sim 4.92$, $P < 0.05$). Although the A value in the SA group was slightly lower than that in the PT group, there was no significant difference between the two treatment groups, suggesting that picroside Ⅱ could inhibit the expression of TLR4 protein and play neuroprotective effects as same as vianic acid A sodium

($t = 1.31$, $P > 0.05$). See Table 5-2 and Figure 5-1.

Table 5-2　Absorbance values (A) of TLR4, NFκB and TNFα expressions (mean ± SD)

Groups	n	TLR4	NFκB	TNFα
SO group	5	0.16 ± 0.09	0.14 ± 0.07	0.14 ± 0.08
IC group	5	$0.46 \pm 0.18^{\Delta}$	$0.65 \pm 0.21^{\Delta}$	$0.51 \pm 0.17^{\Delta}$
SA group	5	$0.28 \pm 0.13^{*}$	$0.26 \pm 0.15^{*}$	$0.30 \pm 0.16^{*}$
PT group	5	$0.24 \pm 0.13^{*\,\#}$	$0.22 \pm 0.08^{*\,\#}$	$0.25 \pm 0.12^{*\,\#}$

$^{\Delta}P < 0.01$ vs the SO group; $^{*}P < 0.01$ vs the IC group; $^{\#}P > 0.05$ vs the SA group.

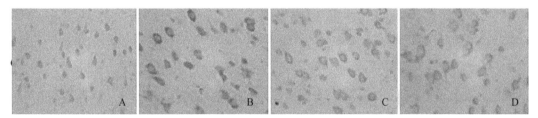

Figure 5-1　TLR4 expression in cortex shown by SABC × 400

(A, B , C, D: SO, IC, SA, PT groups)

Weak NFκB expression was shown in the cortex and the striatum in SO group rats. The number of NFκB positive cells rapidly increased, and its A value was significantly higher than that in the SO group; the expression of NFκB both in the SA group and PT group were apparently lower than that in the IC group ($F = 14.25$, $q = 6.24 \sim 8.17$, $P < 0.01$), but there was no difference between the SA group and the PT group as shown in Table 5-2 and Figure 5-2 ($t = 0.64$, $P > 0.05$).

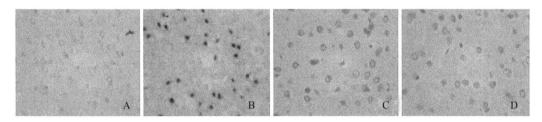

Figure 5-2　NFκB expression in cortex shown by SABC × 400

(A, B , C, D: SO, IC, SA, PT groups)

Ditto, the TNFα expression was very weak in the cortex and the striatum in SO group rats.

TNFα positive cells clearly increased in the IC group, and its *A* value was significantly higher than that in the SO group; the *A* values in the SA and the PT groups were obviously low compared with the IC group ($F = 6.39$, $q = 3.42 \sim 6.03$, $P < 0.05$), and there was no difference between the SA group and the PT group, either ($t = 0.81$, $P > 0.05$). See Table 5-2 and Figure 5-3.

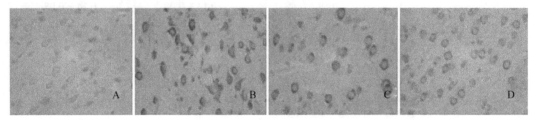

Figure 5-3   TNFα expression in cortex shown by SABC × 400

(A, B , C, D: SO, IC, SA, PT groups)

3.5   The concentrations in brain tissue of TLR4, NFκB and TNF α

The concentrations in brain tissue of TLR4, NFκB and TNFα were low in SO group rats, and increased significantly in the IC group rats; in the SA group and the PT group, the concentrations of TLR4 ($F = 79.42$, $q = 7.20 \sim 21.43$, $P < 0.01$), NFκB ($F = 111.25$, $q = 7.98 \sim 25.27$, $P < 0.01$) and TNFα ($F = 95.29$, $q = 6.89 \sim 23.27$, $P < 0.01$) were obviously lower than those in the IC group, but there was no difference between the SA group and the PT group ($t = 170$, 1.01, 1.69, $P > 0.05$). See Table 5-3.

Table 5-3   The concentrations in brain tissue of TLR4, NFκB and TNFα (mean ± SD)

Groups	*n*	TLR4	NFκB	TNFα
SO group	5	14.26 ± 2.08	11.53 ± 2.13	12.34 ± 2.25
IC group	5	$62.45. \pm 7.26^{\Delta}$	$75.16 \pm 9.12^{\Delta}$	$67.78 \pm 8.37^{\Delta}$
SA group	5	$34.28 \pm 5.04^{*}$	$39.23 \pm 4.38^{*}$	$35.16 \pm 4.71^{*}$
PT group	5	$30.45 \pm 4.32^{*\#}$	$31.64 \pm 4.46^{*\#}$	$28.76 \pm 4.03^{*\#}$

$^{\Delta}P < 0.01$ *vs* the SO group; $^{*}P < 0.01$ *vs* the IC group; $^{\#}P > 0.05$ *vs* the SA group.

4   Discussion

TLR4 is a member of signal transduction family, which combines with the adapter protein MyD88 and then with interleukin-associated kinase (IRAKs) to cause NFκB translocation, to enable the innate immune and inflammatory responses related gene transcription, to activate the

TLR4-MyD88 dependent signal transduction pathway and to induce inflammatory response[1]. Caso et al.[2] found that the cerebral infarction volume in TLR4 deficient rats was smaller than that in normal TLR4 animals after middle cerebral artery occlusion and reperfusion. Hua et al.[22] proved that cerebral infarction size in TLR4 knockout mice was also smaller than the wild-type ones, and its neurological deficit score was lower accordingly. The studies of Yang et al.[23] have shown that the TLR4 positive lymphomonocytes in blood circulation significantly elevated in patients with acute cerebral infarction as compared with that in the control group and the patients with transient ischemic attack, and the expression levels of TLR4 mRNA and TNFα in serum were consistent with IL6. From the data of correlation analysis, they further found that TLR4 and serum cytokine expression levels were closely related to the severity of stroke. Thus they speculated it is TLR4 that activates the downstream signaling protein, evokes the gene transcription associated with the encoding and inflammation-related factor, and induces and aggravates the inflammatory response.

NFκB is an important nuclear transcription factor in eukaryotic cells, which exists in almost all cells. It is located downstream of TLR signaling pathway, regulated by TLRs and involved in immune response and the processes of cell proliferation and differentiation. Cerebral ischemic reperfusion injury not only promotes the innate immune response of the immune system, but also activates TLR4-mediated signal transduction pathway to rapidly translocate NFκB from cytoplasm into nucleus, and combines with specific DNA sequence to stimulate downstream-associated factor (TNFα)-induced inflammation response and ischemia neuronal apoptosis[24]. With the application of MCAO models, Lou et al. [25] confirmed that the increased TNFα protein and its mRNA expression and NFκB DNA-binding-activity could reduce the survival number of spinal cells in the hippocampal CA1 area, suggesting that NFκB activation can lead to neuronal apoptosis in inflammation following cerebral ischemic reperfusion injury. It will become a new treatment target to reduce cerebral ischemic reperfusion injury through efficiently decreasing TNFα protein and mRNA expression and inhibiting NFκB DNA binding-activity. Liu et al. [26] reported that the expression of NFκB enhanced in cytoplasmic or nuclear in brain slices, and the use of Oxymatrine decreased the NFκB expression and the infarction lesions in rats with permanent middle cerebral artery occlusion compared with the sham operation group. Webster et al. [27] found that hypothermy could attenuate the NFκB inhibition factor (IκB) phosphorylation and IκB suppressor kinase, and decrease the expression of NFκB, thereby protect neurons in penumbra against focal ischemic reperfusion damage. Former study had demonstrated that the intracerebroventricular administration of prostaglandin after cerebral ischemia could inhibit the expression of subunit NFκB and play the protection role in ischemia neurons. These results intimate that the inhibition of NFκB expression to reduce apoptosis may be one of the mechanisms to improve the brain ischemic reperfusion injury. Our previous researches proved that picroside II could inhibit the expressions of iNOS [14], NFκB and IκB[15], and reduce the expressions of Caspase-3, PARP and to inhibit the neuronal apoptosis and thus improve the neurological function of rats with cerebral ischemia reperfusion injury[16]. It also reduced brain tissue edema and the aquaporin-4 (AQP4) expression, and the best therapeutic time window was 1 h after cerebral ischemic reperfusion.

This experiment showed that slight expressions of TLR4, NFκB and TNFα could be seen in the cortex and the striatum in the SO group, and their concentrations in brain tissue were very low. After cerebral ischemia 2 h and reperfusion 22 h, the expressions of these proteins, as well as the TUNEL-positive cells and concentrations in brain tissue increased significantly in contrast to the SO group. The data imply that the activation of TLR4 and its downstream NFκB inflammatory factor induce neuronal apoptosis and cerebral ischemic reperfusion injury. In this experiment, NFκB protein inactively expressed in cytoplasm in the SO group. After cerebral ischemic reperfusion, it was mainly located in nuclear, suggesting that the activation of NFκB into nucleus promote the expression of the downstream target genes TNFα, be involved in inflammatory response and induce neuronal apoptosis. Accordingly, the experimental animals appeared cerebral infarction lesions, abnormal morphology and the increased neuronal apoptosis in ischemic ipsilateral, and neurobehavioral dysfunction in contralateral hemisphere. We also found that the injection of picroside II and salvianic acid A sodium via tail vein significantly reduced the amount of apoptotic cells, the concentrations in brain tissue and the expressions of TLR4, NFκB and TNFα proteins in the cortex and the striatum in MCAO/R rats, together with the decreased infarction size and the improvement of cellular structure and neurobehavioral function of rats. In short, the neuroprotective effect of picroside II and salvianic acid A sodium against cerebral ischemic reperfusion injury might be performed by inhibiting TLR4-NFκB signal transduction pathway to reduce inflammatory response-induced apoptosis. However, the concrete differences between the two Chinese drugs need to further elucidated.

References

[1]　Kaushal V, Schlichter L C. Mechanisms of microglia-mediated neurotoxicity in a new model of the stroke penumbra. Journal of Neuroscience, 2008, 28(9): 2221-2230.

[2]　Caso J R, Pradillo J M, Hurtado O, et al. Toll-like receptor 4 is involved in subacute stress-induced neuroinflammation and in the worsening of experimental stroke. Stroke, 2008, 39: 1314-1320.

[3]　Bi X, Yan B, Fang S, et al. Quetiapine regulates neurogenesis in ischemic mice by inhibiting NF-kappaB p65/p50 expression. Neurological Research, 2009, 31(2): 159-166.

[4]　Stuppner H, Wagner H. New cucurbitacin glycosides from Picrorhiza kurrooa. Planta Medica, 1989, 55(6): 559-563.

[5] Wang D Q, He Z D, Feng B S. Chemical constituents from Picrorhiza scrophulariflora. Acta Botanica Yunnanica, 1993, 15: 83-88.

[6] Liu J, Liu B L, Zhang J Q, et al. Hepatoprotective and choleretic action of Picrorhiza scrophulariae flora Pennell. Chin J New Drugs, 2002, 11: 459-461.

[7] Li T, Liu J W, Zhang X D, et al. The neuroprotective effect of picroside II from hu-huang-lian against oxidative stress. American Journal of Chinese Medicine, 2007, 35(4): 681-691.

[8] Cao Y, Liu J W, Yu Y J, et al. Synergistic protective effect of picroside II and NGF on PC12 cells against oxidative stress induced by H_2O_2. Chinese Journal of Clinical Pharmacology & Therapeutics, 2007, 59(5): 573-579.

[9] He L J, Liang M, Hou F F, et al. Ethanol extraction of Picrorhiza scrophulariiflora prevents renal injury in experimental diabetes via anti-inflammation action. J Endocrinol, 2009, 200(3): 347-355.

[10] Li P, Matsunaga K, Yamakuni T, et al. Potentiation of nerve growth factor-action by picrosides I and II, natural iridoids, in PC12D cells. European Journal of Pharmacology, 2000, 406(2): 203-208.

[11] Li P, Matsunaga K, Yamakuni T, et al. Picrosides I and II, selective enhancers of the mitogen-activated protein kinase-dependent signaling pathway in the action of neuritogenic substances on PC12D cells. Life Sciences, 2002, 71(15): 1821-1835.

[12] Tao Y W, Liu J W, Wei D Z, et al. Protective effect of picroside-II on the damage of cultured PC12 cells in vitro. Chinese Journal of Clinical Pharmacology & Therapeutics, 2003, 8: 27-30.

[13] Guo M C, Cao Y, Liu J W. Protective effects of picroside II on glutamate injury of PC12 cells. Chinese Journal of Clinical Pharmacology & Therapeutics, 2007, 12: 440-443.

[14] Yin J J, Zhang W, Du F. Effects of extraction of Huhuanglian on apoptosis and Bcl-2 gene in penumbra area in ischemia reperfusion rats. Shandong Journal of Traditional Chinese Medicine , 2005, 24: 364-366.

[15] Li Q, Guo Y L, Li Z, et al. The interference of picroside II on the expressions of Caspase-3 and PARP following cerebral ischemia reperfusion injury in rats. Chinese Pharmacological Bulletin, 2010, 26(3): 342-345.

[16] Li Z, Li Q, Guo Y L, et al. The interference effect of picroside II on cerebral ischemia reperfusion injury in rats. Acta Anat Sinica, 2010, 41: 9-12.

[17] Longa E Z, Weinstein P R, Carlson S, et al. Reversible middle cerebral artery occlusion without craniectomy in rats. Stroke, 1989, 20(1): 84.

[18] Gao H M, Zhang M Z. Asymmetry in the brain influenced the neurological deficits and infarction volume following the middle cerebral artery occlusion in rats. Behavioral and Brain Functions, 2008, 4(1): 57-61.

[19] Chinese Pharmcopoeia Commission. Chinese Pharmacopoeia, Part I. Beijing: Chemical Industry Press, 2005: 212-213.

[20] Xiao Y J, Jiang Z Z, Yao J C, et al. Investigation of picroside II's impacts on the P450 activities using a cocktail method. Chinese Journal of Natural Medicines, 2008, 6(4): 292-297.

[21]　Bederson J B, Pitts L H, Tsuji M, et al. Rat middle cerebral artery occlusion: evaluation of the model and development of a neurologic examination. Stroke, 1986, 17(3): 472-476.

[22]　Hua F, Ma J, Ha T, et al. Differential roles of TLR2 and TLR4 in acute focal cerebral ischemia/ reperfusion injury in mice. Brain Research, 2009, 1262(1262): 100-108.

[23]　Yang Q W, Li J C, Lu F L, et al. Upregulated expression of toll-like receptor 4 in monocytes correlates with severity of acute cerebral infarction. Journal of Cerebral Blood Flow & Metabolism, 2008, 28(9): 1588-1596.

[24]　Boersma M C, Meffert M K. Novel roles for the NF-kappaB signaling pathway in regulating neuronal function. Science Signaling, 2008, 1(6): pe7.

[25]　Lou H Y, Wei X B, Zhang B, et al. Hydroxyethylpuerarin attenuates focal cerebral ischemia-reperfusion injury in rats by decreasing TNF-alpha expression and NF-kappaB activity. Yao Xue Xue Bao, 2007, 42(7): 710-715.

[26]　Liu Y, Zhang X J, Yang C H, et al. Oxymatrine protects rat brains against permanent focal ischemia and downregulates NF-κB expression. Brain Research, 2009, 1268:174-180.

[27]　Webster C M, Kelly S, Koike M A, et al. Inflammation and NF-κB activation is decreased by hypothermia following global cerebral ischemia. Neurobiol Dis, 2009, 33: 301-312.

Section 4　Words of TCM

1. 滋水涵木 replenishing water to nourish wood

2. 培土生金 reinforcing earth to generate metal

3. 益火补土 tonifying fire to supplement earth

4. 金水相生 mutual generation between metal and water

5. 抑木扶土 inhibiting wood strengthening earth

6. 培土治水 cultivating earth to control water

7. 佐金平木 assisting metal and calming wood

8. 中土五行 five elements with earth as center

9. 土控四方 earth governing four directions

10. 泄南补北 purging south (fire) and nourishing north (water)

11. 子病犯母 disease of son-organ invading mother-organ

12. 母病及子 disease of mother-organ involving son-organ

13. 水火不济 disharmony between water and fire

14. 热因寒用 using warm-natured drugs to treat false heat syndrome

15. 内病外治 external treatment of internal diseases

16. 正治与反治 routine treatment and treatment contrary to the routine

17. 温肾健脾 warming the kidney and strengthening the spleen

18. 平肝和胃 smoothing the liver and harmonizing the stomach

19. 发汗解表 inducing sweating to relieve exterior

20. 输布排泄 distribution and excretion

21. 针灸 acupuncture and moxibustion; acumoxi

22. 进针出针方法 needle-inserting and withdrawing

23. 留针方法 needle-retaining manipulation methods

24. 进针角度、深度 needle-inserting angle, depth

25. 艾灸选穴法 point-selecting methods for moxibustion

26. 瘢痕灸 scar-inducing moxibustion

27. 雀啄灸 sparrow-pecking moxibustion

28. 温针灸 needle heated moxibustion

29. 锋针 lance needle; ensiform needle

30. 投火、闪火法 fir-throwing method, fire-twinkling method

31. 拔罐，起罐法 cupping, cup-withdrawing method

32. 疳积、黄疸 infantile malnutrition, the jaundice

33. 萎黄病 green sickness; chlorosis

34. 忧郁 blue devil; black-browedness; black-facedness; depression; melancholia

35. 六字诀 six-character formula

36. 五禽戏 five animal-mimicked games (tiger, deer, bear, monkey, bird)

37. 八（六）段锦 eight (six)-sectioned games; eight (six)-section brocade

38. 易筋经 tendon-strengthening manipulation

39. 带下医 gynaecologist

40. 室女 virgin; home girl

(Hu Gaojie, Zhai Li)

Chapter 6   Hair Loss

Section 1   Hair Loss Awareness Month

Hair is a protein filament that grows from follicles found in the dermis. Hair is one of the defining characteristics of mammals. The human body, apart from areas of glabrous skin, is covered in follicles which produce thick terminal and fine vellus hair. Most common interest in hair is focused on hair growth, hair types, and hair care, but hair is also an important biomaterial primarily composed of protein, notably alpha-keratin.

Attitudes towards different hair, such as hairstyles and hair removal, vary widely across different cultures and historical periods, but it is often used to indicate a person's personal beliefs or social position, such as their age, sex or religion.

The word hair usually refers to two distinct structures: (1) the part beneath the skin, called the hair follicle, or, when pulled from the skin, the bulb. This organ is located in the dermis and maintains stem cells, which not only regrow the hair after it falls out, but also are recruited to regrow skin after a wound; (2) the shaft, which is the hard filamentous part that extends above the skin surface. A cross section of the hair shaft may be divided roughly into three zones.

Hair fibers have a structure consisting of several layers, starting from the outside: (1) the cuticle, which consists of several layers of flat, thin cells laid out overlapping one another as roof shingles, (2) the cortex, which contains the keratin bundles in cell structures that remain roughly rod-like, and (3) the medulla, a disorganized and open area at the fiber's center.

Each strand of hair is made up of the medulla, cortex and cuticle. The innermost region, the medulla, is not always present and is an open, unstructured region.The highly structural and organized cortex, or second of three layers of the hair, is the primary source of mechanical strength and water uptake. The cortex contains melanin, which colors the fiber based on the number, distribution and types of melanin granules. The shape of the follicle determines the shape of the cortex, and the shape of the fiber is related to how straight or curly the hair is. People with straight hair have round hair fibers. Oval and other shaped fibers are generally more wavy or curly. The cuticle is the outer covering. Its complex structure slides as the hair swells and is covered with a single molecular layer of lipid that makes the hair repel water. The diameter of human hair varies from 0.017 mm to 0.18 mm (0.000 67 ~ 0.007 09 in). There are two million small, tubular glands and sweat glands that produce watery fluids which cool the body by evaporation. The glands at the opening of the hair produce a fatty secretion that lubricates the hair.

Hair growth begins inside the hair follicle. The only "living" portion of the hair is found in the follicle. The hair that is visible is the hair shaft, which exhibits no biochemical activity and is considered "dead". The base of a hair's root (the bulb) contains the cells that produce the hair shaft. Other structures of the hair follicle include the oil producing sebaceous gland that lubricates the hair and the arrector pili muscles, which are responsible for causing hairs to stand up. In humans with little body hair, the effect results in goose bumps.

Root of the hair: The root of the hair ends in an enlargement, the hair bulb, which is whiter in color and softer in texture than the shaft, and is lodged in a follicular involution of the epidermis called the hair follicle. Bulb of hair layers consist of fibrous connective tissue, glassy membrane, external root sheath, internal root sheath composed of epithelium stratum (Henle's layer) and granular stratum (Huxley's layer), cuticle, cortex and medulla of hair.

Natural color: All natural hair colors are the result of two types of hair pigments. Both of these pigments are melanin types, produced inside the hair follicle and packed into granules found in the fibers. Eumelanin is the dominant pigment in brown hair and black hair, while pheomelanin is dominant in red hair. Blond hair is the result of having little pigmentation in the hair strand. Gray hair occurs when melanin production decreases or stops, while poliosis is hair (and often the skin to which the hair is attached), typically in spots, which never possessed melanin at all in the first place, or ceased for natural genetic reasons, generally, in the first years of life.

Human hair growth: Hair grows everywhere on the external body except for mucus membranes and glabrous skin, such as that found on the palms of the hands, soles of the feet, and lips. Hair follows a specific growth cycle with three distinct and concurrent phases: anagen, catagen and telogen phases; all three occur simultaneously — while one strand of hair may be in the anagen phase, another may be in the telogen phase. Each has specific characteristics that determine the length of the hair. The body has different types of hair, including vellus hair and androgenic hair, each with its own type of cellular construction. The different construction gives the hair unique characteristics, serving specific purposes, mainly, warmth and protection.

Hair loss: Hair loss affects 80 million American men and women. It can cause emotional distress while no life-threatening. Disease, genetic predisposition and even poor cosmetic grooming practices all cause hair loss. Even simple changes in your hair care routine can result in healthier hair. Each day, we are bombarded with advertisements for products and services to improve our hair. While some of these products may enhance appearance, they also can contribute to hair loss. August is hair loss awareness month and a good time to take stock of your locks. Breaking through the myths of hair loss and hair care is the first step to maintaining beautiful hair for life.

Myth 1: Dandruff does not contribute to hair loss. Dandruff is caused by a fungus known as malazzesia globosa. This fungus is commonly found floating in the air which is why dandruff can be treated, but not cured. In addition to the scaling which characterizes dandruff, the condition also can lead to hair loss. Studies have shown that with only 90 minutes of continuous scratching by the fingernails, it is possible to remove all of the cuticular scale, a protective covering on individual hairs, off a hair shaft. This loss leaves the hair shaft weakened and permanently damaged, making it easily susceptible to breakage and hair loss. The most effective dandruff shampoos and conditioners contain zinc pyrithione which ingredients leave behind thin plate like pieces of medicine on the scalp to prevent regrowth of the fungus, thus acting as a preventive measure for both dandruff and the hair loss associated with scratching.

Myth 2: Prescription shampoos treat scalp diseases, but also damage hair. The two most common scalp diseases are dandruff and seborrheic dermatitis, which is characterized by both redness and scaling. People often view products that treat these conditions as harsh and medicinal. These misconceptions have led many people to choose to live with the scalp itching rather than treat it with what they fear are harmful chemicals.

Technological advances now allow prescription shampoos to have the necessary medication to treat dandruff and seborrheic dermatitis while also containing the same mild cleansers found in cosmetic shampoos. These potent prescription anti-fungals remain on the scalp, preventing reoccurrence and ultimately helping keep hair healthy.

Myth 3: As hair turns gray, permanent waves and color treatments should be stronger. As people age, they lose melanin, the pigment that gives the hair color. Many people dye their hair to retain a youthful look. Hair dye interacts with the melanin already present in hair to produce the final hair color, but gray hair is less likely to dye as dark as hair that contains more melanin. Also, as hair ages, the hair shaft becomes finer, and thinner hair shafts are more susceptible to chemical damage from permanent waves and coloring.

Aging hair growing slowly means the same hair is often chemically treated multiple times. The more the hair is treated, the more damage is done and the more chances for hair breakage. As hair ages, perming and coloring solutions should be weaker and be left in contact with the hair for as short a period as possible.

Myth 4: Blow drying hair with heat gives the hair body. Blow drying hair is a common morning ritual for many people. While it is a quick, convenient way to dry and style hair, blow drying damages hair as the high heat from a blow dryer can actually boil the water in the hair shaft leaving it brittle. In addition, vigorous towel rubbing or combing of wet hair also can cause hair lose, since wet hair is more elastic and more vulnerable to breakage than dry hair. The hair should be allowed to air dry rather than blow dry, with styling and combing occurring once the hair is partially dry. This will provide excellent body with less opportunity for hair shaft damage.

Hair loss awareness month is a good time to refine your hair care routine. Keep your hair healthy by eating a well-balanced diet, avoiding over-processing with chemicals and using styling tools that are flexible and easily slip through hair.

Section 2　Prognostications of Pulses

In medicine, a pulse represents the tactile arterial palpation of the heartbeat by trained fingertips. The pulse may be palpated in any place that allows an artery to be compressed near the surface of the body, such as at the neck (carotid artery), wrist (radial artery), at the groin (femoral artery), behind the knee (popliteal artery), near the ankle joint (posterior tibial artery), and on foot (dorsalis pedis artery). Pulse (or the count of arterial pulse per minute) is equivalent to measuring the heart rate. The heart rate can also be measured by listening to the heart beat by auscultation, traditionally using a stethoscope and counting it for a minute. The radial pulse is commonly measured using three fingers. This has a reason: the finger closest to the heart is used to occlude the pulse pressure, the middle finger is used to get a crude estimate of the blood pressure, and the finger most distal to the heart (usually the ring finger) is used to nullify the effect of the ulnar pulse as the two arteries are connected via the palmar arches (superficial and deep). The study of the pulse is known as sphygmology.

We come now to another interesting feature of this study, namely, the prognostications of the pulse. Old style physicians profess to be able to predict the result of an illness by its various signs. In cases of apoplexy, the pulse should be superficial and slow; if it is firm, rapid and large there is danger. In typhoid fever if the pulse is superficial, full and overflowing, no anxiety need be felt, but if it is thready, small and soft it is serious. In malaria fever a taut pulse is favorable, if it is taut and slow it indicates heat; if it is taut and quick it indicates chills. It is unfavorable if the pulse is large, scattered and irregular. In cases of diarrhea the pulse is deep, small, slippery and feeble; and if it is strong, large, superficial and quick, there is danger. A good sign in vomiting and regurgitation is a superficial and slippery pulse; when it is deep, quick, fine and small it indicates bleeding in the intestines and the case is hopeless. One should not be alarmed to find an irregular pulse in cholera. It is only when this sign is found together with a curled tongue and shriveled testicles that recovery is very improbable. The pulse in bronchial diseases is generally superficial and small and they are easy to cure; when it is deep, hidden and tense death is near. It is favorable if the pulse in asthma is superficial and slippery; but unfavorable, if it is deep and small especially when the hands and feet are cold. In the case of high fever, a quick and over-flowing pulse is desirable; if it is thready and feeble, accompanied by low spirits, the condition is fatal. In wasting diseases the pulse is weak and quick; if it is thin and small death is certain. In cases of loss of blood no anxiety need to be felt if the pulse is hollow, small and tardy; but if hollow, large and quick danger is apprehended. Where there is pulmonary congestion, a wiry and large pulse is favorable; but few can recover quickly if it is deep, small and thready.

A good sign in diabetes is a large and quick pulse; if it is slender, thready, short and small, a cure is almost hopeless. If the pulse is full and large, the disease is curable, but if slow and small recovery is most difficult. In cases of insanity, if the pulse is superficial and overflowing, it is a good omen; unfavorable if it is deep and quick. The pulse in epilepsy should be superficial and tardy; if it is deep, small and quick it is a sign of death.

There are nine kinds of pain in the abdomen. A slender and large pulse denotes a slow convalescence. Ruptures are due to trouble in the liver and the pulse is always taut. If it is wiry and rapid all is well; if feeble and rapid it is fatal. A favorable indication in jaundice is a full, overflowing and quick pulse; it is bad if the pulse is superficial, large, full and strong; if it is deep, fine and thready no doctor's art is of avail. In accumulation of humors in the system, if the pulse is strong and full no danger exists; but if deep and slender the case is serious. The pulse in diseases caused by evil spirits varies on both wrists; sometimes it is large and sometimes it is small, sometimes quick and sometimes slow. Where obnoxious influences exist and the belly swells up, a tense and fine pulse is hopeful; a large and superficial pulse is serious. In cancer and carbuncle a full, overflowing large pulse before suppuration is good but the same pulse after suppuration is critical. In abscess of the lungs the pulse on the "inch" is quick and full. In both diseases the complexion is white and the pulse short and small. If the pulse is quick and large in compass it means loss of qi and blood. In cancer of the intestines a quick and slippery pulse is favorable, but if deep and slender the patient may as well prepare for the future!

Besides the foregoing, there are even special pulses which indicate impending death. If the pulse resembles the pecking of a bird, water dripping from a roof crack, or the upsetting of a cup it means extinction of the spleen pulse and death may be expected within four days. If the pulse resembles feathers blown by the wind, or feathers brushing against the skin, it indicates serious disease of the lungs and the end will come within three days. It is a sign of fatal kidney trouble and death may happen within four days if the pulse is like the snapping of a cord or like the flipping of the finger against a stone. When the liver ceases to perform its function the pulse is like the string of a new bow or like the blunt edge of a sword, and the patient will die within eight days. If the pulse resembles the rapid rolling of peas death may be expected in a day. A pulse acting like a fish or shrimp darting about in the water or a pulse like water oozing from a spring is a fatal symptom.

An important point, which should also be taken into consideration when taking a pulse test, is the normal variation dependent upon the season of the year, age, constitution and sex of the patient. In spring the pulse is taut and tremulous like a musical string, in summer it is full and overflowing, in autumn it is elastic, and in winter it is deep like a stone thrown into water.

A thin person's pulse is generally superficial and full, while a fat person's pulse is usually deep and quick. Five beats to one cycle of respiration are normal in a hot-tempered person, but four beats to one cycle of respiration in a person of slow temperament mean sickness. In the aged the pulse is mostly empty, in young people it is large, and in infants rapid — about seven beats to one cycle of respiration. Northerners often have strong and full pulses while Southerners soft and weak pulses.

Differentiation is also made between the pulses of the sexes. In man the pulse on the left hand should be large to correspond with the yang principle, but in woman it should be the opposite because the yin principle predominates on the right. Again the "cubit" pulse in man is always slow, weak and compressible while in woman it is usually strong, large and long. Marvelous are the claims made by pulse theorists regarding the diagnostic value of pulse feeling. It is affirmed that one is able to tell whether or not a woman is pregnant, or even to predict the sex and development of uterine fetus by these tests alone. For instance, in a case of cessation of menstruation with no apparent disease, if the three pulses are slippery it indicates pregnancy. If, in addition, they are rapid and scattered it shows three months' conception, if rapid and unscattered five months. If the pulse on the left wrist is rapid a son may be expected, but if the right pulse is rapid it is certain to be a daughter! On the left hand a superficial and overflowing cubit pulse or a large inch pulse denotes a male child; on the right hand a deep and full cubit pulse or a deep and slender inch pulse indicates a female child. If the cubit pulse on both wrists is overflowing it means twin boys; if deep and full twin girls. Triplets may be looked for when the pulses of both wrists are smooth and equal. They will be all of the weaker sex. But if the pulses show the opposite nature all three will be of the stronger sex.

And stranger still are the virtues given to a special kind of pulse called Taisu pulse which, it is said, can reveal the destiny and fortune of a person. According to the secrets of the Taisu pulse by Peng Yingguang of the Ming Dynasty, this method originated from Feng Zhenren of the Eastern Sea. In the Song Dynasty about 963 AD, he came out of a cave and introduced it into practice. The following two examples will serve to give an idea of what it presumes to be: (1) to tell whether a man is noble or common, and will live long or short. As the kidney controls life therefore if the kidney pulse of the left hand is deep and regular it indicates a noble rank; if weak and slender it means poverty at old age. A deep, regular and slippery pulse points to long life; (2) the pulse of the rich and poor. A spleen pulse means honors and riches, but if the beats have no root then this good fortune will not last. A rich and noble man's pulse is slow and regular.

In addition to the above pulse, it is alleged that the pulse feeling can tell whether one is a Monk or a Daoist, clever or stupid, when the disaster comes, the official rank, and even the ability of one's wife. Such, in general, is the sum of what Chinese think of this doctrine of the pulse. Foreign writers, however, usually condemn this as a system of downright and solemn quackery. Perhaps the modern doctor, with so many instruments to aid him in diagnosis, has lost many of his faculties of observation, especially the sense of touch. By constant use and pure concentration the old style physicians may have developed this power to such an extent that they can tell many things imperceptible to the average person. Be that as it may, scientific medicine has made such rapid progress and the various tests — both chemical and instrumental — are so accurate and reliable that this feeling of the pulse as a diagnostic method has lost much of its practical value. At the present time we cannot but relegate this pulse lore of Cathay to the domain of medical history and view it only as one of China's contributions to medicine in the past.

Section 3　Research Article

Interfering effect and mechanism of neuregulin on experimental dementia model in rats

[Abstract] **Objective:** To investigate the effect of neuregulin 1β (NRG1β) on the neuronal apoptosis and the expressions of Bcl-2 and Bax proteins in experimental dementia model rats. **Methods:** Thirty adult healthy male Wistar rats were randomly divided into control group, model group and treated group consisting of ten rats respectively. The experimental dementia models were established by injecting beta-amyloid protein 1-40 (Aβ1-40) stereotactically into the left lateral ventricle, and treated by injecting NRG1β into right lateral ventricle. The cognitive capacity of rats was evaluated with electric Y-maze. The neuronal apoptosis was counted by TUNEL assay. The expressions of Bcl-2 and Bax were determined with immunohistochemistry assay and double immunofluorescence labeling. **Results:** The cognitive ability in model group rats decreased, along with the number of neuronal apoptosis and the expressions of Bcl-2 and Bax increased significantly than those in control group ($P < 0.05$). After treatment with NRG1β, the cognitive ability of rats improved, the number of neuronal apoptosis reduced and the expression of Bcl-2 increased while Bax decreased significantly than those in model group ($P < 0.05$). **Conclusion:** NRG1β could inhibit neuronal apoptosis by regulating the expressions of Bcl-2/Bax to improve the capacity of learning and memory in experimental dementia rats.

Keywords: neuregulin; dementia; beta-amyloid protein; apoptosis; Bcl-2; Bax

1   Introduction

Alzheimer's disease (AD) is the most widespread neurodegenerative disease worldwide [1]. AD accounts for at least 60% of all dementia diagnosed clinically. The major pathological hallmarks of AD are the loss of neurons, occurrence of senile plaques (SPs) as well as neurofibrillary tangles (NFTs) [2]. AD is considered a multifactorial disease [3-4], and the mechanism of neuronal apoptosis in the hippocampus is of importance [5-6]. Although the clinical symptoms of AD are frequently diagnosed in older age, the degenerative process probably starts many years before the clinical onset of the disease [7-8]. Since the diagnosis and therapy of AD is limited, there is no medication to treat or control the disease currently. Neuregulin 1β (NRG1β), an excitomotor of tyrosine kinase receptor (erbB) family, possessed many important regulative effects in the development of nervous system. It can adjust the proliferation, migration, differentiation and survival of various cells, and take part in the formation process of synapse [9]. Previous reports have demonstrated that NRG1β might participate in the neuroprotection during the brain ischemia reperfusion injury [10]. Recent researches indicated that NRG1β attenuated cerebral ischemia reperfusion injury via inhibiting apoptosis and upregulating aquaporin 4 (AQP4) [11], regulating the expressions of signal transducer and activator of transcription (STAT3) to activate JAK/STAT signal transduction pathway [12], inhibiting the activation of matrix metalloproteinase 9 (MMP9) and development of inflammation [13], as well as inhibiting the mitochondrial apoptotic pathway via balancing the activity of X-linked inhibitor of apoptosis protein (XIAP) and the second mitochondrial derived activator of caspases (Smac) proteins to avoid the irreversible neuron death in brain tissue of ischemia/reperfusion rat [14], and thus play a neuroprotective effect on cerebral ischemia reperfusion damage. In this experiment, experimental dementia rats models were induced by intracerebroventricular microinjection of Aβ1-40, so to explore concrete neuroprotective mechanism of NRG1β from neuronal apoptosis and its gene regulation in experimental dementia rats.

2   Materials and methods

2.1   Experimental animals

The total of 40 adult male Wistar rats, weight 200 ~ 220 g, SPF grade, were granted by Experiment Animal Center of Qingdao Drug Inspection Institute [SCXK (LU) 20070010]. The local legislation for ethics of experiment on animals and guidelines for the care and use of laboratory animals were followed in all animal procedures. All animals were adapt the laboratory environment, allowed free access to food and water in room temperature [(23 ± 2)℃]

and humidity-controlled housing with natural illumination for a week.

2.2　Learning and memory detection

Spontaneous alternation behavior in an electric Y-maze was assessed as a spatial working memory task [15-16]. The electric Y-maze (Chinese institute of medicine and pharmacy) consisted of three identical arms. Each rat was placed at the end of one fixed arm and allowed to move freely through the maze during a 3-min session. Rats were initially placed at the end of one arm and allowed to adapt to the light signal for 60 sec. The rats were then exposed to light signals from the two arms, followed by electric stimulation for 2 sec at 60 V, 10 times per second. The correct response was defined if the rats immediately escaped to the safe area. Subsequent to safe escape, the lights continued to turn on and off for an additional 1 min for consolidation of memory, which indicated the end of one exercise. The rat was then shocked in the former safe area to go on a new test, so on and so forth, to alter places of safe areas.

Test of learning capacity: Rats were given 10 trials per day for 7 consecutive days, so as to test the number of electric shocks for right reaction (9/10); the number of trials stood for learning capability. Ruled out slow rats.

Test of memory reoccurrence abilities: The Y-maze test went on 24 h after the learning test, so as to reach 9/10 standard. A stood for the number of times of right reaction (RR); A/10 implied ability of retentive memory, and the higher score, the better memory.

2.3　Establishment of animal models

Beta-amyloid protein 1-40 (Aβ1-40) (Sigma Company, USA) was diluted into 20 g / L solution by the application of 0.1 mol / L PBS sodium, and incubated for 72 h at 37 ℃ to be changed into colloidal state Aβ1-40, then stored at 4 ℃ to be used.

Total of 30 selected rats which own learning and memory abilities were randomly divided into control group, model group and treated group consisting of 10 rats in each group. All surgical procedures were conducted under aseptic conditions, and every effort was made to minimize animal suffering and to reduce the number of animals used. All rats were anesthetized intraperitoneally by 100 g/L chloral hydrate at the dosage of 300 mg/kg. According to Nabeshima [17-19], rats were anesthetized and positioned in a stereotaxic frame (Huamu Agricultural Machinery Factory of Shanghai, Jiangwan-IC). Under sterile conditions, skin incision along of the midline intracerebroventricular microinjection of aggravated Aβ1-40 5 μL.

Under sterile conditions, the skull was exposed, and lambda and bregma were made level. Two small holes were made 3.5 mm posterior to bregma and ± 2.5 mm lateral of the midline, and the dura was exposed. The dura was pierced, and the two electrode arrays were lowered to 1.5 ~ 1.7 mm below dura, one in each hemisphere. Each electrode array comprised four tetrodes. The ground wire from each electrode array was attached to two different skull screws and coated in silver paint. The electrode arrays were then secured in place by using dental acrylic and five small screws affixed to the skull. Rats were then injected with an additional 5 μL of Hartman's solution. The rats were monitored until they awoke and then placed in a modified home cage designed to prevent the microdrive from getting caught on the cage sides. On the day after surgery, an additional dose of carprofen was given. All animals were allowed 1 week to recover before screening for cells began.

2.4   Treatment methods

Recombinant human NRG1β (purity > 97%, R&D Systems, Inc, Catalog number: 396-HB) was diluted into 1 g/L water-solution using 0.1 mol/L phosphate buffered solution (PBS) in advance. Seven days after the experiment, memories were tested by the electric Y-maze. Then, in accordance with 5 μg/kg and injection velocity 1 μL/min, inject NRG1β 5 μL and finished the injection in 5 min, along the coordinate location at AP 0.8 mm, MR 1 mm, DV 3.6 mm, as was on the side of the right cerebral ventricle. Ensure distributed equally and dispersedly and then subsided the needles slowly back, sealed in the skull, the department, skin incision treated by Gentamicin, and then close the incision. Controls and models were injected 0.1 mol/L PBS in equal volume at the same time.

2.5   Evaluating index

2.5.1   Abilities of learning and memory

The abilities of learning and memory of rats was evaluated with electric Y-maze 7 days after treatment with NRG1β.

2.5.2   Sample collection and preparation of paraffin sections

After behavioral evaluation, the rats in each group were deeply anesthetized intraperitoneally by 100 g/L chloral hydrate at the dosage of 300 mg/kg, transcardially perfused with 0.9% sodium chloride and 4% formaldehyde solution 250 mL respectively. The rats were captured, and then brain samples were postfixed by 4% formaldehyde for 2 h. Brain samples were dehydrated in gradient ethanol, transparented in dimethylbenzene and embedded in paraffin. Coronal sections of 5 μm thickness were cut successively with a microtome (LEICA-RM2015, Shanghai Laica Instruments Corporation, China) from the posterior of the optic chiasma, adhered to the slides prepared with poly-L-Lysine, and finally stored at 4 ℃ .

2.5.3   Assessment of apoptosis by TUNEL assay

To observe brain damage, terminal deoxynucleotidyl transference-mediated biotinylated deoxyuridine triphosphate nick end labeling (TUNEL) technique was performed to detect neurocyte apoptosis according to the protocol of TUNEL Detection System (Wuhan Boster Biochemical Techniques Co. Ltd., China). Coronal paraffin sections added DNase Ⅰ at a dose of 1 μg/mL were regarded as positive control samples. Those, with yellow color in nucleus under a microscope, were considered as positive cells. Slices treated without TdT were the negative control ones. Under a 400-fold microscope, four views were detected randomly in hippocampus of the confined areas from four serial slices in each rat. The absorbance (*A*) value of each view was determined with LEICA QWin image processing and analysis system (Leica Company).

2.5.4　Immunohistochemistry assay

A rabbit anti-rat Bcl-2 and Bax multiclonal antibody (Wuhan Boster Biochemical Techniques Co. Ltd., China) was used at a titer of 1∶100 to detect the activity of Bcl-2 and Bax in brain tissue. All procedure was strictly performed in accordance with the manufacture directions. Paraffin sections as described above were dewaxed by xylene, hydrated with gradient alcohol, repaired antigen in a microwave oven, blocked non-specific binding sites with non-immunized animal normal serum for 20 min, and then probed with primary antibody anti-Bcl-2 and Bax (diluted 1∶100 in PBS) for 2 h at 37 ℃, biotin-conjugated secondary antibody (1∶100) and SABC (1∶100) for 30 min at 37 ℃, respectively. Covered with waterborne mount and finally detected directly under a light microscopy. Negative control slides added 0.1 mol/L PBS (containing 1∶100 blocking serum) instead of primary antibody has no immunological reaction. Immunoreactivity was visualized under a 400-fold light microscope; four views were detected randomly in hippocampus of the confined areas from four serial slices in each rat. The absorbance (*A*) value of each view was determined with LEICA QWin image processing and analysis system (Leica Company).

2.5.5　Double immunofluorescence labeling

Double immunofluorescence labeling for Bcl-2 and Bax proteins was performed to assess the associations between these reactions. Before immunofluorescence labeling, four serial sections from the same tissue were reacted with primary antibody of Bcl-2 and Bax, and further stained by different agent, respectively. For example, using laser excitation of 488 nm and reception of 510 ~ 530 nm wavelength, it appears yellow-green light posterior to SABC-FITC addition, while with excitation of 568 nm and reception of 600 ~ 650 nm, it shows red color after SABC-CY3 accession. According to the shade of the coloration, Bcl-2 (SABC-FITC) was definited as the first colorating antibody, and Bax (SABC-CY3) as the second colorating antibody.

Double fluorescence labeling steps: paraffin sections as described above were de-waxed by xylene, hydrated with gradient alcohol, repaired antigen in a microwave oven, blocked non-specific binding sites for 20 min, and then probed with primary antibody anti-Bcl-2 (diluted 1∶200 in PBS) for 2 h at 37 ℃, biotin-conjugated secondary antibody (1∶100) and SABC-FITC (1∶100) for 30 min at 37 ℃, respectively. The sample was added with anti-Bax (1∶200), the secondary antibody IgG (1∶100), SABC-CY3 (1∶100), PBS, successively, covered with waterborne mount and finally detected directly under a fluorescence microscopy. All slides were carried out under a dark circumstance throughout the operation and washed fully in PBS so as to avoid excessive fluorescence residual or degeneration.

2.6　Statistical analysis

SPSS11.5 software was used for statistical analysis. Data were expressed as mean ± standard error (mean ± SD). Multi-group comparison was made by analysis of variance (ANOVA) and students' test, and two-group comparison by t-test. Values were considered to be significant when P is less than 0.05.

3　Results

3.1　The learning and memory abilities of rats

The number of trials were increasing after building the model, and the different was significant between before and after the injection ($P < 0.05$), which meant learning memory ability decreased, but there was no evident difference in the control group ($P > 0.05$). After NRG1β treatment for 7 d, the trial numbers of treated group were less than the model group ($P < 0.05$), as meant learning memory ability of treated group increased significantly; however, the trial numbers were more than control group ($P < 0.05$) (Table 6-1 and Table 6-2).

Table 6-1　The average learning scores evaluated with electric Y-maze of rats (mean ± SD)

Groups	n	Before modeled	After modeled (Before treated)	After treated
Control group	8	60.24 ± 4.46	59.13 ± 7.52	60.18 ± 1.69
Model group	7	58.14 ± 2.52	79.84 ± 6.46 [a, b]	81.22 ± 3.92 [a, b]
Treated group	7	56.56 ± 9.63	81.31 ± 3.31[a, b]	68.54 ± 8.86 [a, b, c]

[a]$P< 0.05$ *vs* before model; [b]$P< 0.05$ *vs* control group; [c]$P < 0.05$ *vs* model group.

Table 6-2　The average memory scores evaluated with Y-electric maze of rats (mean ± SD)

Groups	n	Before modeled	After modeled (Before treated)	After treated
Control group	8	8.1 ± 1.6	7.9 ± 2.2	8.0 ± 2.3
Model group	7	7.8 ± 1.2	4.8 ± 3.1[a, b]	4.6 ± 1.6 [a, b]
Treated group	7	7.5 ± 5.2	5.1 ± 2.5 [a, b]	7.1 ± 1.1 [b, c]

[a]$P< 0.05$ *vs* before model; [b]$P< 0.05$ *vs* control group; [c]$P < 0.05$ *vs* model group.

3.2　Apoptosis

There were a number of apoptosis positive cells and absorbance (A) in control, model and treated groups, while the number and absorbance (A) of apoptotic cells in model group (22.40 ± 4.37 and 0.46 ± 0.17) and treated group (13.60 ± 3.62 and 0.34 ± 0.13) are more than those in control group (5.30 ± 2.12 and 0.14 ± 0.06) ($P < 0.05$), as well as that in treated group less than that in model group ($P < 0.05$). See Table 6-3 and Figure 6-1.

Table 6-3　The number and the expression absorbance (A) of apoptosis cells (mean ± SD)

Groups	n	Positive-cells	A values
Control group	8	5.30 ± 2.12	0.14 ± 0.06
Model group	7	22.40 ± 4.37 [a]	0.45 ± 0.17 [a]
Treated group	7	13.60 ± 3.62 [a, b]	0.34 ± 0.13 [a, b]

[a]$P< 0.05$ *vs* control group; [b] $P < 0.05$ *vs* model group.

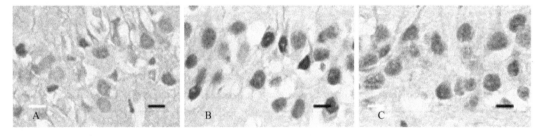

Figure 6-1　The apoptosis cells in hippocampus in control (A), model (B) and
treated (C) groups with TUNEL × 400

Scale bar is 25 μm.

3.3　Immunohistochemical assay

Using a light microscopy, the Bcl-2 and Bax positive cells had irregular shapes and yellow (Figure 6-2 and Figure 6-3) signals and scattered in the hippocampus. There were a few of Bcl-2 and Bax positive cells could be seen in hippocampus in the control group. The number of positive cells and the expression Bcl-2 and Bax proteins increased significantly, as well as the heavier A value in the model group ($P < 0.05$). As expected, the positive cells and the A values of Bcl-2 protein in the treated group were significantly higher, while Bax protein lower than those in the model group ($P < 0.05$). See Table 6-4.

Table 6-4　The number and the expression absorbance (*A*) of Bcl-2 and Bax positive cells (mean ± SD)

Groups	*n*	Bcl-2 cells	Bcl-2 *A* values	Bax cells	Bax *A* values
Control group	8	5.14 ± 0.04	0.16 ± 0.05	6.10 ± 0.04	0.15 ± 0.04
Model group	7	12.56 ± 4.04	0.32 ± 0.14 [a]	30.50 ± 6.15	0.46 ± 0.18 [a]
Treated group	7	32.15 ± 7.06	0.41 ± 0.16 [a, b]	20.34 ± 4.56	0.35 ± 0.14 [a, b]

[a] $P < 0.05$ *vs* control group; [b] $P < 0.05$ *vs* model group.

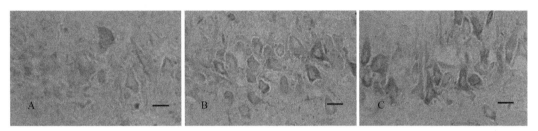

Figure 6-2　The expression of Bcl-2 positive cells in hippocampus (A: Control group, B: Model group, C: treated group) with immunohistochemistry SABC staining × 400

Scale bar is 25 μm.

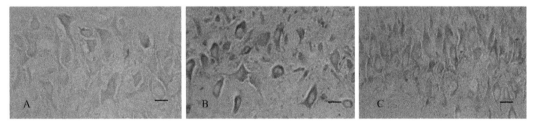

Figure 6-3　The expression of Bax positive cells in hippocampus (A: Control group, B: Model group, C: treated group) with immunohistochemistry SABC staining × 400

Scale bar is 25 μm.

3.4　Double immunofluorescence labeling

Based on immunofluorescent double labeling, we found that almost all the Bcl-2 positive fluorescent signals were co-located in the Bax positive cells in hippocampus. In the treated group with NRG1β, the results demonstrate that exogenous NRG1β could enhance the Bcl-2 and reduce the Bax expressions more than those in the model group.

4　Discussion

4.1　AD and A β

The deposition of beta-amyloid protein (Aβ) is the major reason for the formation of senile plaques (SPs) and it might be the common pathway of Alzheimer's disease caused by all factors [20]. Aβ is composed of 39 ~ 43 amino acid residues formed in the process of modificating amyloid precursor protein (APP) by various cutting methods. The deposition of condensed Aβ in parenchyma starts pathological cascade, results in the formation of neurofibrillary tangles (NFTs), the damage of synapse and neuraxon, and leads to neurocyte denaturation and apoptosis. APP is widely in the cells of all tissues throughout the body, and it is transmembrane glycoprotein with transmembrane receptor protein structure. It mainly locates on neuron synapses, and its functions are unclear until now [21]. Recent studies suggest that lack of APP may result in enhancement of synapse transmission [22]. APP is normally hydrolyzed by α-secretase into soluble secreted APP (β-APP), and it stimulates cells proliferation, promotes adhesion between cells and matrix and protects neurons from the damage caused by excitatory toxin and oxidative stress reaction. β-APP is hydrolyzed into soluble Aβ outside the membrane or at transmembrane location by β-secretase and γ-secretase, and there are usually two types of Aβ ($A\beta_{40}$ and $A\beta_{42}$). Aβ has a strong neurotoxicity, and may lead to huge amounts of neurons death rapidly [23-24]. Besides excessive production of Aβ caused by APP gene mutation, the metabolic disorder of Aβ clearance and degradation is an essential reason for the deposition of Aβ. Aβ may inhibit the activity of high molecular weight protease in brain which will bring about the failure degradation of Aβ and a vicious circle of deposition[25]. More and more evidences have shown that amyloid β_{1-40} ($A\beta_{1-40}$) caused neurons damage mainly by apoptotic pathway[26]. $A\beta_{1-40}$ will lead to oxidative stress and Ca^{2+} overloading, and activate intracellular apoptins and damage mitochondria at the same time, which will result in the disorder of energy supply system, cells dysfunction and neurons apoptosis[27].

Bcl-2 family is important regulators in apoptosis mechanism, and Bcl-2 and Bax will play the role in the form of homodimer or heterodimer. The increase expression of Bax protein will form homodimer to induce apoptosis. Because of cell self-protection mechanism, the expression of Bcl-2 protein will be increased in response which will lead to part of Bax homodimer separation. Heterodimer will be formed by separated Bax homodimer and Bcl-2 protein, and that will inhibit apoptosis[28]. Meng et al.[29] reported that TUNEL positive cells exist in temporal cortex brain of both AD patients and non AD patients, but the number of temporal lobe neurons in AD patients is significantly decreased, the relative amount of TUNEL positive cells is significantly increased. The reason for apoptosis of temporal lobe neurons in AD patients is the increasement of Bax, Caspase expression which is related to apoptosis cascade reaction and the decreasement of Bcl-2 expression with the function of anti-apoptosis, both of these promote apoptosis further. In this experiment, after injecting $A\beta_{1-40}$ into the lateral ventricle of rats, the expression of Bax protein promoting apoptosis is in dominant, and it leads to apoptosis of neurons in specific parts of the brain and significant injures of learning and memory of rats. The rats perform cognitive dysfunction like AD behaviors. This is consistent with previous reports.

4.2　NRG and AD

Researches have proved that in the target region with basal forebrain cholinergic innervation (such as cerebral cortex and hippocampus), there is high concentration expression of NGF mRNA. The expression of NGF mRNA may synthesize nerve growth factor (NGF) which can be absorbed by neuraxon of basal forebrain cholinergic innervation, and be transported to cell body reversely. NGF may induce a series of intracellular information transmission, and finally lead to a series of biological effects including expression of functional protease and growth of neurite in neurons. All of these play an important part in the survival of neurons and neuraxon regeneration[30]. The neuregulins are a family of multipotent growth factors that includes acetylcholine receptor inducing activities (ARIAs), glial growth factors (GGFs), heregulins and neu differentiation factors (NDFs). Neuregulins' effects appear to be mediated by interaction with a class of tyrosine kinase receptors related to the epidermal growth factor (EGF) receptor which includes erbB2, erbB3 and erbB4[31]. In the rat brain, NRG-1, erbB2 and erbB4 are localized in various areas of the cerebral cortex, hippocampus and cholinergic nucleus in the diencephalon primarily in neuronal cell bodies[32]. ErbB4 expression was not seen until 3 days following the injury, suggesting that NRG-1/erbB4 signaling was associated with a delayed neuroprotective or injury promoting response. However in each case, the induction of NRG-1 and erbBs was localized to cells at the edge of the lesion (penumbra) suggesting a role for NRG-1 and erbBs in neural protection and repair[10]. Xu et al.[9] reported that cerebral ischemia rats treated with either vehicle or NRG1β before MCAO, extensive TUNEL staining were found in the nuclei of cells within the ischemic cortical and subcortical areas after reperfusion 24 h. Ischemia-induced TUNEL staining was abolished by NRG1β treatment in the areas within the cortical penumbra. NRG1β-treated tissues showed no TUNEL-positive cells in the cortex. In the striatum, TUNEL-positive cells were seen, although they appeared fewer in number and were lightly stained after NRG1β administration. A large number of these TUNEL-positive cells were co-labeled with antibodies against MAP-2 and neuron specific enolase (NSE) indicating that neurons were protected from apoptosis by NRG1β although many of the TUNEL-positive cells were not neurons.

After the treatment of injecting NRG1β into ventricle, neurons apoptosis is decreased, the positive expression of Bcl-2 is increased while that of Bax is decreased, and Bcl-2/Bax ratio is increased. This suggests that NRG1β might play a role in anti-apoptosis by increasing the expression of Bcl-2, decreasing the expression of Bax, increasing the hereodimer produced by Bcl-2 and Bax, thus reduce the apoptosis caused by amyloid and improve the functions of learning and memory of rats.

5   Conclusion

NRG1β could inhibit neuronal apoptosis by regulating the expressions of Bcl-2/Bax to improve the capacity of learning and memory in experimental dementia rats.

Acknowledgement

This study was supported by grant-in-aids for the Natural Science Fund of Shandong Province (2008BS02026) and the Natural Science Fund of China (30873391).

References

[1]   Hebert L E, Scherr P A, Bienias J L, et al. Alzheimer disease in the US population: prevalence estimates using the 2000 census. Arch Neurol, 2003, 60(8): 1119-1122.

[2]   Selkoe D J. Cell biology of protein misfolding: the examples of Alzheimer's and Parkinson's diseases. Nat Cell Biol, 2004, 6(11): 1054-1061.

[3]   Chen Y, Jia L, Wei C, et al. Association between polymorphisms in the apolipoprotein D gene and sporadic Alzheimer's disease. Brain Res, 2008, 1233(2): 196-202.

[4]   Small G W, Rabins P V, Barry P P, et al. Diagnosis and treatment of Alzheimer disease and related disorders. Consensus statement of the American Association for Geriatric Psychiatry, the Alzheimer's Association, and the American Geriatric Society. JAMA, 1997, 278(13): 63-71.

[5]   Cotman C W, Anderson A J. A potential role for apoptosis neurodegeneration and Alzheimer's disease. Mol Neurobiol, 1995, 10(1): 19-21.

[6]   Shimohama S. Apoptosis in Alzheimer's disease-an update. Apoptosis, 2000, 5(1): 9-16.

[7]   Morris J C. The challenge of characterizing normal brain aging in relation to Alzheimer's disease. Neurobiol Aging, 1997, 18(4): 388-389.

[8]   Morris J C, Price J L. Pathologic correlates of nondemented aging, mild cognitive impairment, and early-stage Alzheimer's disease. J Mol Neurosci, 2001, 17(2): 101-118.

[9]   Xu Z, Jiang J, Ford G, et al. Neuregulin-1 is neuroprotective and attenuates inflammatory responses induced by ischemic stroke. Biochem Biophys Res Commun, 2004, 322(2): 440-446.

[10]   Xu Z, Ford B D. Upregulation of erbB receptors in rat brain after middle cerebral arterial occlusion. Neurosci Lett, 2005, 375(3): 181-186.

[11]   Li Q, Li Z, Mei Y W, et al. Neuregulin attenuated cerebral ischemia-reperfusion injury via inhibiting apoptosis and upregulating aquaporin-4. Neurosci Lett, 2008, 443(3): 155-159.

[12]   Li Q, Zhang R, Ge Y L, et al. Effect of neuregulin on apoptosis and expressions of STAT3 and GFAP in rats following cerebral ischemic reperfusion. J Mol Neurosci, 2009, 37(1): 67-73.

[13]   Li Q, Zhang R, Guo Y L, et al. Effects of neuregulin on expression of MMP-9 and NSE in brain of

ischemia/reperfusion rat. J Mol Neurosci, 2009, 38(2): 207-215.

[14]　Li Q, Zhang R, Zhang H, et al. Impact of neuregulin on the expressions of XIAP and Smac in brain tissue of rats after cerebral ischemic reperfusion injury. Chin Pharmacol Bull, 2009, 25(5): 658-662.

[15]　Wang Y C. Y-electric maze the rational use of learning and memory test in rats. Chin J Beha Med Sci, 2005, 14(1): 69-70.

[16]　Nakamura S, Murayama N, Noshita T, et al. Progressive brain dysfunction following intracerebroventricular infusion of beta(1-42)-amyloid peptide. Brain Res. 2001, 912(2): 128-136.

[17]　Nabeshima T. Trial to produce animal model of Alzheimer's disease by continuous infusion of beta-amyloid protein into the rat cerebral ventricle. Nihon Shinkei Seishin Yakurigaku Zasshi, 1995, 15(5): 411-418.

[18]　Chu J, Li L. The dementia models induced by intracerebroventricular infusion of β-Amyloid peptide in mice. Chin Pharmacol Bull, 2004, 20(7): 827-836.

[19]　Viel T A, Caetano A L, Nasello A G, et al. Increases of kinin B1 and B2 receptors binding sites afterbrain infusion of amyloid-beta 1-40 peptide in rats. Neurobiol Aging, 2008, 29(1): 1805-1814.

[20]　Allsop D, Twyman L J, Davies Y, et al. Modulation of β amyloid production and fibrillization. Biochem Soc Symp. 2001, 67(1): 1-14.

[21]　Tu R B, Ce J. Role and mechanism of β-amyloid in development of senile dementia. J Fourth Mil Med Univer, 2007, 28(1): 91-93.

[22]　Priller C, BauerT, Mitteregger G, et al. Synapse formation and function modulated by the amyloid precursor protein. J Neurosci, 2006, 26(27): 7212-7221.

[23]　Kayed R, Head E, Thompson J L, et al. Common structure of soluble amyloid oligomers implies common mechanism of pathogens. Science, 2003, 300(5618): 486-489.

[24]　Deshpande A, Mina E, Glabe C, et al. Different conformations of amyloid-beta induce neurotoxicity by distinct mechanisms in human cortical neurons. J Neurosci, 2000, 26(22): 6011-6018.

[25]　Chauhan V, Sheikh A M, Chauhan A, et al. Fibrillary amyloid beta-protein inhibits the activity of high molecular weight brain protease and tipsy. J Alzheimer Dis, 2005, 7(1): 37-44.

[26]　Tsukamoto E, Hashimoto Y, Kanekura K, et al. Characterization of the toxic mechanism triggered by Alzheimer's amyloid-beta petides via p75 neurotrophin receptor in neuronal hybrid cells. J Neurosci Res, 2003, 73(5): 627-636.

[27]　Abdul H M, Calabrese V, Calvani M, et al. Acetyl-L-carnitine induced up regulation of heat shock proteins protects cortical neurons against amyloid-beta petide 1-42 mediated oxidative stress and neurotoxicity implications for Alzheimer's disease. J Neurosci Res, 2006, 84(2): 398-408.

[28]　Guo Y L, Gao Y M. The time relationships between apoptosis of neuron and endotheliocyte with the expression of Bcl-2 and Bax after focal cerebral ischemia reperfusion in rats. Acta Anat Sinca, 2002, 33(3): 151-156.

[29]　Meng Y, Wang R, Liu M X, et al. Study on the factors related with mechanism of neuron apoptosis in Alzheimer disease. Chin J Geriat, 2006, 25(4): 245-247.

[30] Levi A. the Mechanism of Action of nerve Growth factor. Anna Rev Pharrnacol Toxic, 1991, 3(1): 205-231.

[31] Buonanno A, Fischbach G D. Neuregulin and ErbB receptor signaling pathways in the nervous system. Curr Opin Neurobiol, 2001, 11(3): 287-296.

[32] Tokita Y, Keino H, Matsui F, et al. Regulation of neuregulin expression in the injured rat brain and cultured astrocytes. J Neurosci, 2001, 21(4): 1257-1264.

Section 4　Words of TCM

1. 阳中之阳（太阳） yang within yang (taiyang/greater yang)

2. 阳中之阴（少阴） yin within yang (shaoyin/less yin)

3. 阴中之阴（太阴） yin within yin (taiyin/greater yin)

4. 阴中之阳（少阳） yang within yin (shaoyang/less yang)

5. 阴中之至阴（厥阴） zhiyin/greatest yin within yin (jueyin)

6. 阳中之至阳（阳明） zhiyang/greatest yang within yang (yangming)

7. 阴阳对立统一 unity and opposition between yin and yang

8. 阴阳互根 interdependence of yin and yang

9. 阴消阳长 waxing of yin and waning of yang; yin waxing and yang waning

10. 阴阳交感 inter-induction between yin and yang

11. 阴阳互藏 inter-containing between yin and yang

12. 阴阳转化 inter-transformation between yin and yang

13. 阴阳自和 spontaneous harmonization of yin and yang

14. 阴阳平秘 / 平衡 balance of yin and yang

15. 阴阳失调 imbalance between yin and yang

16. 阴阳偏盛 excess of yin and yang

17. 阴阳偏衰 deficiency of yin and yang

18. 阴阳互损 inter-impairment between yin and yang

19. 阴阳格拒 repellence between yin and yang

20. 阴阳亡失 exhaustion of yin and yang

21. 体质 / 体格 / 体型 body constitution/physique/body type

22. 气质 / 性格 temperament/character

23. 质化（从化） property transformation

24. 四象体质 four-manifestation (sixiang) constitution

25. 四时五脏阴阳体系 system of four-season five-zang-organ yinyang

26. 心为阳中之太阳 heart pertaining to taiyang (greater yang) within yang

27. 肺为阳中之少阳 lung pertaining to shaoyin (less yin) within yang

28. 肾为阴中之太阴 kidney pertaining to taiyin (greater yin) within yin

29. 肝为阴中之少阳 liver pertaining to shaoyang (less yang) within yin

30. 脾为阴中之至阴 spleen pertaining to zhiyin (greatest yin) within yin

31. 寒性药 cold-natured drugs; drugs with cold nature

32. 凉性药 cool-natured drugs; drugs with cool nature

33. 温性药 warm-natured drugs; drugs with warm nature

34. 热性药 hot-natured drugs; drugs with hot nature

35. 祛湿药 dampness-eliminating drugs

36. 理气药 qi-regulating drugs

37. 平肝药 liver-calming drugs

38. 开窍药 resusciation-inducing drugs

39. 壮阳药 yang-strengthening drugs

40. 清热药 heat-clearing drugs

(Hu Guojie, Zhai Li)

Chapter 7   Nutrition

Section 1   Nutrition and Disease

1   Nutrients needed for memory development

Choline: Choline is an essential nutrient and its primary function within the human body is the synthesis of cellular membranes, although it serves other functions as well. It is a precursor molecule to the neurotransmitter acetylcholine (Ach) which serves a wide range of functions including motor control and memory. Choline itself has also been shown to have additional health benefits in relation to memory and choline deficiencies may be related to some liver and neurological disorders. Because of its role in cellular synthesis, choline is an important nutrient during the prenatal and early postnatal development of offspring as it contributes heavily to the development of the brain. Despite the wide range of foods that choline is found in, studies have shown that the mean choline intake of men, women and children are below the Adequate Intake levels. Women, especially pregnant or lactating women, older people, and infants, are especially at risk for choline deficiency.

Vitamin A: Vitamin A is an essential nutrient for mammals which is taken from either retinol or the provitamin beta-carotene. It helps regulation of cell division, cell function, genetic regulation, helps enhance the immune system, and is required for brain function, chemical balance, growth and development of the central nervous system and vision.

Vitamin B_1 (thiamine): This vitamin is important for the facilitation of glucose use, thus ensuring the production of energy for the brain, and normal functioning of the nervous system, muscles and heart. Thiamine is found throughout mammalian nervous tissue, including the brain and spinal cord. Metabolism and coenzyme function of the vitamin suggest a distinctive function for thiamine within the nervous system. The brain retains its thiamine content in the face of a vitamin-deficient diet with great tenacity, as it is the last of all nervous tissues studied to become depleted.

The lack of thiamine causes the disease known as beriberi. There are two forms of beriberi: wet, and dry. Dry beriberi is also known as cerebral beriberi and characterized by peripheral neuropathy. Thiamine deficiency has been reported in up to 80% of alcoholic patients due to inadequate nutritional intake, reduced absorption, and impaired utilization of thiamine. Clinical signs of B_1 deficiency include mental changes such as apathy, decrease in short-term memory, confusion, and irritability; also increased rates of depression, dementia, falls, and fractures in old age.

The lingering symptoms of neuropathy associated with cerebral beriberi are known as Korsakoff's syndrome, or chronic phase of Wernicke-Korsakoff's. Wernicke encephalopathy is characterized by ocular abnormalities, ataxia of gait, a global state of confusion, and neuropathy. The state of confusion associated with Wernicke's may consist of apathy, inattention, spatial disorientation, inability to concentrate, and mental sluggishness or restlessness. Clinical diagnosis of Wernicke's disease cannot be made without evidence of ocular disturbance, yet these criteria may be too rigid. Korsakoff's syndrome likely represents a variation in the clinical manifestation of Wernicke encephalophathy, as they both share similar pathological origin. It is often characterized by confabulation, disorientation, and profound amnesia. Characteristics of the neuropathology are varied, but generally consist of bilaterally symmetrical midline lesions of brainstem areas, including the mammillary bodies, thalamus, periaqueductal region, hypothalamus, and the cerebellar vermis. Immediate treatment of Wernicke encephalopathy involves the administration of intravenous thiamine, followed with long-term treatment and prevention of the disorder through oral thiamine supplements, alcohol abstinence, and a balanced diet. Improvements in brain functioning of chronic alcoholics may occur with abstinence-related treatment, involving the discontinuation of alcohol consumption and improved nutrition.

2 Age-related macular degeneration

Two studies are suggesting ways to reduce the risk of age-related macular degeneration (AMD), which is the main cause of blindness among older adults. It affects the macula, the part of the eye that lets you see in detail. The disease makes seeing less and less clear and in time leads to blindness.

One study found that cigarette smokers were almost two times as likely to develop AMD as people who did not smoke. The study involved men with twin brothers, almost 700 individuals with an average age of 75 years old. The men were asked questions about their diet and history of cigarette smoking, alcohol use and physical activity. Some of the men already had age-related macular degeneration. The results found that the men who ate more fish, even those who smoked cigarettes, were less likely to develop AMD. Those who ate more than two meals a week containing fish were the least likely to develop the disease. The secondary study produced similar results and found that people who ate at least one meal containing fish each week were 40% less likely to develop AMD.

A prospective study organized by the University of Sydney in Australia studied information on almost 3000 people, aging 49 years or older. They were asked about their diet and medical history, and then tested for the disease after five years. The results of both studies have not yet been confirmed. But they do show a possible link between eating fish and prevention of AMD. The research indicates the best fish are high in omega-three fatty acids, like salmon and mackerel. Some people take fish oil supplements or eat foods, like flax seeds and walnuts, which also have them.

Many people drink coffee to quickly increase their energy levels. There may be another reason to drink coffee that drinking moderate amounts of coffee each day may help protect against some health problems, including heart disease. The findings were published in the *American Journal of Clinical Nutrition* and suggested there may be health reasons for drinking coffee. The researchers also studied the link between coffee drinking and the risk of death from heart disease, cancer and other diseases that involve inflammation of tissue. They used the information of nearly 42 000 women between 55 and 69 years of age when they entered the study. Some of the women were removed from consideration because of their condition (already having heart disease, cancer, diabetes, colitis or liver cirrhosis). As a result, the number of women in this research dropped to 27 300. During a 15-year period, almost 4300 of them died. The results showed a link between the amount of coffee the women reported drinking and their risk of dying from heart disease. Coffee drinking was measured in cups and one cup is equal to about 225 grams. There was a reduced risk of death from heart disease among women who drank 1 ~ 3 cups of coffee each day. A reduction in the risk of death from other inflammatory diseases was also seen. This risk reduction did not decrease among women who drank more coffee. But the risk reduction for death from heart disease did decrease in women who drank more than 3 cups a day. Earlier studies found that coffee has high levels of antioxidants which have been shown to help prevent cancer, heart disease and other conditions. So, the researchers consider that antioxidants in coffee might reduce the risk of heart disease.

In the present, more than 15% of American children and young people weigh too much. This is partly because they eat and drink too many foods of high calories and fat and sugar. Doctors say that extreme overweight in young people can have serious results. Being too fat can lead to high blood pressure, diabetes and liver disease.

Section 2   Vinegar in Chinese Medicine

Vinegar is a liquid consisting of about 5% ~ 20% acetic acid (CH_3COOH), water, and other trace chemicals, which may include flavorings. The acetic acid is produced by the fermentation of ethanol by acetic acid bacteria. Vinegar is now mainly used as a cooking ingredient, or in pickling. As the most easily manufactured mild acid, it has historically had a great variety of industrial, medical, and domestic uses, some of which (such as its use as a general household cleaner) are still commonly practiced today.

Commercial vinegar is produced either by a fast or a slow fermentation process. In general, slow methods are used in traditional vinegar where fermentation proceeds slowly over the course of a few months or up to a year. The longer fermentation period allows for the accumulation of a non-toxic slime composed of acetic acid bacteria. Fast methods add mother of vinegar (bacterial culture) to the source liquid before adding air to oxygenate and promote the fastest fermentation. In fast production processes, vinegar may be produced in 20 hours to three days.

Vinegar has been made and used by people for thousands of years. Traces of it have been found in Egyptian urns from around 3000 BC. In Chinese medicine, there is no hard and fast line between a food and a medicinal. As the well-known Chinese saying goes, food and medicine have a common source. Following on the heels of the popularity of artisanal olive oils, artisanal vinegar is quickly becoming a focus of attention in the world of cooking and cuisine. So far, this attention has mainly centered on these vinegar's extraordinary flavors. However, just as many have discovered the healing benefits of olive oil, vinegar also has its many health benefits and medicinal uses. Source materials for making vinegar are varied, including different fruits, grains, alcoholic beverages or other fermentable materials.

Fruit vinegar is made from fruit wines, usually without any additional flavoring. Common flavors of fruit vinegar include apple, blackcurrant, raspberry, quince, and tomato. Typically, the flavors of the original fruits remain in the final product. Most fruit vinegar is produced in Europe, where there is a growing market for high-price vinegar made solely from specific fruits (as opposed to non-fruit vinegar that is infused with fruits or fruit flavors). Several varieties, however, also are produced in Asia. Persimmon vinegar, called gam sikcho, is popular in South Korea. Jujube vinegar, called zaocu or hongzaocu, and wolfberry vinegar are produced in China.

In Chinese, vinegar is called kujiu, bitter wine, chuncu, pure vinegar, and micu, rice vinegar. It is primarily made in China from fermented millet, wheat, sorghum, and rice. According to Chinese medical theory, vinegar's flavor is sour and bitter and its nature or temperature is warm. It enters the liver and stomach channels, and its functions are scattering stasis, stopping bleeding, resolving toxins, and killing worms. In Chinese professional medicine, various Chinese medicinal is stir-fired in vinegar in order to either help target them to the liver-gallbladder or to increase their functions of moving the qi and quickening the blood. However, in Chinese folk medicine, vinegar is a medicinal in its own right, treating a wide range of disorders and complaints, and including internal medicine, gynecological, dermatological, and traumatological conditions. Below is a selection of folk recipes.

Prevention of common cold: Soak 100 g each of fresh ginger and garlic in 500 mL of vinegar in a tightly sealed jar for 30 days or more. Then drink 10 mL of the resulting liquid after each meal.

Indigestion from overeating: Take 15 mL of vinegar and 1 ~ 3 grams of fine green tea. Put the vinegar and tea leaves in teacup and pour 300 mL of boiling water over it. Allow to steep for 5 minutes. Then divided into three doses and drink one dose at a time as needed.

Viral hepatitis and/or enteritis: Eat (or drink) 30 mL of vinegar each time, 3 times per day.

Bacterial dysentery: Wash a daikon radish in water and slice thinly. Then add a suitable amount of vinegar and sugar to taste. Eat 2 times per day.

High blood pressure: (1) Dry stir-fry 500 g of soybeans till fragrant. Then allow to cool and soak in 1000 mL of vinegar for 10 days. Afterwards, eat the soybeans as one wants. (2) Soak unroasted peanuts in vinegar for 7 days. Do not remove the shells. Then eat 10 peanuts each morning and night. This formula can also be used for arteriosclerosis and coronary artery disease.

Arteriosclerosis: Each day, drink one tablespoon of vinegar.

Angina pectoris: Eat vinegar and garlic on a daily basis.

Diabetes: Wash 100 g of soybeans in water. Then soak in 110 mL of vinegar for 8 days. Eat 3 beans each time, 3 ~ 6 times per day. The constant eating gets the effect.

Thyroid swelling: Soak 60 g of dried seaweed in a suitable amount of vinegar and eat regularly.

Obesity: Eat or drink 15 ~ 40 mL of vinegar per day.

Headache: Boil some vinegar and inhale the fumes.

Edema: (1) Cook 60 g of fresh ginger into soup with 100 mL of vinegar and wash the affected limb with the resulting liquid once each day. (2) Powder a suitable amount of mustard seed and mix with vinegar. Apply to the affected area.

Insomnia: Drink a bowl of hot water mixed with vinegar.

Night sweats: Each night before sleep, wash the chest and upper back with vinegar.

Mouth sores (including thrush): Stir-fry 15 g of Fructus Evodiae Rutecarpae (Wuzhuyu). Then powder and mix into a paste with vinegar. Apply this paste once each evening before going to bed on the bottoms of the feet at the point of Yongquan (KI 1).

Gingivitis: Mix 50 mL of vinegar with 50 mL of hot water and gargle with the resulting liquid 2 times per day for 14 days.

Uterine bleeding: Cook 150 g of tofu with 100 mL of vinegar. Eat once per day for 7 ~ 10 days.

Vaginal candidiasis and itching: Douche with 100 mL of vinegar in 200 mL of water once per day for 10 days.

Nausea and vomiting during pregnancy: Drink a teaspoon of vinegar.

Boils and other inflamed sores: Mix mashed garlic and vinegar and apply to the affected area.

Traumatic injuries: Grind some mung beans into powder and mix with vinegar. Apply to the affected area. This can also be used for nonhealing lower sores, such as diabetic ulcers.

Nosebleed: Soak some sterile cotton in vinegar and insert into the nose.

Flat warts: Boil 200 mL of vinegar down to 100 mL and apply the resulting liquid to the warts 3 times per day.

Common warts: Mash a suitable amount of fresh ginger to obtain the juice. Then mix with a suitable amount of vinegar and apply to the warts several times per day.

Palmar eczema: Soak the hands in warm vinegar for 10 min each time, 2 times per day.

Parenchyomycosis (Fungal nails): With a knife or scissors, cut off as much of the dead nail as possible. Then soak the affected nail in vinegar for 30 min once per day.

Corns: Soak a Chinese preserved plum (Fructus Pruni Mume, Wumei, or umeboshi) in a suitable amount of vinegar. Then apply to the corn once per day.

Itching: Mix some soy sauce and vinegar and apply to the affected area.

Hives: (1) Boil 60 g of brown sugar and 30 g of fresh ginger in 200 mL of vinegar for 5 min. Then apply 20 ~ 30 mL of the resulting liquid mixed with warm water 2 ~ 3 times per day. (2) Mix two parts of the vinegar to one part alcohol and apply to the affected area.

Psoriasis: Apply strong vinegar 3 ~ 4 times per day.

Herpes zoster: Mix vinegar and Realgar (Xionghuang) together and apply externally to the herpes lesion once the blister has ruptured and there is a wet, glistening, slow-healing sore.

Hair loss: Mix 130 mL of vinegar with 200 mL of hot water and rinse the hair with this mixture, massaging it into the scalp, once per day on a regular basis.

Body odor: Soak 5 grams of fennel seeds in 50 mL of vinegar. Then apply the resulting liquid to the underarms 2 times per day.

Sweaty feet: Boil 30 g of Radix Sophorae Flavescentis (Kushen) and 20 g of Fructus Zanthoxyli Bungeani (Huajiao, Sichuan peppercorns) in 50 mL of aged vinegar. Apply the resulting liquid once each evening before going to bed. One should see an effect in 2 ~ 3 days and the full result in 7 days.

Food odor: Mix 15 ~ 20 mL of vinegar in warm water and soak the feet for 15 ~ 20 min, 2 times per day. Do continuously for 7 ~ 10 days and the food odor can be eliminated.

Section 3   Research Article

Buyang Huanwu Decoction alleviated pressure overload induced cardiac remodeling by suppressing Tgf-β/Smads and MAPKs signaling activated fibrosis

[Abstract]Buyang Huanwu Decoction (BHD), a traditional Chinese medicine recipe, is a representative prescription for the treatment of qi-deficiency and blood-stasis syndrome. In this study, the effect of BHD on pressure overload induced cardiac remodeling was investigated and the possible mechanism underlying was explored. Rats were randomly divided into four groups: sham, transverse aorta constriction (TAC) with saline, TAC with telmisartan (TAC + Tel), and TAC with BHD (TAC + BHD) for 16 weeks ($n = 6 \sim 8$ in each group). Cardiac morphological and functional changes were evaluated by echocardiography and histological methods, and the molecular alterations were detected by western blotting. Our results revealed that pressure overload prominently induced cardiac dysfunction, dilated and atrophied left ventricle, and decreased cardiomyocyte cross-sectional area and fibrosis. However, BHD, similar to Tel, greatly reversed cardiac dysfunction, left ventriculardilation, and fibrosis, together with increased left ventricular wall thickness and size of cardiomyocyte. Furthermore, activated classical profibrotic signaling of Tgf-β/Smads and MAPKs after TAC was dramatically suppressed by BHD or Tel treatment. Taken together, it was demonstrated in this study that BHD exerted a cardioprotective effect against pressure overload induced cardiac remodeling via inactivation of Tgf-β/Smads and MAPKs signaling triggered fibrosis.

Keywords: Buyang Huanwu Decoction; cardiac remodeling; fibrosis; transformation growth factor-β; smads; mitogen-activated protein kinases

1   Introduction

Cardiovascular disease, the first leading cause of death, is now severely threatening the whole world[1]. Cardiac remodeling, triggered by inflammation, pressure overload, oxidative stress and other stimuli, participates in the development of almost every kind of heart disease, and even leads to heart failure[2]. The pathogenesis of cardiac remodeling includes not only cardiomyocyte hypertrophy, apoptosis and necrosis, but also extracellular fibrosis which is a main predictor of mortality in patients with cardiac dysfunction[3].

In traditional Chinese medicine (TCM), heart failure is considered to be in virtue of qi-deficiency and blood-stasis syndrome[4-6]. Characterized by shortness of breath, light colored tongue, and hemorheological disorders, this syndrome commonly exhibits in various courses of cardiovascular and cerebrovascular diseases[7]. According to TCM theory, Buyang Huanwu Decoction (BHD), recorded in *Yilin Gaicuo* (*Correction on Errors in Medical Classics*), is a classical prescription of qi-tonifying and stasis-eliminating method[8]. It is composed of Radix Astragali (Huangqi), Radix Angelicae Sinensis (Danggui), Radix Paeoniae Rubra (Chishao), Rhizoma Ligustici Chuanxiong (Chuanxiong), Semen Persicae (Taoren), Flos Carthami (Honghua), and Lumbricus (Dilong), in the ratio of 120 : 6 : 4.5 : 3 : 3 : 3 : 3 on a dry weight basis, respectively, recorded in the *Chinese Pharmacopoeia*. BHD is widely used for stroke in China, which has been clinically and experimentally reported to be neuroprotective by multiple target[9-10]. Moreover, BHD has also showed to protect myocardial from ischemic injuries[7, 11]. In our previous finding, BHD significantly alleviated pressure overload induced heart failure via sarcoplasmic reticulum calcium uptake[12]. However, the effect of BHD on cardiac remodeling, especially cardiac fibrosis, was not explored.

Therefore we focused the protective effect of BHD on pressure overload induced cardiac remodeling by a rat transverse aortic constriction (TAC) model and further explored the mechanism underlying in this study.

2　Materials and methods

2.1　Animals and drugs

Male adult Wistar rats [8 weeks, mean body mass (180 ± 10) g] were purchased from Shanghai Laboratory Animal Center (Shanghai, China). All procedures in this study were approved by the Animal Care and Use Committee of Shanghai University of Traditional Chinese Medicine, which is in accordance with the National Institutes of Health Guide for the Care and Use of Laboratory Animals (NIH Publications No. 8023, revised 1978). The animals were housed in cages under standard conditions at 25 °C with a 12/12 h light-dark cycle and allowed free access to water and standard diet.

BHD (Xiaoshuan granule) was purchased from Harbin Pharmaceutical Group Co., Ltd. (Heilongjiang, China), which was composed of Radix Astragali (Huangqi), Radix Angelicae Sinensis (Danggui), Radix Paeoniae Rubra (Chishao), Rhizoma Ligustici Chuanxiong(Chuanxiong), Semen Persicae (Taoren), Flos Carthami (Honghua), and Lumbricus (Dilong) as a granule. Telmisartan (Tel) was purchased from Sigma Aldrich (MO, USA). Before using, they were dissolved in saline at a final concentration of 2.0 g/mL and 5 mg/mL, respectively.

2.2　Transverse aortic constriction

TAC surgery was used to generate pressure overload induced cardiac hypertrophy and heart failure. Briefly, general anesthesia was induced with 5% isoflurane in 95% oxygen and 5% carbondioxide by a calibrated vaporizer (Surgivet Inc, WI, USA), and maintained by mechanical ventilation (60 bpm, 1.5 ~ 2.0 mL tidal volume, 2% isoflurane in 95% oxygen and 5% carbon dioxide) (Harvard Inspira-ASV, Harvard Apparatus, MA, USA). Rats were placed supine on a warm electric pad (World Precision Instruments Inc, FL, USA) to keep at approximately 37 °C. After thoracotomy, the aortic arch was carefully dissected free of surrounding tissues, and a bended and blunted style from a 18 G intravenous catheter was tightly tied to the aorta between the brachiocephalic trunk and the left common carotid artery using 4–0 silk, and then removed to create partial aortic constriction. The sternum and the skin incision were closed with 5–0 sutures. The sham group underwent all operation procedures except the ligation of aorta. Postoperative animals were kept in separated cages and allowed free access to water and standard diet. Analgesia with buprenorphine 0.05 mg/kg was subcutaneously provided every 12 h for 48 h.

2.3　Medication treatment

After 3 days of operation, animals were randomly divided into sham, TAC, TAC plus telmisartan (TAC + Tel), and TAC plus BHD (TAC + BHD) group ($n = 6 \sim 8$ in each group), and the whole duration for this study lasted for 16 weeks. The sham and TAC groups were treated with saline, while the TAC + Tel and TAC + BHD groups were treated with telmisartan [5 mg/kg, a selective angiotensin II type 1 receptor (AT1R) antagonist as positive control] and BHD (2 g/kg), respectively, once a day by oral gavage.

2.4　Echocardiography

Echocardiography was performed using a high resolution ultrasound imaging system (Vevo 2100, Visualsonics Inc, Toronto, Canada). The animals were anesthetized with 2.5% isoflurane in 95% oxygen and 5% carbon dioxide, and the hair was removed with depilatory cream. M-mode recordings were obtained from the parasternal short axis views. The internal dimensions of left ventricular (LV) cavity, left ventricular posterior wall (LVPW) and interventricular septal wall (IVS) thickness, LV fractional shortening (FS), and LV ejection fraction (EF) were measured and recorded.

2.5　Histological procedure

Tissue samples were fixed in 4% paraformaldehyde overnight at 4 °C, rinsed, transferred to phosphate buffer saline (PBS), and embedded by paraffin. Hematoxylineosin (H&E) and Masson's trichrome staining were performed. The sections were examined by light microscopy and photographed. LV wall thickness and mean cross sectional area were quantified by the Image J, and collagen deposition was quantitatively analyzed by collagen volume fraction via Image Pro Plus (Media Cybernetics Inc, MD, USA).

2.6　Western blotting

Protein lysates from heart samples were loaded on and separated by a 10% SDS-

PAGE, and then transferred to PVDF membranes (Millipore, MA, USA). The membranes were probed overnight with primary antibodies overnight at 4 °C after blocking with 5% milk in tris-buffered saline with 0.1% Tween (TBST). The primary antibodies were: anti-transformation growth factor β1 (Tgf-β1) (Santa Cruz, MA, USA), anti Tgf-β receptor I (Tgf RI) (Cell Signaling Technology, MA, USA), anti Tgf-β receptor II (Tgf R II) (Cell Signaling Technology, MA, USA), anti phosphorylated Smad 2/3 (Cell Signaling Technology, MA, USA), anti Smad 2/3 (Cell Signaling Technology, MA, USA), anti Smad 4 (Santa Cruz, MA, USA), anti phosphorylated c-Jun N-terminal kinase (JNK) (Cell Signaling Technology, MA, USA), anti JNK (Cell Signaling Technology, MA, USA), anti phosphorylated extracellular signal regulated kinase 1/2 (ERK1/2) (Cell Signaling Technology, MA, USA), anti ERK1/2 (Cell Signaling Technology, MA, USA), anti phosphorylated P38 (Cell Signaling Technology, MA, USA), anti P38 (Cell Signaling Technology, MA, USA) and anti glyceraldehyde-3-phosphate dehydrogenase (GAPDH) (Multi Sciences, Zhejiang, China). Membranes were washed by TBST for 3 times and then incubated with appropriate secondary antibody for 1 h at room temperature. After another 3 times wash by TBST, the signal was detected on Fluor Chem E (Protein Simple, CA, USA). The densities of bands were quantified by using an Image J Analysis System and expressed as ratios to GAPDH.

2.7 RNA analysis

Total RNA was extracted from heart tissue with Trizol reagent (Invitrogen, CA, USA), and reverse transcribed with SuperScript reverse transcriptase kit (Invitrogen, CA, USA). Gene expression was analyzed by quantitative real-time polymerase chain reaction (PCR) using SYBR® dye (LightCycler® 96 Real-Time PCR System). Transcript level was determined relative to the signal from GAPDH and normalized to the mean value of samples from the sham group. The primers encoding rattus tumor necrosis factor α (TNF-α), interleukin 1(IL-1), IL-6, collagen type I (Col I), collagen type III (Col III), and GAPDH were as follows (Table 7-1).

Table 7-1　The primers encoding rattus TNF-α, IL-1, IL-6, Col I , Col II and GAPDH

TNF-α	F	TTCCAATGGGCTTTCGGAAC	Col I	F	GACATGTTCAGCTTTGTGGACCTC
	R	AGACATCTTCAGCAGCCTTGTGAG		R	AGGGACCCTTAGGCCATTGTGTA
IL-1	F	CCCTGAACTCAACTGTGAAATAGCA	Col III	F	TTTGGCACAGCAGTCCAATGTA
	R	CCCAAGTCAAGGGCTTGGAA		R	GACAGATCCCGAGTCGCAGA
IL-6	F	ATTGTATGAACAGCGATGATGCAC	GAPDH	F	GGCACAGTCAAGGCTGAGAATG
	R	CCAGGTAGAAACGGAACTCCAGA		R	ATGGTGGTGAAGACGCCAGTA

2.8 Statistical analysis

All values were analyzed with SPSS18.0 and results were presented as means ± SEM. The data were analyzed with one-way analysis of variance (one-way ANOVA) followed by Tukey's post hoc analysis, and P value less than 0.05 was considered statistically significant.

3 Results

3.1 BHD attenuated pressure overload induced cardiac functional remodeling

To evaluate the effect of BHD on TAC induced cardiac functional alteration in vivo, a rat model of TAC induced cardiac hypertrophy was introduced, and echocardiography was applied to assess the dynamic changes of the heart. In general, there were no differences in the bodyweight, tibia length, heart rate and death rate of those four groups after 16 weeks' treatments (Table 7-2). As shown in Figure 7-1(A) ~ (C) and Table 7-2, 16 weeks of TAC resulted in significantly reduced left ventricular function, as evidenced by decreased LV EF and FS compared with those in the sham group (P < 0.05). This was further supported by dilated left ventricle and thinned left ventricular posterior wall [P < 0.05 vs the sham group, Figure 7-1 (D) ~ (F) and Table 7-2]. However, BHD or telmisartan, a selective AT1 antagonist, treatment exhibited beneficial effect on TAC induced left ventricular dysfunction, which was verified by increased LV EF and less dilated LV [P < 0.05 vs the TAC group, Figure 7-1 (B) ~ (E) and Table 7-2]. Moreover, BHD treatment also reversed LV posterior wall atrophy at diastolic period [P < 0.05 vs the TAC group, Figure 7-1 (F) and Table 7-2].

Table 7-2   Summary of general and cardiac phenotypes of each group after 16 weeks of different treatments

Group phenotypes	Sham	TAC + sal	TAC + Tel	TAC + BHD
body weight / g	433.60 ± 9.62	407.60 ± 3.66	408.40 ± 3.54	420.00 ± 17.10
heart weight / g	1.10 ± 0.01	1.01 ± 0.02[*]	0.99 ± 0.02[*]	1.02 ± 0.03[*]
lung weight / g	1.52 ± 0.06	1.51 ± 0.05	1.25 ± 0.02[*#]	1.20 ± 0.03[*#]
tibia length / mm	54.51 ± 0.89	54.12 ± 0.95	54.71 ± 0.35	55.06 ± 0.21
HR / bpm	324 ± 15.65	318 ± 17.28	323 ± 20.76	316 ± 14.93
Death rate / %	0	0	0	0
LVIDd / mm	7.46 ± 0.16	8.28 ± 0.27[*]	7.28 ± 0.25[#]	7.46 ± 0.15[#]
LVIDs / mm	4.01 ± 0.26	5.06 ± 0.27[*]	3.85 ± 0.20[#]	4.32 ± 0.18[#]
LVPWd / mm	1.62 ± 0.05	1.36 ± 0.08[*]	1.54 ± 0.06	1.59 ± 0.01[#]
LVPWs / mm	2.66 ± 0.07	2.55 ± 0.12	2.58 ± 0.14	2.57 ± 0.12
IVSd / mm	1.49 ± 0.03	1.38 ± 0.06	1.55 ± 0.1	1.51 ± 0.05
IVSs / mm	2.50 ± 0.12	2.63 ± 0.11	2.50 ± 0.14	2.54 ± 0.14
FS / %	46.22 ± 2.54	37.56 ± 1.87[*]	47.61 ± 1.44[#]	44.86 ± 2.11
EF / %	77.67 ± 2.06	63.60 ± 2.43[*]	75.58 ± 1.78[#]	74.34 ± 2.25[#]

The data were expressed as the mean ± SEM. $^*P < 0.05$ versus the sham group; $^#P < 0.05$ versus the TAC group; $n = 6 \sim 8$ in each group; TAC, transverse aortic constriction; sal, saline; Tel, telmisartan; BHD, Buyang Huanwu Decoction; HR, heart rate; LVIDd, left ventricular internal dimension at diastolic period; LVIDds, left ventricular internal dimension at systolic period; LVPWd, left ventricular posterior wall thickness at diastolic period; LVPWs, left ventricular posterior wall thickness at systolic period; IVSd, interventricular septal wall thickness at diastolic period; IVSs, interventricular septal wall thickness at systolic period; EF, left ventricular ejection fraction; FS, left ventricular fractional shortening.

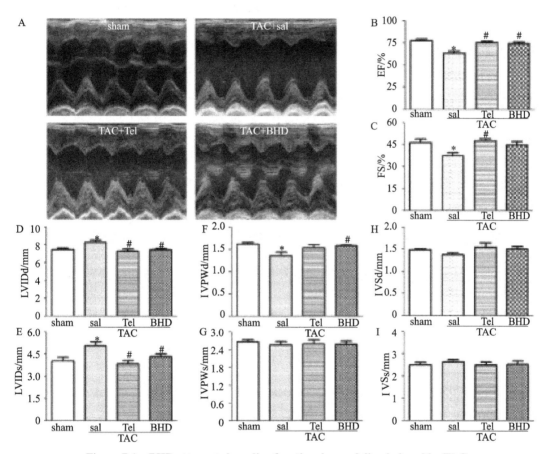

Figure 7-1 BHD attenuated cardiac functional remodeling induced by TAC

A: Representative M-mode tracings of echocardiography; B ~ I: Quantification echocardiographic parameters ($n = 10$ in each group). B: left ventricular ejection fraction (EF); C: left ventricular fractional shortening (FS); D: left ventricular internal dimension at diastolic period (LVIDd); E: left ventricular internal dimension at systolic period (LVIDds); F: left ventricular posterior wall thickness at diastolic period (LVPWd); G: left ventricular posterior wall thickness at systolic period (LVPWs); H: interventricular septal wall thickness at diastolic period (IVSd); I: interventricular septal wall thickness at systolic period (IVSs).

Echocardiography was recorded and measured at 16 weeks after surgery. The data were expressed as the mean ± SEM. $^*P < 0.05$ *vs* the sham group; $^#P < 0.05$ *vs* the TAC group; $n = 6 \sim 8$ in each group; TAC, transverse aortic constriction; sal, saline; Tel, telmisartan; BHD, Buyang Huanwu Decoction.

3.2 BHD alleviated pressure overload induced cardiac morphological remodeling and pulmonary congestion

To further explore the effect of BHD, heart and lung samples were collected for the following observations. The TAC group after 16 weeks pressure overload exhibited pulmonary congestion, as evidenced by significant elevated lung weight to body weight and lung weight to tibia length ratios ($P < 0.05$ vs the sham group), but with no differences in heart weight to body weight and heart weight to tibia length ratios. Microscopic examination of HE sections at papillary muscle level revealed a slight atrophy of the left ventricular wall and smaller cross sectional area of cardiomyocyte after TAC ($P < 0.05$ vs the sham group). The treatment of BDH or Tel, nevertheless, significantly reduced lung weight to body weight and lung weight to tibia length ratios ($P < 0.05$ vs the TAC group). In addition, reversed left ventricular wall atrophy ($P > 0.05$ vs the sham group, $P < 0.05$ vs the TAC group) and markedly increased cross sectional areas of cardiomyocyte ($P < 0.05$ vs the sham group, $P < 0.05$ vs the TAC group), but not elevated heart weight to body weight or heart weight to tibia length ratios, were observed after BDH or Tel administration, indicating that the two medications improved TAC induced cardiac dysfunction by compensatory cardiomyocyte hypertrophy.

3.3 BHD suppressed pressure overload induced myocardial fibrosis

Considering fibrosis is an important factor for cardiac remodeling, cardiac collagen deposition was then measured by Masson's trichrome staining. Histological findings revealed that TAC induced significant interstitial and perivascular fibrosis compared with the sham group ($P < 0.05$). On the contrary, BHD or Tel treatment significantly suppressed cardiac fibrosis elicited by TAC ($P < 0.05$ vs the TAC group).

3.4 BHD alleviated pressure overload induced cardiac fibrosis by down-regulation of Tgf-β /Smads and MAPKs signaling

The pro-fibrotic process in the development of cardiac remodeling is mainly through activation of phosphorylation of Smads, which is under the control of Tgf-β and Ang Ⅱ activated mitogen-activated protein kinases (MAPKs)[13-15]. Therefore, the following signals were focused to illustrate the mechanism involving in the anti-fibrotic effect of BHD. Western blotting results demonstrated that myocardial Tgf R Ⅰ, but not the level of Tgf-β1 and Tgf R Ⅱ, was significantly up-regulated in the TAC group compared to the sham group ($P < 0.05$). In parallel with this, activated Smads and MAPKs were observed after pressure overload, as evidenced by increased Smad 4 and phosphorylation of Smad 3, ERK1/2, JNK, and P38 ($P < 0.05$, vs the sham group). However, administration of BHD or Tel significantly down-regulated Tgf R Ⅰ, inactivated Smad 3 and dephosphorylated MAPKs ($P < 0.05$ vs the TAC group), and slightly decreased Smad 4 ($P > 0.05$ *vs* the TAC group).

4   Discussion

Cardiac remodeling represents physiological and pathophysiologic adaption of the heart in response to different stimuli such as pressure overload, inflammation, reactive oxygen stress, etc.. This study demonstrated that BHD treatment, a TCM classical prescription, provided a cardioprotective effect against pressure overload induced cardiac functional and morphological remodeling via suppressing Tgf-β/Smads and MAPKs signaling activated fibrosis.

BHD is a well-known classic traditional Chinese herbal prescription for stroke, which is still widely used throughout China and elsewhere in the world. Both clinical trials and animal model experiments indicated that BHD therapy appears to be beneficial to cerebrovascular diseases[9]. According to the theory of treating different diseases with the same method, BHD has also been applied and proved to be effective in heart diseases, such as ischemic heart disease and heart failure which exhibit the qi-deficiency and blood-stasis syndrome similar to cerebrovascular diseases [7,11,16-18]. Based on these findings and theories, we focused on the effect of BHD on cardiac remodeling after pressure overload, and it was demonstrated in this study that the administration of BHD, as well as telmisartan, ameliorated TAC induced cardiac remodeling and pulmonary congestion by compensatory cardiomyocyte hypertrophy, less dilated chamber, and inhibition of cardiac fibrosis, which ultimately resulted in improved heart function. This is in accordance with the clinical study by Liu et al. that BHD effectively lowered blood pressure and plasma lipid, and improved hemorrheological parameters in patients with hypertension[19]. Moreover, our previous study in a rat model of abdominal aortic constriction also revealed that BHD mitigated cardiac dysfunction and hypertrophy via improvement of sarcoplasmic reticulum calcium uptake capacity [12].

Recent literatures have illustrated that BHD possesses multiple target in the interventions of cerebrovascular diseases and cardiovascular diseases[20]. Zhang et al. have revealed the corresponding relations between vascular targets and effective components in BHD by networked pharmacological method [21]. According to this, the main bioactive components of BHD targeting at vascular diseases includes isoimperatorin, isorhamnetin, paeonol, kaempferol, palmitic acid, thymol, o-cresol, angelicin, z-ligustilide, butylphthalide, juglone, catechin, gallocatechin, epigallocatechin, etc.. Both clinical and experimental studies have demonstrated the BHD exhibits multi-target protective effect by improvement of microcirculation and capillary permeability, reduction of calcium overload, oxidative stress and nitration stress, inhibition of inflammation and apoptosis, and promotion of angiogenesis[9, 20]. Thus it is not surprising that BHD exerted an anti-pathophysiologic cardiac remodeling effect in this study.

The mechanism of pressure overload induced cardiac remodeling is sophisticated, and much attention has focused on myocardial and endothelial biology. However, cardiac fibrosis is another active research area, which indicates not only increased mechanical stiffness with diastolic dysfunction but poor prognosis as well [3, 22]. Accordingly, our finding illustrated that TAC elicited prominent cardiac fibrosis, accompanied with decreased cardiac function. On the contrary, BHD, at least partially, reversed cardiac fibrosis with improved cardiac function. Therefore, we targeted the underlying mechanism of BHD.

Fibrosis in hypertensive cardiomyopathy is driven by profibrotic molecules, particularly the rennin-angiotensin-aldosterone system (RAAS) and cytokines such as Tgf-β[23]. Persistent elevation of Ang II activates MAPKs, which thereafter stimulates fibroblasts to produce collagen type I and collagen type III, leading to progressive derangement of cardiac structure[15]. Moreover, extensive evidence suggests that Tgf-β1 acts as downstream of Angiotensin II, which mediates fibroblast proliferation and production of collagen and extracellular matrix via its receptor (Tgf R I and Tgf RII) activated Smads [13, 14, 15, 24]. In consistence with this, our study demonstrated that blockage of AT1R by telmisartan efficiently suppressed TAC induced up-regulation of Tgf R I, phosphorylation of MAPKs and Smad 3, and cardiac fibrosis, which was similar to the effect of BHD treatment. Besides this, pressure overload induced elevation of pro-inflammatory cytokines, including IL-6 and TNF-α, were also suppressed by BHD or Tel treatment, implying that BHD exerted the beneficial effect against pathophysiologic cardiac remodeling by alleviating myocardial inflammatory stress. However, the specific intracellular anti-fibrotic target of BHD requires more detailed proofs by in vivo and in vitro experiments.

Smads are intracellular signaling effector necessary for the mediation of cardiac fibrosis, hypertrophy, atherogenesis, and even for the regulation of cardiac structural development in embryos[25]. The distinct role of Smads in fibrosis depends on their transcriptional activity[26]. Nuclear translocations of Smad 2/3 and Smad 4 after the phorsphorylation of Smad 2/3, which thereafter form a complex directly binds to gene promoters to induce transcription of pro-fibrotic molecules, including α-smooth muscle actin (α-SMA), collagen and tissue inhibitor of matrix metalloproteinases (TIMP), and ultimately initiates myofibroblast activation and matrix deposition[26]. Coincidently, our data revealed that elevations of collagen III mRNA and myocardial fibrosis after TAC were accompanied with activation of Smad 3 and increased Smad 4. More importantly, BHD or telmisartan treatment markedly dephosphorylated Smad 3 and slightly decreased Smad 4 expression, leading to the reduction of myocardial fibrosis. This further provided the molecular mechanism of BHD in modulating pressure overload induced cardiac remodeling.

In conclusion, the study demonstrated that the traditional Chinese medical recipe BHD exerted a cardioprotective effect against pressure overload induced cardiac remodeling via suppressing myocardial Tgf-β/Smads and MAPKs signal activated fibrosis, which provide a direct experimental proof for the application of BHD in the clinical practice.

Source of funding

This work was supported by the following grants: National Natural Science Foundation of China No. 30973821 and 81373858.

References

[1] Roth G A, Huffman M D, Moran A E, et al. Global and regional patterns in cardiovascular mortality from 1990 to 2013. Circulation, 2015, 132 (17): 1667-1678.

[2] Konstam M A, Kramer D G, Patel A R, et al. Left ventricular remodeling in heart failure: current concepts in clinical significance and assessment. Jacc Cardiovascular Imaging, 2011, 4(1): 98-108.

[3] López B, González A, Ravassa S, et al. Circulating biomarkers of myocardial fibrosis: the need for a reappraisal. Journal of the American College of Cardiology, 2015, 65(22): 2449-2456.

[4] Miao Y, Zhao W J, Jing L. Retrospective analysis on integrative medicinal treatment of chronic heart failure. Chinese Journal of Integrated Traditional & Western Medicine, 2008, 28(5): 406-409.

[5] Zhu B Q, Dai R H. Use of qi-replenishing and stasis-removing herbs in treating patients with heart failure of qi deficiency and blood stasis type. Chinese Journal of Integrated Traditional & Western Medicine, 1987, 7(10): 591.

[6] Wu Q Y, Hu X P, Li D X. Qi deficiency and blood stasis and circulatory renin-angiotensin system as well as plasminogen activator inhibitor activity in rats with cardiac qi deficiency syndrome. Chinese Journal of Integrated Traditional & Western Medicine, 2001, 21(5): 367-369.

[7] Wang W R, Lin R, Zhang H, et al. The effects of Buyang Huanwu Decoction on hemorheological disorders and energy metabolism in rats with coronary heart disease. Journal of Ethnopharmacology, 2011, 137(1): 214-220.

[8] Zhang Z Q, Tang T, Luo J K, et al. Effect of qi-tonifying and stasis-eliminating therapy on expression of vascular endothelial growth factor and its receptors Flt-1, Flk-1 in the brain of intracerebral hemorrhagic rats. Chinese Journal of Integrative Medicine, 2007, 13(4): 285-290.

[9] Wei R, Teng H, Yin B, et al. A systematic review and meta-analysis of buyang huanwu decoction in animal model of focal cerebral ischemia. Evidence-based complementary and alternative medicine: eCAM, 2013, 2013(2): 138484.

[10] Li H Q, Wei J J, Xia W, et al. Promoting blood circulation for removing blood stasis therapy for acute intracerebral hemorrhage: a systematic review and meta-analysis. Acta Pharmacol Sin, 2015, 36(6): 659-675.

[11] Zhou Y C, Liu B, Li Y J, et al. Effects of buyang huanwu decoction on ventricular remodeling and differential protein profile in a rat model of myocardial infarction. Evidence-Based Complementary and

Alternative Medicine, 2012, 2012(2): 385247.

[12] Gu Y P, Liao Y L, Zhang C, et al. Effects of buyang huanwu decoction on the sarcoplasmic reticulum calcium uptake in abdominal aortic constriction induced myocardial hypertrophic rats. Chinese Journal of Integrated Traditional & Western Medicine, 2013, 33(33): 627-631.

[13] Teekakirikul P, Eminaga S, Toka O, et al. Cardiac fibrosis in mice with hypertrophic cardiomyopathy is mediated by non-myocyte proliferation and requires Tgf-β. Journal of Clinical Investigation, 2010, 120(10): 3520-3529.

[14] Moustakas A, Heldin C H. The regulation of TGFbeta signal transduction. Development, 2009, 136(22): 3699-3714.

[15] Sciarretta S, Paneni F, Palano F, et al. Role of the renin-angiotensin-aldosterone system and inflammatory processes in the development and progression of diastolic dysfunction. Clinical Science, 2009, 116(6): 467-477.

[16] Liu Y, Lin R, Zhang H, et al. Protective effect of buyanghuanwu decoction on myocardial ischemia induced by isoproterenol in rats. Journal of Chinese Medicinal Materials, 2009, 32(3): 380-383.

[17] Liu Y, Lin R, Shi X, et al. The Roles of buyang huanwu decoction in anti-inflammation, antioxidation and regulation of lipid metabolism in rats with myocardial ischemia. Evidence-Based Complementary and Alternative Medicine, 2011(4): 561396.

[18] Jiang M, Zhang C, Zheng G, et al. Traditional Chinese medicine zheng in the era of evidence-based medicine: a literature analysis. 2014, 2012(3): 409568.

[19] Liu H, Zhou J F. Xianbai buyang huanwu decoction used for treating hypertension with kidney qi deficiency and blood stasis. Chinese Journal of Integrated Traditional and Western Medicine, 1993, 13(12): 714-717.

[20] Li J H, Liu A J, Li H Q, et al. Buyang huanwu decoction for healthcare: evidence-based theoretical interpretations of treating different diseases with the same method and target of vascularity. Evidence-Based Complementary and Alternative Medicine, 2014, 2014: 506783.

[21] Zhang W, Gao K, Liu J, et al. A review of the pharmacological mechanism of traditional Chinese medicine in the intervention of coronary heart disease and stroke. African Journal of Traditional Complementary & Alternative Medicines Ajtcam, 2013, 10(6): 532-537.

[22] Chaturvedi R R, Herron T, Simmons R, et al. Passive stiffness of myocardium from congenital heart disease and implications for diastole. Circulation, 2010, 121(8): 979-988.

[23] Díez J. Mechanisms of cardiac fibrosis in hypertension. Journal of Clinical Hypertension, 2007, 9(7): 546-550.

[24] Rosenkranz S. TGF-beta1 and angiotensin networking in cardiac remodeling. Cardiovascular Research, 2004, 63(3): 423-432.

[25] Dobaczewski M, Chen W, Frangogiannis N G. Transforming growth factor (TGF)-β signaling in cardiac remodeling. Journal of Molecular & Cellular Cardiology, 2011, 51(4): 600-606.

[26] Meng X M, Nikolic-Paterson D J, Lan H Y. TGF-β: the master regulator of fibrosis. Nature Reviews

Section 4　Words of TCM

1. 相生相克 mutual promotion and restriction

2. 相乘相侮 mutual over-restriction and counter-restriction

3. 生中有制 restriction within promotion

4. 制则生化 restriction resulting in generation and changes

5. 木曰曲直 wood being characterized by bending and straightening

6. 火曰炎上 fire being characterized by heating and ascending

7. 土爱稼穑　earth being characterized by planting and harvesting

8. 金曰从革 metal being characterized by changes

9. 水曰润下 water being characterized by moistening and descending

10. 五行胜复 resistance of oppressed elements

11. 腐熟水谷 digesting food

12. 胃气下降 stomach qi descending

13. 胃气降浊 stomach qi lowering the turbid

14. 受盛化物 containing and digesting

15. 泌别清浊 separating clear from turbid

16. 心肾相交 coordination between heart and kidney

17. 水火相济 regulation between water and fire

18. 升降相因 inter-dependence between ascending and descending

19. 纳运相得 inter-promotion between containing and digesting

20. 燥湿相济 inter-dependence between drying and moistening

21. 寒凉派 school of cold- and cool-natured drugs

22. 攻下派 purgation-applying school

23. 补土派 spleen-strengthening school; school of strengthening spleen

24. 滋阴派 yin-nourishing school; school of nourishing yin

25. 吐法 emesis-inducing method

26. 下法 purgation-inducing method

27. 汗法 diaphoresis method

28. 清法 heat-reducing method

29. 行气法 qi-promoting method

30. 降气法 qi-decreasing method

31. 治未病 prevention of diseases

32. 调养 recuperation

33. 传变 transmission and changes

34. 推拿按摩 pushing, grasping, pressing and rubbing manipulation

35. 理脾功 spleen-regulating qigong

36. 回春功 life-recuperating qigong

37. 阴盛则阳病 excessive yin leading to yang diseases

38. 阳盛则阴病 excessive yang resulting in yin diseases

39. 肾阴不足 deficiency of kidney yin

40. 肝阴不足 yin deficiency of the liver

(Liu Tianwei, Liu Yingjuan)

Chapter 8　Acupuncture

Section 1　Acupuncture Therapy

Acupuncture is a form of alternative medicine in which thin needles are inserted into the body. It is a key component of traditional Chinese medicine (TCM). TCM theory and practice are not based upon scientific knowledge, and acupuncture is a pseudoscience. There is a diverse range of acupuncture theories based on different philosophies, and techniques vary depending on the country. The method used in TCM is likely the most widespread in the United States. It is most often used for pain relief, though it is also used for a wide range of other conditions. Acupuncture is generally used only in combination with other forms of treatment.

Ear acupuncture therapy promotes rehabilitation by applying the methods such as acupuncture, needle-embedding therapy and electrotherapy to puncture the corresponding acupoints of the specific sites of the auricle according to certain acupoint selection principles. The auricle is like an inverted fetus with the corresponding sites of the internal organs, limbs and other tissues and organs of the fetus on it. The location and nomenclature of auricular acupoints mostly correspond with such a distribution and have certain regularity. The auricular acupoint, also called positive sensitive point or sensitive spot, pressure pain point, good conducting point, etc., has double value in diagnosis and treatment. The commonly-used methods of ear acupuncture therapy include needle-embedding therapy, seed-pressing method, needling method with the filiform needle, electrotherapy, warming needle therapy, etc.. Ear acupuncture therapy is commonly applicable to various painful diseases as well as many dysfunctional diseases in TCM health preservation and rehabilitation such as hemicrania, trigeminal neuralgia, toothache, ischia, hypertension, insomnia, aphasia, numbness of limbs, indigestion, gallstone, chronic tracheitis, chronic enteritis, chronic pelvic inflammation, impotence and menopausal syndrome.

Strict measures should be taken for antisepsis during ear acupuncture therapy. Needling is contraindicated on the site with frostbite or inflammation and immediate treatment is required in case of infection. Besides, needling is contraindicated in pregnant women with a history of habitual abortion; patients with sprain or disturbance of limb movement should move the affected part to improve the rehabilitation effects when the feeling of congestion and fever appears on the auricle after the insertion of the needle.

Scalp acupuncture therapy treats diseases or promotes the somatopsychic rehabilitation of the patient by needling the specific areas of the scalp. The specific stimulation areas of the scalp are established on the basis of the location theory of cortico-cerebral functions. Two standard lines (the antero-posterior midline of the scalp and the eyebrow-occiput line) should be firstly established in order to delimit the stimulation areas of the scalp acupuncture precisely, and on which the specific stimulation areas can be determined respectively. The division of the stimulation areas of the scalp acupuncture may be determined with the help of flexible rule in general. The location may be determined by the experience with the mastery of the skill. Finger measurement may be applicable to patients of different age groups and different scalp types. Generally, the middle finger of an adult measures $2.0 \sim 2.5$ cm. The division of stimulation areas of scalp acupuncture is very strict. Each stimulation area corresponds accurately to the indications it controls. Therefore, all the areas and their corresponding indications should be mastered and correctly used in TCM health preservation and rehabilitation.

In scalp acupuncture therapy, the stimulation area opposite to the diseased limb is mostly selected for the disease of the unilateral limb in the stimulation area selection; the bilateral stimulation areas are selected for diseases of bilateral limbs; the bilateral stimulation areas are selected for visceral diseases, and diseases of which the right and left cannot be easily differentiated. In addition, other stimulation areas may be cooperatively selected in accordance with the accompanying symptoms besides the selection of the stimulation area corresponding to the disease. For example, the foot motor sensory area may be cooperatively selected for paralysis of lower limbs besides the selection of the motor area of lower limbs. Quick speed and a wide range are advisable to twirl the needle in scalp acupuncture (200 times / min). When twirling and retaining the needle, let or help the patient move the limbs and enhance training. This helps to improve the therapeutic effects.

Scalp acupuncture therapy is applicable to the rehabilitation of cerebrogenic diseases such as hemiplegia, aphasia, facial distortion, tinnitus, numbness, vertigo and cholera; it also has better therapeutic effects on the treatment of cardiovascular diseases, and diseases of digestive system as well as many types of neuralgia and enuresis. The head with hair is susceptible to infection, and accordingly strict sterilization should be done during scalp acupuncture therapy. The therapy is not advisable for the patients with apoplexy; it is not applicable to the patients with accompanying high fever and heart failure, either. In addition, the stimulation of scalp acupuncture is more severe, so needling fainting should be particularly prevented. The scalp with rich blood vessels is subject to hemorrhage. When withdrawing the needle, press the punctured site with the cotton ball.

Section 2   Chinese Acupuncture

Though relatively new to the west, acupuncture and moxibustion is a highly developed medical science in China, which is the important component of traditional Chinese medicine (TCM), and a summary of experience of ordinary Chinese people in the struggle against disease over thousands of years. As the valuable contributions to medicine, acupuncture and moxibustion is the focus of people's attention from all parts of the world. These techniques are characterized by their amazingly rapid attainment of the desired results, their wide indications, simple equipment, and easy manipulation. They have therefore been widely accepted by the general population. According to incomplete statistics analysis, more than 120 countries and regions across the world have their own acupuncture and moxibustion doctors. A great upsurge in the application and study of acupuncture and moxibustion is now in the ascendant all over the world. Acupuncture and moxibustion have become an essential component of world medicine, providing a great service for human health and playing an increasingly important role in the world. They will become one of the methods for the effective prevention and treatment of disease in support of "health and care for all by the year 2000" statement put forward by the WHO. Even so, a lot of people are still not familiar with acupuncture and moxibustion. They may have questions, even doubts or negations. Therefore, this study aims to introduce some popular knowledge regarding acupuncture and moxibustion, and hopes that it will help people to understand further these therapies and their benefits.

What is acupuncture? The term acupuncture is derived from the Latin words acus, which means needle, and puncture, which means to puncture. Acu plus puncture is acupuncture, which means needling.

What is acupuncture therapy? The acupuncture therapy is a therapeutic method which prevents or treats diseases by applying needles to stimulate certain superficial parts of body.

What is moxibustion? Moxibustion means the use of a moxa as a cautery by igniting it on the skin. Moxa, a soft woolly mass prepared from the young leaves of various wormwoods of eastern Asia and applied especially in Chinese and Japanese popular medicine as a cautery by being ignited on the skin; any of various substances applied and ignited like moxa as a counterirritant.

What is moxibustion therapy? The moxibustion therapy is a therapeutic method which applies heat produced by ignited moxa wool or roll over the skin surface to stimulate certain points of body for the prevention or treatment of disease.

Why do we often call acu-moxibustion? Acupuncture and moxibustion are general names for acupuncture therapy and moxibustion therapy. The two therapies are commonly applied in combination. They have the same therapeutic theory and use the same stimulating points, though the equipment and materials used in the two methods are different. Therefore, together they are called acu-moxibustion, zhenjiu in Chinese, which literally means needling-moxibustion. For convenience of calling, the acupuncture and moxibustion are often termed as acu-moxibustion.

What is a broad sense and narrow sense of acu-moxibustion? Acu-moxibustion in a broad sense includes many techniques for stimulating points on the body using various physical or chemical methods, the application of various needles or stimulating instruments, and needling on various part of body according to TCM theory. Of the needling methods, the filiform needle is the most common. In the narrow sense, however, acu-moxibustion refers mainly to body-needling-moxibustion.

What is basis of scientific definition of acu-moxibustion? Acupuncture and moxibustion is a summary of experience by ordinary Chinese people in the struggle against disease over thousands of years, which are important components of TCM. Nowadays, acu-moxibustion is a highly developed medical science in China. Following the modern science development in the world, acu-moxibustion has rapidly established its own modern science system in China as well as in the world. Based on the clinic practice and experimental research, they have been greatly developed and have their own systematic theories, independent practice, systematic education, broad scientific researches, specific books and magazines, independent academic organizations and scientific meetings, numerous varied specific teams and specialists or experts, etc.. Therefore, they are not only stayed on therapy or therapeutic method stage, but also are independent scientific discipline, which is called science of acu-moxibustion. For the sake of shortness and standardization, the term has been suggested as acupunctology (i.e., acupuncture plus -ology).

What is the content of acupunctology? Acupunctology belongs to a branch of TCM which has very extensive and substantial contents. The contents of acupunctology include three aspects：(1) The basic theories of acu-moxibustion. Because acupunctology is a branch of TCM, the basic theories of acu-moxibustion are the same as basic theories of TCM mentioned above. (2) The techniques of acu-moxibustion. Acu-moxibustion in a broad sense includes many techniques such as stimulation of points with various physical or chemical methods, or application of various needles or stimulating instrument, or needling on various part of the body according to different TCM theories. (3) The treatment of acu-moxibustion. It includes the general principles and methods of treatment, basic principles for prescription and selection of points. It also includes applying basic theory of acu-moxibustion to differentiate, analyze and diagnose diseases or disorders of the body, and treat them with the therapies of acu-moxibustion.

With the development of the acupunctology, many secondary branches have been derived from this general acupunctology, such as medical history of acupunctology, doctrines of various historical schools in acupunctology, literature of acupunctology, science of meridian and collateral, science of acupuncture points, diagnostics based on meridians and points, technology of needling and moxibustion, formulas of acu-moxibustion, therapeutics of acu-moxibustion, acupuncture anesthesiology, science of experimental acu-moxibustion, science of acu-moxibustion in micro-systems, acupuncture psychology, etc., and all of them still belong to the category of broad sense of acupunctology.

How did acu-moxibustion originate? The initiation of the acu-moxibustion has undergone a long historical process. As early as the Stone Age, in primitive society before metallurgy was known, acupuncture was administered with needles fashioned from pieces of sharp stone. This is known as Bian which is a rudiment of acupuncture. According to *Shuowen Jiezi* (a dictionary of characters), compiled during the Han dynasty (206 BC ~ 220 AD), Bian means the curing of diseases by pricking with a stone. A cure was affected by pressing or pricking a certain section of the body. As social production developed, Bian was replaced first by needles made of stone, bone or bamboo. When human society entered the Bronze and then the Iron Age, as metals were discovered, needles were made of copper, iron or silver. With the development of social productive technique, needling instruments were constantly improved which provided conditions for the further refinement of acupuncture. Today, acupuncture is done with fine needles of stainless steel. From the study of unearthed artifacts we can assess that Bian was initiated at the end of the New Stone Age (the Neolithic Age), and metallic needles might have been initiated in the Xia dynasty (21st ~ 16th century BC) or the Shang dynasty (16th ~ 11th century BC). Moxibustion originated after the introduction of fire into man's life. It is assumed that while warming themselves by the fire, ancient people accidentally found relief or disappearance of certain pain or illness when definite areas of the skin were subjected to burning. Moxa leaves were later chosen as the material for cauterization as they are easily lit, and the heat produced is mild and effective in removing obstruction of meridians and collaterals. Thus the moxibustion was established. According to the research of archaeology, the Peking Men applied fire 500 thousand years ago. Recently, it has been reported by two archaeologists of South Africa that humans utilized fire as early as 1.2 million years ago. The moxibustion should be initiated after that when man invented utilization of fire. It should be initiated at least before the Spring-Autumn Period (700 BC ~ 476 BC) or the Warring States (475 BC ~ 221 BC) according to some literature of this period which mentioned moxibustion or moxa.

In the early 1980s, *Outline of Chinese Acupuncture & Moxibustion* was published by the Foreign Languages Press. This was the first English language exposition of contemporary

Chinese acupuncture as taught and practiced in the People's Republic of China，and，for many of us, it was the first introduction with what has come to be known (rightly or wrongly) as TCM. For many of us struggling to reconcile a blend of disparate theories and practices, TCM was a revelation. Here was a complete, self-consistent system of Chinese medicine laid out in a very logical, methodological way. In short order, this book gave way to the new and improved essentials of Chinese acupuncture & moxibustion which eventually gave way to the even better Chinese acupuncture & moxibustion, commonly known by students as CAM. Most of the schools which sprang up in the early and mid-80s based their curriculum on TCM and used these books as their main acupuncture texts. Following suit, the State of California and the NCCAOM also based their acupuncture exams mostly on these books for many years.

However, at the same time as many American schools and practitioners adopted TCM and its contemporary Chinese acupuncture as their standards, there were also a number of critics of this style. Probably the earliest and most vociferous of these critics were the Worsleyan five element practitioners. These were some of the very first non-Asian practitioners of acupuncture in England and North America. According to their teachers, TCM acupuncture was symptomatic, eight principle acupuncture. It was not the real, kingly, orally transmitted acupuncture. It only treated the body, not the spirit, and even then, it didn't treat the root, the Worsleyans' causitive factor (CF).

Eventually, in the mid 1990s, all these various criticisms of TCM acupuncture gained currency or critical mass within the profession. It became harder and harder to sell books and classes on standard Chinese acupuncture, while classes on Japanese acupuncture became more and more popular, with Japanese-style needles eventually displacing Chinese-style needles from the marketplace. Japanese-style acupuncturists are among some of the most popular teachers on the postgraduate circuit. The only Chinese acupuncture teachers to hold on to national followings are those who teach non-TCM styles. To some extent, these criticisms have become the "conventional wisdom" within our profession.

According to many students, their Chinese teachers' acupuncture is not very good because these teachers only use the "same-old same-old" points on each and every patient, such as hegu (LI4), quchi (LI11), zusanli (St36), etc.. According to these students' point of view, it would seem that really great acupuncture should use esoteric, little known points — especially points with the word spirit in their names — and arcane point selection methods based on Taoist mysticism.

In Chinese, there is a saying that young practitioners use many formulas and old practitioners use only a few. In fact, there are many famous old Chinese doctors who treated most of their patients with only a single formula. This is because, as one gains more and more clinical experience, one comes to understand that there are only a handful of key Chinese medical disease mechanisms at work in the majority of chronic conditions. If one understands these key, core disease mechanisms and how to reliably spot them in a host of seemingly different patients, then one only needs to use the same core or key treatment principles over and over again in slightly varying combinations. Further, over 2000 years of recorded clinical experience, Chinese doctors have winnowed through all the potential acupoints on the body to identify those that are the most therapeutically reliable. The most famous acupoints of Chinese acupuncture, the ones even the rankest beginner knows, are the most famous because they are the ones that time has shown work the best and the most dependable. To look for other, lesser known points in the hope of finding ones that hundreds of generations of Chinese doctors before have overlooked or failed to find is arrogance of the first order and possibly even racism. If Chinese acupuncturists use the same points over and over again, it is because, in real life, patients present the same patterns over and over again (albeit in different combinations), and those acupuncturists choose to treat these same patterns with the points that are empirically most reliable to treat them. This is not simplistic treatment; it is the highest level of masterly simplicity.

Section 3　Research Article

Investigation on correlation between metabolic syndrome and constitution types in senior military ex-service personnel of the People's Liberation Army

[Abstract] This research had investigated the incidence of metabolic syndrome (MS) and the distribution of constitutional pattern in elderly ex-service personnel of the People's Liberation Army. Adopting the method of cross-sectional field investigation, from June to December in 2008, the investigation questionnaires were completed by the retired cadres over 60 and collected from 69 military cadre sanatoriums in the four cities of Shanghai, Nanjing, Hangzhou and Qingdao. Other data, including demographic characteristics, physiological characteristics, life style and former medical history were collected and analyzed by the tests on biochemical indexes. The database for statistical analysis was drawn up by the software Epidata 3.0. A total of 4502 elderly ex-service personnel were included in this study and 35.3% of them were diagnosis with MS. There was no obvious difference in morbidity among ages (60 ~ 69, 70 ~ 79 and over 80, $P > 0.05$). Referring to the MS patients in the 70s age group, both the phlegm-dampness and damp-heat constitutional types are evidently higher than those in 60s age group ($P < 0.01$, $P < 0.01$); while MS patients in 80s and older showed a significantly lower incidence of dampness-heat consitition than in the 60s ($P = 0.00$) and qi-deficiency constitution was obviously higher in the 80s age group than in the other two groups ($P = 0.00$). The top 3 constitutions occurring in MS people were, respectively, phlegm-dampness, dampness-heat and qi-deficiency constitution; while in non-MS people, the top 3 constitutions were gentleness, qi-deficiency and phlegm-dampness. When the patient's body mass index was more than 25 kg/m², the rate of phlegm-dampness and dampness-heat constitution significantly increased, while the rate of qi-deficiency constitution declined, the discrepancy was significant ($P = 0.00$). The prevalence rate of MS in military senior people is 35.5%, which does not vary between the three age groups. Phlegm-dampness, dampness-heat and qi-deficiency constitution are the three modal constitutional types seen in MS patients. The distribution of constitution formation is different in MS people and non-MS people. For different dimensions of BMI, the proportion of each kind of constitutions is varied.

Keywords: aged; metabolism syndrome; body constitution; clinical trial; cross-sectional studies

1 Introduction

The term metabolic syndrome dates back to at least the late 1950s, but came into common usage in the late 1970s to describe various associations of risk factors with diabetes that had been noted as early as the 1920s. The Marseilles physician Dr. Jean Vague, in 1947, observed that upper body obesity appeared to predispose to diabetes, atherosclerosis, gout and calculi. Avogadro, Crepaldi and coworkers described six moderately obese patients with diabetes, hypercholesterolemia, and marked hypertriglyceridemia, all of which improved when the patients were put on a hypocaloric, low-carbohydrate diet. In 1977, Haller used the term metabolic syndrome for associations of obesity, diabetes mellitus, hyperlipoproteinemia, hyperuricemia, and hepatic steatosis when describing the additive effects of risk factors on atherosclerosis. The same year, Singer used the term for associations of obesity, gout, diabetes mellitus, and hypertension with hyperlipoproteinemia. In 1977 and 1978, Gerald B. Phillips developed the concept that risk factors for myocardial infarction concur to form a constellation of abnormalities (i.e., glucose intolerance, hyperinsulinemia, hypercholesterolemia, hypertriglyceridemia, and hypertension) associated not only with heart disease, but also with aging, obesity and other clinical states. He suggested there must be an underlying linking factor, the identification of which could lead to the prevention of cardiovascular disease; he hypothesized that this factor was sex hormones. In 1988, in his Banting lecture, Reaven proposed insulin resistance as the underlying factor and named the constellation of abnormalities syndrome. Reaven did not include abdominal obesity, which has also been hypothesized as the underlying factor, as part of the condition.

Metabolic Syndrome (MS) is a cluster of metabolic disorders for which the central link is insulin resistance (IR). A broad range of epidemiological investigations indicate that MS is highly related to the occurrence of diabetes, cardiovascular disease and nephrosis[1-2], and it significantly increases the risk of death in cardiovascular disease[3]. Therefore, MS has become one of the biggest hidden dangers which threatens the life and well-being of the elderly. Senior military ex-service personnel are a special group among the elderly. They worked extremely hard in their early life while enjoying superior living conditions in their later years, which may result in the even higher rate of MS incidence. Most MS patients are not definitively diagnosed, leading to challenges in Western medicine when adopting effective measure to prevent the condition. However, the constitution is a relatively stable variable in the life process, and constitutes a key element which can determine and influence the occurrence, development and variation of disease. Therefore, understanding the correlation between constitution and MS in order to deliver constitutionally based care may have a significant effect on MS prophylaxis and treatment. In China, there have already been extensive investigations and reports on MS[4-5], but there rarely has been data on the correlation between the prevalence and constitution in 4502 senior ex-service personnel; the results are reported as follows.

2　Materials and methods

2.1　Investigation subjects

The investigation subjects were retired cadres who were over 60 years old and from 69 military cadre sanatoriums in the four cities of Shanghai, Nanjing, Hangzhou and Qingdao. The following circumstances resulted in exclusion: (1) those with mental disease or behavioral disorders; (2) those whose condition is too severe to express thoughts correctly; (3) those without informed consent. From June to December in 2008, total of 4502 valid paper was collected, which had reached 92% of the total population of the senior ex-service personnel above 60 from the 69 retired cadre sanatoriums. Among them, 3789 were male and 713 were female. Between the ages of 60 and 69, there were 352 subjects; from 70 to 79, there were 2294; above the age of 80, there were 1856 people; and the average age was (77.0 ± 6.8) years.

2.2　Investigation methods

Diagnostic criteria of MS: The Chinese Diabetes Society of Chinese Medical Association issued MS diagnostic criteria in 2004[6] which includes 4 terms. Those who meet at least 3 of these criteria can be confirmed as a MS patient. (1) Overweight and/or obese, with a body mass index (BMI) $\geqslant$ 25.0 kg/m^2; (2) Hyperglycemia: fasting blood glucose $\geqslant$ 6.1 mmol/L, and/or 2 hours after meal blood glucose $\geqslant$ 7.8 mmol/L, and/or confirmed and treated as diabetes; (3) Hypertension: systolic pressure $\geqslant$ 140 mmHg and/or diastolic pressure $\geqslant$ 90 mmHg, and confirmed and treated for hypertension; (4) Dyslipidemia: triacylglycerol (TAG) $\leqslant$ 1.7 mmol/L, and/or fasting high density lipoprotein cholesterol (HDL-C) $<$ 0.9 mmol/L (male) or $<$ 1.0 mmol/L (female).

Classification of traditional Chinese medicine constitution: According to the *Constitution in Chinese Medicine Questionnaire*[7-8] compiled by Wang Qi and evaluated by *Classification and Determination of Constitution in TCM*[9] which is issued by Chinese Medical Association, there are 9 types of constitution: gentleness, qi-deficiency, yang-deficiency, yin-deficiency, phlegm-dampness, dampness-heat, blood-stasis, qi-depression, and a special constitution.

2.3   Data collection

Adopting a cross-sectional investigation method, and based on the subject's informed consent, the qualified investigator conducted field investigation by using questionnaires. The investigation content included 6 aspects: (1) general demographic characteristics; (2) physiological characteristics, such as body height, body weight, blood pressure and pulse, etc.; (3) living habits, including diet, smoking, alcohol consumption and exercise, etc.; (4) medical history and family history, referring to some content of the *Cadre Health Examination Booklet* edited by Ministry of Public Health; (5) biochemical parameters, including liver function, fasting blood glucose, TAG, total cholesterol, HDL-C and low-density lipoprotein cholesterol (LDL-C), etc., measured by the oxide method (the reagents were provided by Shanghai Kehua Dongling Diagnosis Products Co., Ltd. and the testing instruments — automatic biochemical analyzer Wlcyon-300 produced by France Biochem Co. Ltd.); (6) constitutional types of traditional Chinese medicine. Initially, the respondents filled out their part of the questionnaire and then the investigator completed the interviewing section, which including four diagnostic methods of TCM, symptom diagnosis and health status judgment.

2.4   Quality control

During the execution of the field investigation process, professional staff were engaged in quality control. Concrete procedures were established for the concept and judgment standards in investigation contents and targets. The database was developed using Epi-Data 3.0 software and data were double entered, compared to correct information and checked automatically. 10% of the subjects were randomly picked for repeating investigation, and the data qualified only when its coincidence rate was more than 85%. Recalling bias was controlled by checking additional medical document records and relevant examination data. The investigator objectively collected data, questioned in details, so as to avoid and reduce subjective questioning bias. To control subjects' bias, the investigator routinely made inquiries of the subjects and data were checked by his/her spouse, when necessary it was supplemented and checked by neighbors and then verified and proofread by doctors in cadre sanatoriums. Finally the investigator checked and signed all data.

2.5   Statistical analysis

Data inputting adopted the SPSS 13.0 software. Continuous variables meeting normal distribution were represented as mean ± SD, and a *t*-test was used to compare the differences of two groups; the comparison of proportion used a χ^2 test; and ordered grouped data was analyzed by the linear trend test.

3   Results

3.1   MS prevalence in senior ex-service personnel

Of the 4502 respondents, 1589 respondents met the MS diagnosis standard, which constituted 35.3% of the total proportion. The MS prevalence rate of the ex-service personnel aged 60 ~ 69 was 33.8% (119/352); the rate of those aged 70 ~ 79 was 37.0% (849/2294); and the rate of those who were 80 and above was 33.5% (621/1856). Statistical analysis demonstrated that the comparative discrepancy in MS prevalence rate of the three different age groups had no statistical significance ($P > 0.05$).

3.2   Comparison of constitutions between MS patients and non-MS patients in elderly ex-service personnel

Among the MS group, the top three constitutions were phlegm-dampness (53.8%), qi-deficiency (16.5%) and dampness-heat (16.2%) respectively; in the non-MS group, the top three constitutions were gentleness (34.6%), qi-deficiency (14.8%) and phlegm-dampness (10.4%). According to the statistical analysis, there were differences in constitution type distribution in the two groups ($P < 0.05$, Table 8-1).

Table 8-1   Constitutional types of MS or non-MS in elderly ex-service personnel of the People's Liberation Army

Constitutional types	Metabolic syndrome (MS)		Non-metabolic syndrome(non-MS)	
	n	Percentage / %	n	Percentage / %
Gentleness	79	5.1	1008	34.6
Qi-deficiency	262	16.5	431	14.8
Yang-deficiency	89	5.6	298	10.2
Yin-deficiency	11	0.7	65	2.2
Phlegm-dampness	855	53.8	302	10.4
Dampness-heat	258	16.2	262	9.0
Blood-stasis	12	0.7	274	9.4
Qi-depression	21	1.3	256	8.8
Special diathesis	2	0.1	17	0.6
Total	1589	100	2913	100

3.3　Correlation between MS prevalence features and constitutions

The results illustrated that the constitutions of phlegm-dampness, dampness-heat and qi-deficiency accounted for the main constitution types in MS patients in different age groups. In the age group of 70 ~ 79, 56.8% of MS patients presented with a phlegm-dampness constitution, which was evidently higher than 45.4% in the 60 ~ 69 group ($P < 0.01$); in the age group over 80, the phlegm-dampness constitution reached 51.4%, which has no statistical significance in comparison to the other two groups. In the MS group of ages 70 ~ 79, the dampness-heat constitution reached 17.4%, which in the over 80 group was only 12.9%, but both of these two rated lower than that of ages 60 ~ 69, which was 25.2% ($P < 0.01$, $P = 0.00$); the qi-deficiency constitution trended to be more evident with the increase of age; the occurrence of this constitution in the over 80 group was 22.4%, which was obviously higher than that of the other groups ($P = 0.00$).

According to the grouping by BMI status, a qi-deficient constitution showed the most statistical significance (38.1%) and was most prevalent in elderly MS people with a BMI less than 18; following this were phlegm-dampness constitution (20.6%), gentleness constitution (16.1%) and dampness-heat constitution (11.6%). When the BMI was more than 25 kg/m^2, the phlegm-dampness constitution in MS prevalence reached 57.9%, the dampness-heat constitution was 19.3%, while the qi-deficient constitution reduced to 13.6%, simultaneously, and the incidence of gentleness and qi-deficient constitutions were significantly lower. Compared with the data from those with a BMI less than 18 kg/m^2, the conditional differences in the above had statistical significance ($P = 0.00$). Compared with the BMI less than 18 kg/m^2 group, the prevalence of phlegm-dampness in BMI 18 ~ 25 kg/m^2 evidently increased (56%), while the occurrence of qi-deficiency gradually reduced (15.6%); this difference also has statistical significance (Table 8-2).

Table 8-2　Relationships between constitutional types and ages and BMI in elderly ex-service personnel of the People's Liberation Army with MS

Unit: n (%)

Constitutional types	Distribution according to age			Distribution according to BMI		
	60 ~ 69 years	70 ~ 79 years	≥ 80 years	<18 kg/m^2	18 ~ 25 kg/m^2	>25 kg/m^2
Gentleness	10 (8.4)	38 (4.5)	31 (5.0)	25 (16.1)	38 (9.7)	16 (1.5) [△]
Qi-deficiency	12 (10.1)	111 (13.1)	139 (22.4)[*]	59 (38.1)	61 (15.6) [△]	142 (13.6) [△]
Yang-deficiency	8 (6.7)	47 (5.5)	34 (5.5)	9 (5.8)	18 (4.6)	62 (5.9)
Yin-deficiency	1 (0.8)	6 (0.7)	4 (0.6)	5 (3.2)	4 (1.0)	2 (0.2) [△]

Constitutional types	Distribution according to age			Distribution according to BMI		
	60 ~ 69 years	70 ~ 79 years	≥ 80 years	<18 kg/m²	18 ~ 25 kg/m²	>25 kg/m²
Phlegm-dampness	54 (45.3)	482 (56.8)*	319 (51.4)	32 (20.6)	219 (56) △	604 (57.9) △
Dampness-heat	30 (25.2)	148 (17.4)*	80 (12.9)*	18 (11.6)	39 (10)	201 (19.3) △
Blood-stasis	2 (1.7)	5 (0.6)	5 (0.8)	2 (1.3)	2 (0.5)	8 (0.8)
Qi-depression	2 (1.7)	11 (1.3)	8 (1.3)	4 (2.6)	10 (1)	7 (0.7)
Special diathesis	0(0)	1 (0.1)	1 (0.2)	1 (0.6)	0 (0)	1 (0.0)

*$P < 0.05$ vs aged from 60 to 69; △ $P < 0.05$ vs BMI < 18. Data were analyzed by Linear-by-Linear Association. BMI: body mass index; MS: metabolic syndrome.

4   Discussions

Metabolic syndrome, sometimes known by other names, is a clustering of at least three of the five following medical conditions: abdominal obesity, high blood pressure, high blood sugar, high serum triglycerides and low high-density lipoprotein (HDL) levels. Metabolic syndrome is associated with the risk of developing cardiovascular disease and type 2 diabetes. In the US about a quarter of the adult population has metabolic syndrome, and the prevalence increases with age, with racial and ethnic minorities being particularly affected. Insulin resistance, metabolic syndrome and prediabetes are closely related to one another and have overlapping aspects. The syndrome is thought to be caused by an underlying disorder of energy utilization and storage. The cause of the syndrome is an area of ongoing medical research.

It is common for there to be a development of visceral fat, after which the adipocytes (fat cells) of the visceral fat increase plasma levels of TNFα and alter levels of a number of other substances (e.g., adiponectin, resistin, and PAI-1). Tumor necrotic factor α (TNFα) has been shown not only to cause the production of inflammatory cytokines, but also possibly to trigger cell signaling by interaction with a TNFα receptor that may lead to insulin resistance[10]. An experiment with rats fed a diet with 33% sucrose has been proposed as a model for the development of metabolic syndrome. The sucrose first elevated blood levels of triglycerides, which induced visceral fat and ultimately resulted in insulin resistance. The progression from visceral fat to increased TNFα to insulin resistance has some parallels to human development of metabolic syndrome. The increase in adipose tissue also increases the number of immune cells present within, which plays a role in inflammation. Chronic inflammation contributes to an increased risk of hypertension, atherosclerosis and diabetes[11].

The involvement of the endocannabinoid system in the development of metabolic syndrome is indisputable[12-14]. Endocannabinoid overproduction may induce reward system dysfunction[13] and cause executive dysfunctions (e.g., impaired delay discounting), in turn perpetuating unhealthy behaviors. The brain is crucial in development of metabolic syndrome, modulating peripheral carbohydrate and lipid metabolism[12-13].

The metabolic syndrome can be induced by overfeeding with sugar or fructose, particularly concomitantly with high-fat diet[15]. The resulting oversupply of omega-6 fatty acids, particularly arachidonic acid (AA), is an important factor in the pathogenesis of metabolic syndrome. Arachidonic acid (with its precursor — linoleic acid) serve as a substrate to the production of inflammatory mediators known as eicosanoids, whereas the arachidonic acid-containing compound diacylglycerol (DAG) is a precursor to the endocannabinoid 2-arachidonoylglycerol (2-AG) while fatty acid amide hydrolase (FAAH) mediates the metabolism of anandamide into arachidonic acid[16]. Anandamide can also be produced from N-acyl-phosphatidylethanolamine via several pathways. Anandamide and 2-AG can also be hydrolized into arachidonic acid, potentially leading to increased eicosanoid synthesis.

Metabolic syndrome is a risk factor for neurological disorders[17]. Metabolomic studies suggest an excess of organic acids, impaired lipid oxidation by products, essential fatty acids and essential amino acids in the blood serum of affected patients. However, it is not entirely clear whether the accumulation of essential fatty acids and amino acids is the result of excessive ingestion or excess production by gut microbiota.

The first line treatment is change of lifestyle (e.g., Dietary Guidelines for Americans and physical activity). However, if in three to six months of efforts at remedying risk factors prove insufficient, then drug treatment is frequently required. Generally, the individual disorders that compose the metabolic syndrome are treated separately. Diuretics and ACE inhibitors may be used to treat hypertension. Cholesterol drugs may be used to lower LDL cholesterol and triglyceride levels if they are elevated, and to raise HDL levels if they are low. Use of drugs that decrease insulin resistance, e.g., metformin and thiazolidinediones, is controversial; this treatment is not approved by the US Food and Drug Administration. Weight loss medications may result in weight loss[18]. As obesity is often recognized as the culprit behind many of the additional symptoms, with weight loss and lifestyle changes in diet, physical activity, the need for other medications may diminish.

MS is a cluster of conditions including obesity, hypertension, hyperglycemia, blood lipid abnormality and insulin resistance. In the formation of factors related to MS, apparently obesity is the original element which leads to the disorders of blood pressure, blood glucose and blood lipid. It has been demonstrated[10] by contemporary research that, in China, the incidence of stroke reduces to 15% in males and 22% in females if the BMI is reduced to 24.0 kg/m^2. Therefore, besides the investigation based on the correlation between MS and the constitutional types, this research also discussed, in particular, the correlation between BMI and the constitution.

The investigation results illustrate that among 4502 military retired cadres who were above the age of 60, the MS incidence rate was 35.3%. Gu et al.[11] selected 15 540 individuals from the age 35 to 74 in a nationwide study to conduct a cross-sectional investigation, and indicated that the MS prevalence rate of Chinese adults was 16.5%, clearly lower than that seen in elderly ex-service personnel. The reduction of the incidence of MS would play a significant role in decreasing the danger of cardio-cerebrovascular disease and improving the overall quality of life. The constitution is the common soil of many kinds of disease and different constitutions carry specific predispositions to disease occurrence. By evaluating the constitution of MS patients, individual measures particular to each patient to prevent the occurrence of MS can be adopted. This not only embodies the ideology of preventive treatment of disease central to Chinese medicine, but also prevents MS at its source, and furthermore remedies the shortcomings in Western medicine for effective systematical preventive measures on MS.

The investigation also indicated that the phlegm-dampness constitution was the main type among the different ages, and was obviously predominant in the group of BMI > 18 kg/m^2. This relates to and supports some Chinese medical theories for instance, if the diet is too fatty, sweet or rich it will harm the spleen and stomach, as well as weakening the vessels so that it can breed dampness and heat, brew phlegm, and combine them within the body. In clinical epidemiological investigation, it also indicated that there are certain correlations between phlegm-dampness constitution and obesity, diabetes, coronary heart disease and cardio-cerebrovascular disease, which constitute the main perspectives of MS. This demonstrates that clinic practice should pay more attention to adopting methods of removing phlegm and dampness to adjust constitution, and to prevent MS.

In MS patients with BMI < 18 kg/m^2 and over the age of 80, qi-deficiency constitution is evidently higher, because most people in this group have debilitating conditions, such as loss in vital energy, or deficiency in qi and blood. The method of conditioning the constitution in this circumstance is mainly by invigorating qi, nourishing blood, and strengthening and consolidating the body's resistance. The dampness-heat constitution was more prevalent in the MS group between the ages of 60 ~ 69 and BMI > 25 kg/m^2, and its constitutional adjustment mainly requires clearing heat and removing dampness, and additionally on eliminating phlegm and turbid liquid.

This investigation is based on the cross-sectional method; it is, therefore, hard to estimate the morbidity, leading to a limit on causal reasoning. Moreover, in senior ex-service personnel, the male population is larger than that of the female; therefore it may contain certain bias compared with other elderly groups. However, this investigation focuses on ex-service personnel — a specific group as the objective, and discovers a MS incidence rate much higher than a normal social cross section; furthermore, the high incidence is somehow related to constitution. This indicates significant clinic materials under the guidance of Chinese medical theories, and illustrates the possibility of adjusting the constitution in order to prevent the special group from MS. Furthermore, it also lays a solid foundation for further in-depth study in this field.

References

[1]   Executive summary of the third report of the National Cholesterol Education Program (NCEP) expert panel on detection. Evaluation, and treatment of high blood cholesterol in adults (Adult Treatment Panel Ⅲ). JAMA. 2001, 285(19): 2486-2497.

[2]   Isomaa B, Almgren P, Tuomi T, et al. Cardiovascular morbidity and mortality associated with the metabolic syndrome. Diabetes Care. 2001, 24(4): 683-689.

[3]   Trevisan M, Liu J, Bahsas F B, et al. Syndrome X and mortality: a population-based study. Am J Epidemiol. 1998, 148(10): 958-966.

[4]   Wu G X, Wu Z S, Liu J, et al. A study on the incidence of cardiovascular disease on the metabolic syndrome in 11 provinces in China. Zhonghua Liu Xing Bing Xue Za Zhi. 2003, 24(7): 551-553.

[5]   Gu D, Reynolds K, Wu X, et al. Prevalence of the metabolic syndrome and overweight among adults in China. Lancet, 2005, 365(9468): 1398-1405.

[6]   Wang Q, Zhu Y B, Xue H S, et al. Primary compiling of Constitution in Chinese Medicine Questionnaire. Chinese Journal of Clinical Rehabilitation. 2006, 10(3): 12-14.

[7]   Zhu Y B, Wang Q, Xue H S, et al. Preliminary assessment on performance of Constitution in Chinese Medicine Questionnaire. Chinese Journal of Clinical Rehabilitation, 2006, 10(3): 15-17.

[8]   Gu D F, Reynolds K, Yang W J. The prevalence of metabolic syndrome in the general adult population aged 35-74 years in China. Chinese Journal of Diabetes, 2005, 13(3): 181-186.

[9]   Zhu Y B, Wang Q, Wu C Y, et al. Logistic regression analysis on relationships between traditional Chinese medicine constitutional types and overweight or obesity. Journal of Chinese Integrative Medicine, 2010, 8(11): 1023-1028.

[10]   Hotamisligil G S. The role of TNF alpha and TNF receptors in obesity and insulin resistance. J Inter Med. 1999, 245 (6): 621-625.

[11]   Whitney E N, Rolfes S R. Understanding Nutrition. Belmont, CA: Wadsworth Cengage Learning, 2011.

[12]   Blandine G C, Daniela C. Endocannabinoids and metabolic disorders. Handbook of Experimental Pharmacology, 2015, 231: 367-391.

[13]   Vemuri V K, Janero D R, Makriyannis A. Pharmacotherapeutic targeting of the endocannabinoid

signaling system: drugs for obesity and the metabolic syndrome. Physiol Beha, 2008, 93 (4-5): 671-686.

[14]   Turcotte C, Chouinard F, Lefebvre J S, et al. Regulation of inflammation by cannabinoids, the endocannabinoids 2-arachidonoyl-glycerol and arachidonoyl-ethanolamide, and their metabolites. J Leuk Biol, 2015, 97 (6): 1049-1070.

[15]   Fukuchi S, Hamaguchi K, Seike M, et al. Role of fatty acid composition in the development of metabolic disorders in sucrose-induced obese rats. Exp Biol Med, 2004, 229 (6): 486-493.

[16]   Di Marzo V, Fontana A, Cadas H. Formation and inactivation of endogenous cannabinoid anandamide in central neurons. Nature. 1994, 372 (6507): 686-691.

[17]   Farooqui A A, Farooqui T, Panza F, et al. Metabolic syndrome as a risk factor for neurological disorders. Cell Mol Life Sci, 2012, 69 (5): 741-762.

[18]   Garvey W T. Phentermine and topiramate extended-release: a new treatment for obesity and its role in a complications-centric approach to obesity medical management. Expert Opinion on Drug Safety, 2013, 12 (5): 741-756.

Section 4   Words of TCM

1. 水谷精微 food essence
2. 储藏精气 storing essence and qi
3. 藏而不泻 storing without eliminating
4. 泻而不藏 eliminating without storing
5. 喜湿恶燥 preference to dampness and aversion to dryness
6. 形体诸窍 build and orifices
7. 胃主受纳 the stomach controlling reception and digestion
8. 消食化滞 promoting digestion, resolving food to dispel food retention
9. 通调水道 dredging water passage
10. 活血化瘀 activating blood to remove blood stasis
11. 滋阴活血 nourishing yin and promoting blood stasis
12. 益气补血 invigorating qi to benefit blood
13. 软坚散结 softening hard lumps and dispelling the nodes
14. 固肾涩精 strengthening the kidney to astringe renal essence
15. 男子不育，女子不孕 infertility (in men), sterility (in women)
16. 七情内伤 internal injury caused by seven emotions
17. 怒则气上 rage causing qi to flow upwards
18. 喜则气缓 joy causing qi slack
19. 悲则气消 grief causing qi depression

20. 思则气结 contemplation causing qi stagnation

21. 惊则气乱 terror causing qi disorder

22. 恐则气下 fear causing qi collapse

23. 饮食不节 / 洁 improper diet / dirty diet

24. 饮食偏嗜 diet preference

25. 劳则气耗 over-strain causing qi exhaustion

26. 虚实错杂 mixture of asthenia and sthenia

27. 虚实转化 inter-transformation between asthenia and sthenia

28. 虚实真假 pseudo or true manifestation of asthenia and sthenia

29. 大实有羸状 excessive sthenia manifesting as excessive asthenia

30. 至虚有盛候 excessive asthenia manifesting as excessive sthenia

31. 正盛邪退 healthy qi expelling pathogen

32. 邪去正虚 pathogen retreating with asthenic healthy qi

33. 邪盛正虚 prosperous pathogen with asthenia healthy qi

34. 正邪相持 struggle between healthy qi and pathogen

35. 正虚邪恋 asthenic healthy qi with pathogen lingering

36. 满而不实 full of essence without foodstuff

37. 内邪 endopathogen; endoogenous factor causing diseases

38. 外邪 exopathogen; exogenous factor causing diseases

39. 外（表）邪入里 external pathogen invading interior

40. 内（里）邪出表 internal pathogen reaching exterior

(Liu Tianwei, Liu Yingjuan)

Chapter 9　Death

Section 1　When Death Is Approaching

In caring for a loved one who has advanced cancer you may be present at the time of death. The following is intended to help with some of the anxiety that surrounds the end of life by looking at the process of dying. This section lists some signs that death may be close. People often take advantage of this time to gather the family to say goodbye to their loved one. They may take turns with the patient, holding hands, talking to the patient, or just sitting quietly. It can also be a time to perform any traditional religious rituals and other activities surrounding death. It is a chance for many families and friends to express their love and appreciation for the patient and for each other.

It is important to have a plan for what to do after death, so that the family can know what to do during a very emotional time. If the patient is in hospice, the hospice nurse and social worker will help you. If the patient is not in hospice, talk with your doctor about it so that you will know what to do at the time of death.

Not all of the following symptoms will happen, but it may be comforting to know about them. Profound weakness, the patient is usually unable to get out of bed, and requires help with nearly everything he or she does. They are less and less interest in food, often with very little food and fluid intake. More drowsiness, the patient may doze or sleep much of the time. If pain is relieved, they may restless and pick or pull at bed linens, and hard to rouse or wake. Anxiety, fear, restlessness and loneliness may worsen at night. The patient cannot concentrate and has short attention span. The patient may be confusion about time, place, or people, have trouble swallowing pills and medicines, and have limited ability to cooperate with caregivers.

The possible changes in body function include: (1) Weakness, having trouble moving around in bed. (2) Unable to change positions without help. (3) Having trouble swallowing food, medicines, or even liquids. (4) Involuntary movement of any muscle, jerking of hands, arms, legs, or face.

For these conditions, the caregivers can: (1) Help the patient turn and change positions every hour or two. (2) Avoid sudden noises or movements to lessen the startle reflex. (3) Speak in a calm, quiet voice to reduce chances of startling the patient. (4) If the patient has trouble swallowing pain medicines, ask the doctor or hospice nurse about getting liquid pain medicines or pain patch. (5) If the patient is having trouble swallowing, avoid solid foods. Give ice chips or sips of liquid. (6) Do not push fluids. Near the end of life, some dehydration is normal, and is more comfortable for the patient. (7) Apply cool, moist wash cloths to head, face and body for comfort.

The possible changes in consciousness include: (1) More sleeping during the day. (2) Hard to wake or rouse from sleep. (3) Confusion about time, place, or people. (4) Restlessness; may pick or pull at bed linen. (5) May talk about things unrelated to the events or people present. (6) May have more anxiety, restlessness, fear, and loneliness at night. (7) After a period of sleepiness and confusion, may have a short time when he or she is mentally clear before lapsing back into semi-consciousness.

For these conditions, the caregivers can: (1) Plan your times with the patient when he or she is most alert or during the night when your presence may be comforting. (2) When talking with the patient, remind her or him who you are and what day and time it is. (3) Continue pain medicines up to the end of life. (4) If the patient is very restless, try to find out if he or she is having pain. If it appears so, give breakthrough pain medicines as prescribed, or check with the doctor or hospice nurse if needed. (5) When talking with a confused person, use calm, confident tones to reduce chances of startling or frightening the patient. (6) Touching, caressing, holding, and rocking are all appropriate and comforting.

The possible changes in metabolism include: (1) Lost interest in food, as needs for food and drink decrease. (2) Mouth may dry out. (3) May no longer need some of his or her medicines, such as vitamins, chemotherapy, replacement hormones, blood pressure medicines, and diuretics (unless they help make the patient more comfortable).

For these conditions, the caregivers can: (1) Apply lubricant or petroleum jelly (vaseline) to the lips to prevent drying. (2) Ice chips from a spoon, or sips of water or juice from a straw may be enough for the patient. (3) Check with the doctor to see which medicines may be stopped. Medicines for pain, nausea, fever, seizures or anxiety should be continued to keep the patient comfortable.

The possible changes in secretions include: (1) Mucus in the mouth may collect in the back of the throat (This may be a very distressing sound to hear, but doesn't usually cause discomfort to the patient). (2) Secretions may thicken and build up due to a lower fluid intake and inability to cough.

For these conditions, the caregivers can: (1) Keep them loose by adding humidity to the room with a cool mist humidifier if mouth secretions increase. (2) If the patient can swallow, ice chips or sips of liquid through a straw may thin secretions. (3) Change the patient's position, turning to the side may help secretions drain from the mouth. Continue to perform good mouth care with a soft toothbrush. (4) Certain medications may help. Ask the hospice or home-care nurse.

The possible changes in circulation and temperature include: (1) Arms and legs may feel cool to the touch as circulation decreases. (2) Skin of arms, legs, hands and feet may darken in color and appear mottled. (3) Other areas of the body may become either darker or pale. (4) Skin may feel cold and either dry or damp. (5) Heart rate may become fast, faint or irregular. (6) Blood pressure may get lower and become hard to hear.

For these conditions, the caregivers can: (1) Keep the patient warm with blankets or light bed coverings. (2) Avoid the use of electric blankets, heating pads, etc..

The possible changes in senses and perception include: (1) Vision may become blurry or dim. (2) Hearing may decrease, but most patients are able to hear you even after they can no longer speak.

For these conditions, the caregivers can: (1) Leave indirect lights on as vision decreases. (2) Never assume the patient cannot hear you. (3) Continue to speak with and touch the patient to reassure him or her of your presence. (4) Your words of endearment and support are likely to be understood and appreciated.

The possible changes in breathing include: (1) Breathing may speed up and slow down due to less blood circulation and build up of waste products in the body. (2) Rattling or gurgling with each breath may happen due to mucus in the back of the throat. (3) 10 ~ 30 seconds may occur with periods of no breathing.

For these conditions, the caregivers can: (1) Put the patient on his or her back, or slightly to one side. (2) Raising the patient's head may give some relief. (3) Use pillows to prop head and chest at an angle or raise the head of a hospital bed. (4) Any position that seems to make breathing easier is okay, including sitting up with good support. A small child may be more comfortable in your arms.

The possible changes in elimination include: (1) Urine may become darker and decrease in amount. (2) Loss of control (incontinence) of urine and stool may occur when death is near.

For these conditions, the caregivers can: (1) Pad bed beneath the patient with layers of disposable waterproof pads. (2) If the patient has a catheter, the home health nurse will teach you to care for it.

The signs that death has occurred include: Breathing stops, pulse stops, eyes stop moving, pupils of the eye stay large, even in the light, and the control of bowels or bladder is lost as the muscles relax. For the caregivers, it is okay to sit with your loved one for a while at this time. There is no rush to get anything done immediately. Many families find this is an important time to pray or talk together and reconfirm your love for each other as well as for the person who has passed away. If the patient dies in the home, caregivers are responsible for calling the proper people. Regulations concerning proper notifications and the removal of the body differ from one community to another, and the doctor or nurse can get this information for you. If you have a hospice or home-care agency involved, give them a call. If you have completed funeral arrangements, notifying the funeral director and doctor is necessary.

Preparing for approaching death: When a person enters the final stage of the dying process, two different dynamics are at work which are closely interrelated and interdependent. On the physical plane, the body begins the final process of shutting down, which will end when all the physical systems cease to function. Usually this is an orderly and undramatic progressive series of physical changes which are not medical emergencies requiring invasive interventions. These physical changes are a normal, natural way in which the body prepares itself to stop, and the most appropriate kinds of responses are comfort enhancing measures. The other dynamic of the dying process at work is on the emotional-spiritual-mental plane, and is a different kind of process. The spirit of the dying person begins the final process of release from the body, its immediate environment, and all attachments. This release also tends to follow its own priorities, which may include the resolution of whatever is unfinished of a practical nature and reception of permission to "let go" from family members. These events are the normal, natural way in which the spirit prepares to move from this existence. The most appropriate kinds of responses to the emotional-spiritual-mental changes are those which support and encourage this release and transition.

Section 2　XiaoChaiHu Tang

XiaoChaiHu Tang (XCHT) is also called Xiaochaihu Tang or Minor Bupleurum Decoction. It is a traditional Chinese medicine formula consisting of seven medicinal plants and has been used in the treatment of various diseases. In Japan, it is named as Shosaiko-to Decoction. Clinically, this formula has very extensive application. In addition to shaoyang syndrome, it can be applied by proper modifications to malaria, jaundice, wind attacking on woman after delivery or during menstruation or heat invading the blood-compartment due to cold-attack. Because bupleurum root has the properties of ascending and dispersing, this formula is not suitable to cases of hyperactivity of yang due to deficiency. In the United States of America (USA), traditional Chinese materia medica (TCMM, known as herbal medicine) is still officially considered as dietary supplement but not formal medicine. Therefore, no matter who and whether he or she is educated in traditional Chinese medicine (TCM) or not, including someone who was only educated modern medicine, can practice or prescribe herbal formula. Furthermore, the patients themselves can purchase herbal medicine in the herbs store without any restriction.

Ingredients and analysis of formula: This formula consists of Bupleurum root 12 g, Scutellaria root 9 g, Ginseng 6 g, Pinellia tuber 9 g, Roasted licorice 9 g, Fresh ginger 9 g, and Chinese date 4 pcs. It is a representative formula for harmonizing shaoyang. As the main herb, Bupleurum root clears heat from shaoyang and soothes the liver for relieving depression, so as to disperse the evil out from the half exterior. Scutellaria root acts as the assistant herb to clear away heat from the half interior of shaoyang. The cooperation of these two herbs plays role of exteri-or-expelling and interior-clearing so as to mediate shaoyang. Ginseng, Chinese date and Licorice root can invigorate qi and regulate the middle to expel evil and prevent its invasion by means of supporting the genuine-qi. Pinellia tuber and Fresh ginger can harmonize stomach to lower the rebellious qi; Fresh ginger and Chinese date can harmonize the nutrient and defensive qi as well as mediate cold and heat. They all act as the adjuvant herbs. Licorice root as the dispatcher herb harmonizes all components of the formula.

The application of TCMM must be performed or directed by a traditional Chinese medical doctor. If the herbal medicine does not fit the disease, not only can the disease not be cured, but may also have harmful side effect, and may even be fatal to the people. But in a ginseng store or herbal store, the customer probably purchased several packages of XCHT for treating hepatitis. The TCMM could be sold, bought and applied without prescription according to the policy of TCM in USA. Unless the TCMM policy in USA can be changed and the practice of TCM would be restricted in the people who are educated by TCM. Otherwise, it would be useless trying to make the people change their mind.

In March of 1996, the Ministry of Public Health in Japan released the information that because XCHT was used in the treatment of chronic hepatitis, 88 patients had suffered from interstitial pneumonia, and among them 10 patients died. Over 40 newspapers and televisions in Japan including Asahi Newspaper reported this information as the important news. Strong repercussions were evoked in countrywide of Japan. After this happened, some Japanese scholars wrote to Chinese experts to discuss this accident. They asked why XCHT could cause the patient death, and how to restrict the side effect of Chinese herbal medicine.

In fact, this accident was caused because the doctors who prescribed XCHT did not receive formal education and training in TCMM. Those people prescribed the herbal formula based on the advertisements and propaganda material. They did not follow the TCMM theories and methods to apply TCMM in the treatment. Hepatitis is a term of modern medicine and has several clinical types based on the patient constitution and the stage of hepatitis according to the theories and experience of TCM. If the clinical type of hepatitis is consistent with the indications of XCHT, it could have no such toxicity or side effect. Otherwise, it could cause a serious problem to the hepatitis patients. Moreover, the type of herbs, the procedure of preparing herbs and the compatibility of the herbal formula should also be taken into consideration. In short, TCM is an independent branch of human medicine and only can be applied by the doctor who has received formal education in TCM. It is just like that if someone has no modern medical knowledge, he or she should not prescribe western materia medica to the patients. Such monstrous absurdity somehow exists in the USA which has an advanced scientific level. In some areas of the USA, people including modern medical doctors who are not properly educated in TCM can legally practice herbal medicine and /or acupuncture, and TCM practitioner and /or acupuncturist can practice without the supervision of modern medical doctor. It is clear that no good result could be attained by doing this way. However, any negative results caused by this improper way are usually considered as the evidence to doubt the scientific sense of TCM.

This mismanagement of herbs in Japan will probably give a hope that Americans could draw a lesson from the death of patients caused by the abusive application of herbal formula XCHT. If they once didn't shed a tear until seeing the coffin, now it is the time to face the problem. There is no scientific sense that anyone can practice TCM and acupuncture in USA. Also, it is not right that a medical doctor who is not trained in TCM can apply TCM or supervise TCM practitioner and/or acupuncturist. TCM will be given a proper scientific evaluation and management in very soon future.

Renal protective effect of XCHT on diabetic nephropathy: Increasing prevalence of nephropathy and/or end-stage renal disease (ESRD) in diabetic patients is becoming a serious social and health problem worldwide. Hyperglycemia is considered as the main factor to induce diabetic nephropathy (DN), and clinical strategies for management of DN include glycemic control and blood pressure regulation. However, current therapeutic effect for DN remains unsatisfactory, thus resulting a year-by-year increase in the number of diabetic patients with nephropathy. Pathological changes of DN are characterized by structural abnormalities including renal-cell hypertrophy, increase in thickness of glomerular basement membranes, and progressive accumulation of extracellular matrix components.

Due to hyperglycemia, diabetes exhibits high oxidative stress which depletes the activity of antioxidative defense system and in turn promotes free radicals generation; thus, strategies to reduce oxidative stress in diabetes mellitus may exert favorable effects on the progression of diabetic glomerulosclerosis. Hyperglycemia and oxidative stress during DN induce abnormal production and stimulation of transformation growth factor-1 (TGF-1) resident renal cells. TGF-1 causes augmented deposition of extracellular matrix proteins, such as collagen IV and fibronectin, in the glomeruli, thus inducing mesangial expansion and glomerular basement membrane thickening. The renal protective protein, bone morphogenetic protein-7 (BMP-7), can reduce glomerular and tubulointerstitial fibrosis and prevent the pathogenesis in diabetic nephropathy. Expression or treatment with recombinant BMP-7 has been shown to improve renal damage from hyperglycemia-induced oxidative stress in the kidney of diabetic animals.

XCHT is a herbal drug formula widely used in traditional Chinese medicine and Japanese kampo medicine. XCHT consists of a mixture of seven different medicinal plants and has several experimentally proven pharmacological activities, including the prevention of experimental hepatotoxicity, immunomodulatory effect, antineoplastic activity and promotion of liver regeneration. XCHT has also been documented to decrease fibrogenic protein expression, including TGF-1 and collagen, to inhibit hepatic fibrosis.

The recent search for new antifibrotic drugs has refocused on herbal medicine. XCHT is widely prescribed to patients with liver cirrhosis for over a millennium in Asia, and the formula is established based on traditional clinical experience and practice. TGF-1 is involved in mediating the development of diabetic renal hypertrophy and is up-regulated in diabetic kidney. Hyperglycemia-induced up-regulation of TGF-1 stimulates mesangial cell proliferation and ECM induction (increased fibronectin and collagen production), which contributes to the major pathological changes observed in DN. Thus, TGF-1 has been considered as a therapeutic target in DN and other chronic kidney diseases. XCHT has been documented to inhibit hepatic expression of TGF-1 mRNA and protein in many experimental fibrogenic animal models.

Oxidative stress induced by hyperglycemia is implicated in the development of DN. ROS generated from high-glucose condition can stimulate a number of growth factors and cytokines, including TGF-1, and lead to excessive production and accumulation of ECM proteins. The vitro studies have shown that mesangial cells are the major source of free radicals after the exposure to high-glucose concentrations.

BMP-7 helps to maintain normal renal structure and physiological function, and its expression is decreased in damaged kidney. During the development of DN, hyperglycemia causes oxidative stress and leads to BMP-7 expression decrease in renal cells. Exogenous and overexpression of BMP-7 has been shown to improve renal function and prevent glomerular sclerosis in diabetic rats. The medicinal plant Angelica sinensis could also prevent STZ-diabetic rat from DN through increasing renal BMP-7 expression.

In conclusion, XCHT could prevent renal functions through augmenting BMP-7 expression and reducing ROS and ECM production. It is suggested that XCHT could be applied for handling diabetic nephropathy and merits further study for its clinical application in diabetic nephropathy.

Section 3　Research Article

The effect of kelp on serum lipids of hyperlipidemia in rats

[Abstract] We conducted this study to investigate the reducing effect and mechanism of kelp on serum lipid in rats with hyperlipidemia induced by a fat-rich diet. The levels of serum lipid including the triglyceride

(TG), total cholesterol (TC), low-density lipoprotein (LDL), and high-density lipoprotein (HDL) were detected by biochemical assay. Enzyme-linked immunosorbent assay (ELISA) was applied to determine the level of oxidized LDL (ox-LDL). The activity of lipoprotein lipase (LPL) and hepatic lipase (HL) were determined by chemical colorimetry. The concentrations of malondialdehyde (MDA) and nitric oxide (NO) were respectively measured by thiobarbituric acid assay and nitrate reductase assay. The activities of superoxide dismutase (SOD) and glutathione peroxidase (GSH-Px) were respectively determined by xanthine oxidase assay and chemical colori metry. After treated with kelp feeds, the tested rat serum levels of TG, TC and LDL decreased while HDL increased significantly compared to those of model groups ($P < 0.05$). The value of ox-LDL of treated groups were much lower than those of model groups ($P < 0.05$). The activities of LPL and HL in serum and hepatic tissue in treated groups were significantly higher than those of model groups ($P < 0.05$). The levels of MDA and NO in serum and hepatic tissue were lower than those of model groups ($P < 0.05$), while the activities of SOD and GSH-Px were significantly higher than those of model groups ($P < 0.05$). Our study indicated that kelp may correlate with the metabolism of TG, TC, LDL and HDL by enhancing the activities of LPL and HL, and regulate the levels of serum lipids by increasing the activities of SOD and GSH-Px to reduce the levels of MDA and NO.

Keywords: kelp; hyperlipidemia; lipoprotein lipase; hepatic lipase; oxidized LDL; oxidative injury; rats

1   Introduction

Hyperlipidemia is one kind of common and frequently-occurring syndromes in metabolic diseases and closely related to cardiovascular and cerebrovascular diseases (Iversen et al., 2009). Since hyperlipidemia is one of the main factors causing atherosclerosis, the lowering of serum cholesterol levels is very important for the prevention of cardiovascular diseases (Yoon et al., 2008). Currently, the fibrates (Li et al., 2008), statins (Newman, 2009), cholesterol amide (Adaramoye et al., 2008) and so on used clinically could reduce serum values of triglyceride (TG) and total cholesterol (TC) through the adjustment natural metabolism.

Lipoprotein lipase (LPL) is a key enzyme in the process of lipid metabolism, which may lead the TG and very low-density lipoprotein (VLDL) to advance when its flaw or activeness reduce, and may further cause the metabolism disorder of other lipoprotein and apolipoprotein (Huang et al., 2007). Hepatic lipase (HL) is another key enzyme during vivo fat metabolism, because it decomposes of lipoprotein microparticle and affects the conversion process of LDL and HDL, and the HL synthesis or activeness exceptionally can initiate the metabolic disorder (Van Haperen et al.,2009). As known to all, superoxide dismutase (SOD) is an enzyme to seize the free radicals and can weaken it to the cell membrane extent of damage by getting rid of superoxide anion radical and reducing the production of lipid peroxides (LPO) (Aguilar et al., 2007). GSH-Px is a kind of significant catalyze enzyme which was extensively existed inside of the body. SOD and GSH-Px are a group of important enzymes in eliminating oxygen free radicals; when the activeness drops they can cause the oxygen free radical metabolite in vivo stack. Malondialdehyde (MDA) is the degradation product that the oxygen free radical oxidation biomembrane multi-unsaturated fatty acid produces, which can reflect the content of oxygen radicals' metabolites by the MDA gallery level.

Kelp, called *Laminaria japonica* popularly in China, belongs to the genus *Laminaria* and is classified into an entire-blade group and a palmately split-blade group (Zhu et al., 2005). It is a common kind of seafood and important economical brown alga in China and many other countries. It has been documented as a drug in traditional Chinese medicine for over 1000 years and is considered effective in removing phlegm, inducing diuresis, alleviating edema, eliminating carbuncle, and clearing heat (Huang et al., 2010). To the best of our knowledge, *Laminaria japonica* contains more than 40 kinds of functional components which composed mainly kelp polysaccharide, laminine, mannitol, vitamins, amino acids and many trace elements (Yang et al., 2007). Many *Laminaria japonica* polysaccharides (LJPS) extracted from kelp have some physiological functions of enhancing organism immunity, anti-senile biological activity, anti-tumor and so on (Zhou et al., 2009). Nonetheless, few researches on the reducing blood lipid levels and anti-oxidation were reported (Wang et al., 2007). We are currently conducting intensive studies on the potential utilization of kelp which regulates effects on blood lipids and explores the potential application of kelp with the treatment of hyperlipidemia in rats.

2　Experimental section

2.1　Animal models

40 healthy female Wistar rats, weighted 150 ~ 170 g, SPF grade [SCXK (LU) 200900100], were purchased from Experiment Animal Center of Qingdao Drug Inspection Institute. The local legislation for ethics of experiment on animals and guidelines for the care and use of laboratory animals were followed in all animal procedures. All animals were acclimatized for 7 days and allowed free access to food and water in a temperature and humidity-controlled housing with natural illumination. The room temperature was maintained at $(23 \pm 2)\,°C$. Before the experiment, blood sample (0.5 mL) was collected from tail vein and separated serum for determining the TG, TC, LDL and HDL levels. Then 10 ($n = 10$) of these experimental animals were randomized as control group which were fed basically with general forage, and the rest 30 rats were fed with fat-rich forage (it was composed of general forage 59%, sucrose 20%, pig fat oil 10%, egg yolk powder 10% and cholic acid sodium 1%, well-mixed and made up granular-like forage at room temperature) for 4 weeks to established hyperlipidemia models (Zhang et al., 2007). 4 weeks later, blood sample (0.5 mL) was collected from tail vein and separated serum for determination of TG, TC, LDL and HDL. The experimental rats, which the

triglyceride (TG) > 1.5 mmol/L, total cholesterol (TC) > 1.5 mmol/L, low-density lipoprotein (LDL) > 1.0 mmol/L and high-density lipoprotein (HDL) < 0.2 mmol/L, were considered as successful hyperlipidemia rat models. 10 of the 30 experimental rats were excluded due to unsuccessful reaching in the standard, therefore, the remaining 20 rat models each considered as an experimental unit in the succeeding experiments, and then divided randomly into model (hyperlipidemia) group and treatment (kelp powder) group, 10 rats respectively.

2.2 Plant materials and treatments

The good variety kelp (Laminaria japonica) powder Zhongke No. 1, which is originally selected and harvested from Rongcheng city of Shandong Province, is used as feeder for the rats. Its main components are dietary fiber 26.1%, protein 8.5%, lipid 0.39%, the total amino acid 10.49 mg/100 g, Vitamin A 273 μg/100 g, and Vitamin C 3 μg/100 g. The general forage 90% and the kelp powder 10% are blend and mixed into lump forage, and aired at room temperature. The rats in the control group and the model group were fed with normal forage for two weeks. The rats in the treatment group were fed with the kelp forage for two weeks, each rats consumed about 2 g of kelp (equal to 10 g/kg body weight) per day and about 28 g of kelp in total.

2.3 Sample collection

Serum: At the end of this experiment, all rats were forbidden food for 12 h, and then injected heparin sodium (1.0 mg/kg, Qilu Pharmacy Co., Ltd.) from tail vein to collect blood 4 mL from eye artery using heparinized capillary tubes. The blood sample was centrifugalized for 10 minutes at 4000 r/min to separate the serum and then stored at 4 ℃ before use.

Hepatic tissue: At the end of this experiment, we used cervical dislocation to sacrifice animals and collect hepatic tissue 0.2 g immediately, washed the rudimental blood with normal saline and grinded fully at –4 ℃ ice bath. The hepatic tissue sample was centrifugalized for 10 minutes at 12 000 r/min to separate the supernatant and then stored at –20 ℃ before use.

2.4 Examination indexes

The levels of TG, TC, LDL and HDL were detected by the biochemical assay (the kits were provided by DiaSys Co., Ltd.). Before the determination, samples were redissolved at room temperature and centrifugalized for the collection of supernatant. Usually, about 100 μL of serum was collected and put into an automatic chemistry analyzer (Beckman CX-7, USA) for the detection. The sensitivity is mmol/L.

Enzyme-linked immunosorbent assay (ELISA) was applied to determine the level of oxidized LDL (ox-LDL). Usually 100 μL of serum or hepatic tissue supernatant was used to determine ox-LDL with the kits (QnSsytems™ Co., Ltd.). Standardization was conducted before the detection, and the selected wavelength was 450 nm for the Enzyme Labelling Apparatus (Bio-Rad 550, USA). The sensitivity is ng/mL.

The activities of lipoprotein lipase (LPL) and hepatic lipase (HL) were detected by chemical colorimetry with the kits (Jiancheng Institute of Biomedical Technology, Nanjing). Before the determination, samples were redissolved at room temperature and were centrifugalized for the collection of supernatant. Usually, 100 μL of serum or hepatic tissue supernatant was used for determination the free fat acid and calculating the activities of LPL and HL. Standardization was conducted before the detection, and the selected wavelength was 550 nm for the ultraviolet spectrophotometer (Bechmann DU640, USA). The sensitivity is U/mL.

The values of MDA and NO were detected by thiobarbituric acid and nitrate reductase method with the kits (Jiancheng Institute of Biomedical Technology, Nanjing China), respectively. Standardization was conducted on the ultraviolet spectrophotometer and the selected wavelength were 532 nm for MDA and 550 nm for NO respectively. The sensitivity is nmol/L (MDA) and μmol/L (NO) respectively.

The activities of SOD and GSH-Px were detected by xanthinoxidase method and chemical colorimetry with the kits (same as MDA and NO), respectively. Standardization was conducted on the ultraviolet spectrophotometer and the selected wavelength were 550 nm (SOD) and 412 nm (GSH-Px) respectively. The sensitivity is U/mL.

2.5 Statistical Analysis

SPSS17.0 software was used for statistical analysis. Data were expressed as mean ± standard difference (mean ± SD). Multi-group comparison was made by analysis of variance (ANOVA) and students' test, and two-group comparison by t-test. Values were considered to be significant when P is less than 0.05.

3 Results and discussion

3.1 The body weight of rats

All rat weights have no difference before switching rats to the fat-forage ($P > 0.05$) and increase significantly after switching rats to the fat-forage ($P < 0.05$), while the rat weights in the model group and the treated group are significantly higher than those in the control group ($P < 0.05$). After switching rats to the kelp forage in the treated group and general forage in the control and modeled groups, the rat weights of all groups increase significantly than those before switching kelp diet and control diet ($P < 0.05$), while the rat weights in the modeled group and the treated group are also significantly higher than those in the control group ($P < 0.05$), but there is no difference between the modeled group and the treated group ($P > 0.05$)

(Table 9-1).

Table 9-1　The rat weights before and after experiment (mean ± SD)

Unit: g

Groups	n	Before modeled	After modeled (Before treated)	After treated
Control group	10	161.15 ± 4.34	193.75 ± 6.26 [a]	205.66 ± 6.17 [c]
Model group	10	160.24 ± 4.23	201.67 ± 7.04 [a, b]	213.54 ± 7.23 [b, c]
Treated group	10	160.16 ± 4.31	203.18 ± 7.25 [a, b]	214.23 ± 6.18 [b, c]

[a]$P < 0.05$ *vs* before modeled; [b]$P < 0.05$ *vs* control group; [c]$P < 0.05$ *vs* before treated.

3.2　The serum levels of TG

After modeled, the serum level of TG was sharply increased due to feeding fat-forage ($P < 0.05$) and was higher than that of the control group ($P < 0.05$). The serum levels of TG decreased after switching control diet in the model group and kelp diet in the treated group ($P < 0.05$). After treated by kelp forage, the serum level of TG in the treated group was significantly lower than that in the model group ($P < 0.05$), while no difference between the treated and control groups ($P > 0.05$) (Table 9-2).

Table 9-2　The serum levels of TG before and after treated with kelp (mean ± SD)

Unit: mmol/L

Groups	n	Before modeled	After modeled (Before treated)	After treated
Control group	10	0.96 ± 0.22	0.98 ± 0.19	0.89 ± 0.18
Model group	10	0.95 ± 0.14	2.23 ± 0.17 [a, b]	1.83 ± 0.29 [b, c]
Treated group	10	0.98 ± 0.20	2.25 ± 0.14 [a, b]	0.97 ± 0.26 [c, d]

[a]$P < 0.05$ *vs* before modeled; [b]$P < 0.05$ *vs* control group; [c]$P < 0.05$ *vs* before treated; [d]$P < 0.05$ *vs* model group.

3.3　The serum levels of TC

After modeled, the serum level of TC was sharply increased due to feeding fat-forage ($P < 0.05$) and was higher than that of the control group ($P < 0.05$). The serum levels of TC decreased after switching control diet in the model group and kelp diet in the treated group ($P < 0.05$). After treated by kelp forage, the serum level of TC in the treated group was significantly lower than that in the model group ($P < 0.05$), while no difference between the treated and control groups ($P > 0.05$) (Table 9-3).

Table 9-3 The serum levels of TC before and after treated with kelp (mean ± SD)

Unit: mmol/L

Groups	n	Before modeled	After modeled (Before treated)	After treated
Control group	10	1.29 ± 0.11	1.30 ± 0.17	1.43 ± 0.10
Model group	10	1.30 ± 0.14	2.25 ± 0.19 [a, b]	1.93 ± 0.20 [b, c]
Treated group	10	1.32 ± 0.16	2.27 ± 0.15 [a, b]	1.43 ± 0.18 [c, d]

[a]$P < 0.05$ vs before modeled; [b]$P < 0.05$ vs control group; [c]$P < 0.05$ vs before treated; [d]$P < 0.05$ vs model group.

3.4 The levels of LDL and ox-LDL

The levels of LDL increased sharply after modeled. In contrast, the levels of HDL was with a decreasing due to feeding fat-forage ($P < 0.05$). However, the levels of LDL decreased again whereas the levels of HDL increased after treating by kelp ($P < 0.05$). See Table 9-4.

The value of ox-LDL in the hepatic tissue in the model group was much higher than that in the control group ($P < 0.05$). After treated with kelp forage, the value of ox-LDL of the treated group was much lower than that of the model group ($P < 0.05$), and no difference to the control group ($P > 0.05$). The value of ox-LDL was too low to be detected by ELISA (Table 9-4).

Table 9-4 The levels of LDL, HDL and ox-LDL in serum after treatment (mean ± SD)

Groups	n	LDL/ (mmol/L)	HDL/ (mmol/L)	ox-LDL/ (ng/mL)
Control group	10	0.93 ± 0.19	0.30 ± 0.08	21.85 ± 1.75
Model group	10	1.21 ± 0.12[a]	0.17 ± 0.09[a]	29.54 ± 2.72[a]
Treated group	10	0.93 ± 0.17[b]	0.30 ± 0.13[b]	23.58 ± 3.29[b]

[a]$P < 0.05$ vs control group; [b]$P < 0.05$ vs model group.

3.5 The activities of LPL and HL

In the model group, the activities of LPL and HL of serum were more significantly decreased than those in the control group ($P < 0.05$), and then increased slightly after switching kelp forage in the treated group ($P < 0.05$). The variations of LPL and HL activities in hepatic tissue were similar to those in the serum (Table 9-5).

Table 9-5　The activities of LPL and HL after treatment (mean ± SD)

Groups	n	LPL / (U/mL)		HL / (U/mL)	
		Serum	Hepatic tissue	Serum	Hepatic tissue
Control group	10	0.53 ± 0.06	1.56 ± 0.15	0.46 ± 0.05	1.42 ± 0.16
Model group	10	0.39 ± 0.05^{a}	1.10 ± 0.14^{a}	0.37 ± 0.04^{a}	1.03 ± 0.10^{a}
Treated group	10	0.70 ± 0.08^{b}	2.04 ± 0.18^{b}	0.59 ± 0.08^{b}	1.76 ± 0.25^{b}

[a]$P < 0.05$ *vs* control group; [b] $P < 0.05$ *vs* model group.

3.6　The values of MDA and NO

It is showed that the serum values of MDA and NO of model groups were significantly higher than those of control groups ($P < 0.05$), while the levels of MDA and NO of treatment groups were sharply lower than those of model groups ($P < 0.05$). The variations of MDA and NO activities of hepatic tissue were similar to those of the serum (Table 9-6).

Table 9-6　The levels of MDA and NO after treatment (mean ± SD)

Groups	n	MDA / (nmol/L)		NO / (μmol/L)	
		Serum	Hepatic tissue	Serum	Hepatic tissue
Control group	10	6.73 ± 0.83	5.58 ± 0.37	20.94 ± 2.91	21.45 ± 3.68
Model group	10	9.69 ± 0.89^{a}	6.81 ± 0.78^{a}	26.10 ± 2.33^{a}	26.14 ± 3.72^{a}
Treated group	10	6.19 ± 0.82^{b}	5.71 ± 0.35^{b}	21.28 ± 2.49^{b}	21.46 ± 3.28^{b}

[a]$P < 0.05$ *vs* control group; [b]$P < 0.05$ *vs* model group.

3.7　The activities of SOD and GSH-Px

It is indicated that the activities of SOD and GSH-Px of the model group were significantly lower than those of control groups ($P < 0.05$), whereas the activities of SOD and GSH-Px of treatment groups were sharply higher than those of model groups ($P < 0.05$). The variations of SOD and GSH-Px activities of hepatic tissue were similar to those of the serum (Table 9-7).

Table 9-7   The activities of SOD and GSH-Px after treatment (mean ± SD)

Groups	n	SOD / (U/mL)		GSH-Px / (U/mL)	
		Serum	Hepatic tissue	Serum	Hepatic tissue
Control group	10	241.95 ± 9.95	609.89 ± 49.30	291.54 ± 8.26	429.15 ± 28.12
Model group	10	219.28 ± 7.79[a]	502.28 ± 53.48[a]	255.37 ± 7.95[a]	345.77 ± 22.56[a]
Treated group	10	247.36 ± 7.70[b]	588.86 ± 40.35[b]	286.96 ± 9.32[b]	394.65 ± 34.13[b]

[a]$P < 0.05$ *vs* control group; [b]$P < 0.05$ *vs* model group.

4   Discussion

Hyperlipidemia is an umbrella term which refers to any of several acquired or genetic disorders that result in a high level of lipids (fats, cholesterol and triglycerides) circulating in the blood. These lipids can enter the walls of arteries and increase your risk of developing atherosclerosis (hardening of the arteries), which can lead to stroke, heart attack and the need to amputate. The risk of atherosclerosis is higher if you smoke, or if you have or develop diabetes, high blood pressure and kidney failure. More than 3 million people have this genetic disorder in the United States and Europe. It is extremely common for those who live in developed countries and follow a Western high-fat diet.

Hyperlipidemia is abnormally elevated levels of any or all lipids or lipoproteins in the blood. It is the most common form of dyslipidemia (which includes any abnormal lipid levels). Lipids (water-insoluble molecules) are transported in a protein capsule. The size of that capsule, or lipoprotein, determines its density. The lipoprotein density and type of apolipoproteins it contains determines the fate of the particle and its influence on metabolism. Hyperlipidemias are divided into primary and secondary subtypes. Primary hyperlipidemia is usually due to genetic causes (such as a mutation in a receptor protein), while secondary hyperlipidemia arises due to other underlying causes such as diabetes. Lipid and lipoprotein abnormalities are common in the general population and are regarded as modifiable risk factors for cardiovascular disease due to their influence on atherosclerosis. In addition, some forms may predispose to acute pancreatitis.

Hyperlipidemias may basically be classified as either familial (also called primary) caused by specific genetic abnormalities, or acquired (also called secondary) when resulting from another underlying disorder that leads to alterations in plasma lipid and lipoprotein metabolism. Also, hyperlipidemia may be idiopathic; that is, without a known cause. Hyperlipidemias are also classified according to which types of lipids are elevated; that is hypercholesterolemia, hypertriglyceridemia or both in combined hyperlipidemia. Elevated levels of Lipoprotein (a) may also be classified as a form of hyperlipidemia.

Hyperlipidemia is usually chronic, requiring ongoing statin medication to control blood lipid levels. Lipid metabolic disorder has been considered as a crucial risk factor to the occurrence of hyperlipidemia (Diehm et al., 2004). Therefore, it is as soon as possible to carry on the treatment of reducing TG, TC, LDL and enhancing HDL regarding the patients with lipid metabolic disorder (Zhong et al., 2007), and controlling other hazard factors positively in order to reduce the occurrence of cardiovascular diseases which were caused by hyperlipidemia (Kügler et al., 2003). In the lipid metabolism, lipoprotein lipase (LPL) and hepatic lipase (HL) were the key enzymes (Tian et al., 2005). The LPL mainly decomposed TG in chylomicron (CM) and very low density lipoprotein (VLDL), and transferred TC, phospholipids (PHL) and apolipoprotein (Apo) among the lipoproteins. The HL existed in the surface of the hepatic endothelial cell and participated in the transformation of IDL and LDL. It can also decompose PHL and TG contained in HDL-2 selectivity, and cause HDL-2 transforming into HDL-3. Finally the activited LPL and HL could reduce the levels of TG, TC and LDL in serum (Moen et al., 2007).

The dynamic cholesterol balance in cells is mainly dependent on two kinds of regulating mechanisms: exogenousc cholesterol ingesting by the extra-cellular LDL receptor and endogenous cholesterol synthesis. Oxidized LDL (ox-LDL) is not only a real factor injured vascular endothelial cells, but a most important factor induced atherosclerosis (Puddu et al., 2005). Ox-LDL is a special component in atherosclerosis spots. The LDL could be oxidized and modified to transform into ox-LDL by endothelium, smooth muscles and macrophages in arterial walls (Rao et al., 2008). Ox-LDL could be toxic to vascular endothelium, enhance proliferation of smooth muscle, absorbed by macrophages, and stimulate organism to produce special antibody inducing immune reactions (Chen et al., 2007).

In this experiment, the serum levels of TG, TC and LDL in kelp forage group declined remarkably while the HDL was obviously higher than those in the model groups. The results indicated that the kelp could reduce the TG, TC and LDL values and increase the HDL values. Enzymatic activities tests showed that the activity of LPL and HL of serum and hepatic tissue in the kelp group were obviously higher than those in the model groups. It is suggested that the kelp may affect TG, TC, LDL and HDL metabolism and adjust blood lipid values through strengthening enzyme activeness.

It is reported that Laminaria japonica polysaccharides (LJPS) had obviously effects on anti-coagulation, spasmolysis, depolymerization and hypotensive, hypolipemic, reducing blood viscosity, expanding vessels and improving microcirculation in connection with cardiovascular and cerebrovascular disease (Wang et al., 2007). Animal experiment indicated that LJPS can directly eliminate the oxygen anion free radicals (O_2^-) and hydroxyl free radicals (OH^-) ex vitro, and also strengthen obviously antioxidant enzymes activities in vitro (Wang et al., 2009).

In this experiment, the ox-LDL levels in serum and hepatic tissue of the model group increased significantly than those of the control group, while decreased in kelp treated group than those in the model group. It is suggested that kelp could reduce the ox-LDL levels by antioxidant effect to regulate the lipid metabolism.

MDA was the last substance during the lipid per oxidation, which could yield oxygen radical in organisms and accelerate oxygen radical generation (Surapaneni et al., 2007). Nitric oxide (NO) is an important messenger member and effective molecule of organism (Stoyanova et al., 2005). If NO was exceptional or the homeostasis in the system oxidize/anti-oxidation, it would result in the consistency of oxygen radical abnormally high, aggravate oxygen radical pathologically and accelerate the cell senescence, and finally produce a premium on disease. Here in our study, we found that the MDA and NO values in model groups increased obviously than those in normal groups. It is indicated that hyperlipemia could generate massive lipid peroxidation in rats, while the content of MDA and NO of the treated groups obviously dropped. It can be concluded that the kelp exhibited effects of anti-oxidation to lighten lipid peroxidation and regulate lipoprotein metabolism caused by the hyperlipemia.

Superoxide dismutase (SOD), which is a natural antioxidant enzyme capturing free radical, could eliminate the ultra oxygen anion free radical $[O_2 \cdot]^-$ to protect the cell to be exempt from the damage (Li et al., 2007). GSH-Px can interdict the chain reaction of lipid per oxidation, and then protect the structure and function (Chung et al., 2009). In the present experiment, the activities of SOD and GSH-Px in kelp treatment groups were obviously raised up than those of model groups. It could be concluded that kelp can enhance anti-oxidative enzyme activities, and then reduce lipid peroxidation. GSH-Px has the function of returning to original state peroxide, and may reduce the lipid peroxidation damage and cause the content of MDA to reduce. Therefore, further studies should be conducted to characterize the mechanism underlying the regulation of serum lipid levels by kelp.

5　Conclusions

This study suggested that kelp may correlate with the metabolism of TG, TC, LDL and HDL, and regulate the levels of serum lipids by enhancing the activities of LPL and HL, and by increasing the activities of SOD and GSH-Px to reduce the levels of MDA and NO.

Acknowledgement

This study was supported by grant-in-aids for the Natural Science Foundation of China (grant No. 40976085).

References

[1]　Iversen A, Jensen J S, Scharling H, et al. Hypercholesterolaemia and risk of coronary heart disease in the elderly: impact of age: the Copenhagen City Heart Study. European Journal of Internal Medicine, 2009, 20(2): 139-144.

[2]　Yoon N Y, Kim H R, Chung H Y, et al. Anti-hyperlipidemic effect of an edible brown algae, Ecklonia stolonifera, and its constituents on poloxamer 407-induced hyperlipidemic and cholesterol-fed rats. Archives of Pharmacal Research, 2008, 31(12): 1564-1571.

[3]　Li C, Grillo M, Badagnani I, et al. Differential effects of fibrates on the metabolic activation of 2-phenylpropionic acid in rats. Drug Metabolism & Disposition, 2008, 36(4): 682-687.

[4]　Newman D H. The statins in preventive cardiology. New England Journal of Medicine, 2009, 360(5): 541-542.

[5]　Adaramoye O A, Olajumoke A, Jonah A, et al. Lipid-lowering effects of methanolic extract of Vernonia amygdalina leaves in rats fed on high cholesterol diet. Vascular Health & Risk Management, 2008, 4(1): 235-241.

[6]　Huang L, Guo H W, Huang Z Y, et al. The association of lipoprotein lipase gene polymorphism with hyperlipidemia and dietary predisposition of obesity. Acta Nutrimenta Sinica, 2007, 29(3): 228-231.

[7]　Van H R, Samyn H, Van G T, et al. Novel roles of hepatic lipase and phospholipid transfer protein in VLDL as well as HDL metabolism. Biochimica Et Biophysica Acta, 2009, 1791(10): 1031-1036.

[8]　Aguilar A, Alvarez-Vijande R, Capdevila S, et al. Antioxidant patterns (superoxide dismutase, glutathione reductase, and glutathione peroxidase) in kidneys from non-heart-beating-donors: experimental study. Transplantation Proceedings, 2007, 39(1): 249-252.

[9]　Zhu L, Zhang Q, Wang Y F, et al. Determination of polysaccharide from Ecklonia kurome. Chinese Journal of Marine Drugs, 2005, 24: 47-48.

[10]　Huang L, Wen K, Gao X, et al. Hypolipidemic effect of fucoidan from Laminaria japonica in hyperlipidemic rats. Pharmaceutical Biology, 2010, 48(4): 422-426.

[11]　Yang H T, Yao L, Wang C F, et al. Study on the abstraction about active component of Laminaria japonica. The Food Industry, 2007, 3: 9-11.

[12]　Zhou Q F, Li M Y, Na G S, et al. Progress in research of antitumor mechanisms of marine polysaccharides. Chinese Pharmacological Bulletin, 2009, 25(8): 995-997.

[13]　Wang T X, Wang T X, Pang J H. Study on the hypoglycemic and hypolipidemic effect of laminarina japonica polysaccharides. Acta Nutrimenta Sinica, 2007, 29(1): 99-100.

[14]　Dong Z, Hai-Jun W U, Chen S P, et al. Comparison of the five models on experimental hyperlipidemia rats. Chinese Pharmacological Bulletin, 2007, 23(9): 1254-1256.

[15]　Diehm C, Lange S, Trampisch H J, et al. Relationship between lipid parameters and the presence of peripheral arterial disease in elderly patients. Current Medical Research & Opinion, 2004, 20(12): 1873-1875.

[16]   Zhong Q Q, Zhao S P, Dong J, et al. Effect of high density lipoprotein on adipocytes stimulated by lipopolysaccharide. Chin Pharmacol Bull, 2007, 23: 896-898.

[17]   Kügler C F, Rudofsky G. The challenges of treating peripheral arterial disease. Vascular Medicine, 2003, 8(2): 109-114.

[18]   Tian Y, Zhang R, Long S Y, et al. Relationship between subclasses of serum HDL and LPL gene Hind Ⅲ polymorphism in hyperlipidemia. Chinese Journal of Pathophysiology, 2005, 21(7): 1359-1363.

[19]   Moen C J, Tholens A P, Voshol P J, et al. The Hyplip2 locus causes hypertriglyceridemia by decreased clearance of triglycerides. Journal of Lipid Research, 2007, 48(10): 2182-2192.

[20]   Puddu G M, Cravero E, Arnone G, et al. Molecular aspects of atherogenesis: new insights and unsolved questions. Journal of Biomedical Science, 2005, 12(6): 839-853.

[21]   Rao J, Digiandomenico A, Unger J, et al. A novel oxidized low-density lipoprotein-binding protein from Pseudomonas aeruginosa. Microbiology, 2008, 154(Pt 2): 654-665.

[22]   Chen X J, Gong A P. The significance of plasma lysophosphatidic acid and low density lipoprotein in patients with stroke. Prevention and Treatment of Cardio-Cerebral-Vascular Disease, 2007, 7: 148-150.

[23]   Wang J, Wang F, Zhang Q, et al. Synthesized different derivatives of low molecular fucoidan extracted from Laminaria japonica and their potential antioxidant activity in vitro. International Journal of Biological Macromolecules, 2009, 44(5): 379-384.

[24]   Surapaneni K M, Venkataramana G. Status of lipid peroxidation, glutathione, ascorbic acid, vitamin E and antioxidant enzymes in patients with osteoarthritis. Indian Journal of Medical Sciences, 2007, 61(1): 284.

[25]   Stoyanova I I, Lazarov N E. Localization of nitric oxide synthase in rat rigeminal primary afferent neurons using NADPH diaphorase histochemistry. Mol Histol, 2005, 36: 187-193.

[26]   Li D L, Wang X Y, Han H, et al. The effect of progesterone on the activities of SOD and GSH-Px in brain tissue of hypoxic ischemia entepholopathy in infant rats. Chin Pharmacol Bull, 2007, 23: 276-277.

[27]   Chung S S, Kim M, Youn B S, et al. Glutathione peroxidase mediates the antioxidant effect of peroxisome proliferator-activated receptor in human skeletal muscle cells. Mol Cell Biol, 2009, 29: 20-30.

Section 4 Words of TCM

1. 气机调畅 harmonious functional activities of qi
2. 气郁化热 qi stagnation transforming heat
3. 气不摄血 qi failing to keep blood circulation within vessels
4. 气不固精 qi failing to consolidate essence
5. 气随血脱 qi exhaustion resulting from hemorrhage

6. 元气虚衰 decline of primordial qi

7. 精气两虚 asthenia of essence and qi

8. 气滞精瘀 qi stagnation and essence stasis

9. 血瘀精阻 blood stasis and essence obstruction

10. 气逆、闭、陷 qi adverseness, blockage and collapse

11. 气随津脱 qi exhaustion resulting from body fluid loss

12. 水停气阻 water retention causing qi stagnation

13. 津枯血燥 body fluid depletion causing blood dryness

14. 津亏血瘀 body fluid depletion causing blood stasis

15. 血瘀水停 blood stasis causing water retention

16. 风气内动 disturbance of endogenous wind

17. 热极生风 extreme heat causing wind

18. 阴虚风动 yin asthenia causing wind

19. 寒从中生 cold originating from interior

20. 湿浊内生 dampness originating from interior

21. 津伤化燥 body fluid impairment causing dryness

22. 火热内生 heat or fire originating from interior

23. 阳亢化火 excessive yang causing fire

24. 感邪即发 acute onset after affected

25. 伏而后发 latent onset

26. 重感致复 re-affectedness causing recurrence

27. 情志致复 emotion recurrence

28. 合病、并病 simultaneous onset, following onset

29. 继发、徐发 secondary onset, chronic onset

30. 食复、劳复 diet recurrence, overstrain recurrence

31. 益肝明目 liver-nourishing manipulation for improving sight

32. 强肾聪耳 kidney-reinforcing manipulation for improving hearing

33. 宣肺通鼻 pulmonary qi-promoting manipulation for removing nasal obstruction

34. 润肺清音 lung-moistening manipulation for improving the voice

35. 输布排泄 distribution and excretion

36. 五志化火 five emotions causing fire

37. 六经传变 six channels transmission

38. 三焦传变 sanjiao (tri-energizer) transmission

39. 脏腑传变 visceral transmission

40. 寒热转化 cold and heat inter-transformation

(Xu Yingjie, Li Shan)

Chapter 10   Pregnancy

Section 1   Pregnancy Diet and Diseases

You are what you eat. That's old news. So is the fact that your diet during pregnancy affects your newborn's health. But the new news is that what you eat in the next nine months can impact your baby's health, as well as your own, for decades to come. Here are 10 easy nutrition rules that will benefit you both.

1. Get enough folic acid: Ideally, you need 400 μg of vitamin B daily before conceiving. Because sufficient intake in the first trimester reduces neural-tube defects such as spinabifida by 50% ~ 70%, you should increase the dose to 600 μg when pregnancy is confirmed. Recent research suggests that supplementing with folic acid for a year before pregnancy and in the second trimester may also reduce the risk of preterm delivery.

2. Don't "eat for two": As many as half of women gain too much weight during pregnancy. The upshot: an increased risk for preclampsia, gestational diabetes and delivery of either a preterm or a too-large baby. Talk to your doctor.

3. Eat your fish: Getting enough DHA (found in abundance in seafood and flaxseed) is one of the most important things you can do for your and your developing baby's health, according to nutritionists. DHA is the omega-3 fatty acid that can boost your baby's brain development before birth, leading to better vision, memory, motor skills and language comprehension in early childhood. Eat at least 12 ounces a week of low-mercury fish, or take a DHA supplement (both are safe).

4. Avoid alcohol: There may be behavior problems, learning disabilities, attention deficit disorder, hyperactivity and aggressive behavior in children when mom drinks during pregnancy. No amount of alcohol has been shown to be safe.

5. Get adequate iron: During pregnancy, your iron needs nearly double, to about 30 mg per day, to support your 50% increase in blood volume and promote fetal iron storage. Iron transports oxygen, and your baby benefits from a healthy supply. To boost absorption, combine iron-rich foods with vitamin C; for example, load your chicken burrito with salsa.

6. Ban bacteria: Protect your baby from harmful bacteria such as Listeria, Salmonella and E. coli (any of which can, in severe cases, cause miscarriage or preterm delivery), steer clear of soft cheeses made with unpasteurized milk, as well as raw or undercooked meat, poultry, seafood or eggs. Keep your fridge below 40° F, and dump leftover food that's been sitting out for more than two hours.

7. Limit caffeine: About 300 mg of caffeine per day, the amount in about two cups of coffee, has long been considered acceptable during pregnancy. But a Kaiser Permanente study found that consuming 200 mg of caffeine per day increased the risk of miscarriage. "There's no magic cut-off point, but the less the better," says the study's lead author, perinatal epidemiologist De-Kun Li, M.D., Ph.D..

8. Trash junk food: If you constantly indulge in fries and shakes now, your child might clamor for Dairy Queen in the future. "Somehow a salty, sugary, high-fat, low nutrient diet seems to program a baby's taste preference," says Elizabeth Somer, M.A., R.D., author of *Nutrition for a Healthy Pregnancy* (Holt Paperbacks).

9. Bone up on calcium: Aim to get at least 1000 mg a day; your baby needs it for tooth and bone development in the second and third trimesters. Plus, if you don't get enough calcium in your diet the fetus will leach it from your bones, which may increase your osteoporosis risk later in your life.

10. Focus on fiber: A diet high in fruits, vegetables and whole grains helps prevent constipation and hemorrhoids and keeps you feeling full so you are less likely to overeat. High-fiber foods also are packed with vitamins, minerals and phytochemicals essential to your baby's development. Aim to get at least $25 \sim 35$ mg of fiber a day, which is about twice what most Americans consume.

Two years ago, the United States government advised pregnant women to limit fish in their diet to 340 g per week. Women in some other countries get the same advice too. The aim is to reduce the risk that mercury pollution in fish could harm the developing nervous system in children. But now, it is reported that women following this advice may be harming their children instead of protecting them, because of the value to brain development from the omega-3 fatty acids in fish oil outweighs the risk from mercury.

"My belly is not a chemical location" is the message of these pregnant women in Germany, protesting against industrial pollution. Yet a researcher suggests that the risk to fetuses from mercury in fish may be overstated. The information came from a retrospective health study known as the Children of the Nineties Project, based at the University of Bristol. The research looked at the records of 9000 pregnant women. The information included the amount of seafood their members ate while pregnant.

The researchers compared families that ate plenty of fish against those ate less than 340 g per week and also compared the development of the children at different ages. The results showed an important difference between the children of women who ate a lot of fish and the children of women who did not. The scientists based their observations on 31 different tests. These are some of the reported findings: By around 2 years old, children whose mother ate no fish had lower scores in tests for motor, communication and social skills. At the age of 7, they had more problems dealing with other children. And by 8 they were more likely to do poorly on intelligence tests of language skills. Mothers who had the most omega-3 acids in their diet had the children with the best fine-motor skills at 3.5 years old.

Nearly all fish contains some amount of mercury, a metallic element. Some kinds contain more than others. It gets into the environment from the burning of coal and other fossil fuels and also comes from the use of mercury in electronics and other products. The advisory in 2004 came jointly from the Food and Drugs Administration and the Environment Protection Agency. They said eating seafood is not a health concern for most people. But they had advice for young children and three groups of women consisting of pregnant women, women who might become pregnant and those who breastfeed their babies. The women and children were advised not to eat shark, swordfish, king mackerel or tilefish because they contain high levels of mercury.

Most researches are responsible for the health advisory looking only at the study of the effects of eating whale meat with high mercury, but not consider the risk of restricting the nutrients that pregnant women can get from fish. There are five of the most commonly eaten fish that are low in mercury (shrimp, canned light tuna, salmon, pollock and catfish). Albacore or "white" tuna has more mercury than canned light tuna. The women and children were also told to be very careful about the safety of fish caught in local waterways.

Omega-3 fatty acids have been in the news for years. Some of them may reduce the risk of heart attacks by reducing the risk of blockages in the blood system. Countries with the highest rate of eating fish have lower rates of depression, and even lower rates of murder. Walnuts and seed oil also contain omega-3 acids, but fish oil, or fish oil supplements are the best way to get them. There may be limits to the power of fish oil, though. It does not appear to reduce the risk of cancer.

More than 2400 years ago, Athens was struck by a sickness which was said to have killed up to 1/3 of all Athenians, including their leader Pericles. The huge loss of life helped to change the balance of power between Athens and its enemy, Sparta, in the ancient world. Historians say the sickness began in what is now Ethiopia. It passed through Egypt and Libya before it entered Greece. Knowledge of the disease has come mainly from the writings of the ancient Greek historian Thucydides survived. The diseases have been suggested anthrax, bubonic plague, measles and smallpox. Now, a study based on genetic testing indicated it was probably typhoid fever. Researchers from the University of Athens tested human remains from an ancient burial place in the Greek capital. They collected genetic material from teeth and found genetic evidence similar to the modern-day organism Salmonella enterica serovar Typhi. This finding throws light on one of the most debated mysteries in medical history.

Typhoid fever is a life-threatening disease that is common today in developing countries. There are more than 21 million cases each year. Typhoid can be spread by food or drink which has been handled by a person infected with the bacteria that causes it. Bacteria expelled in human waste can pollute water supplies. So water used for drinking or to wash food can also spread the infection. Hand washing is important to reduce the spread of typhoid and the vaccines can help prevent it. People with typhoid fever usually develop a body temperature as high as 40℃ and can usually be treated with antibiotics. Some people recover but continue carrying the bacteria and these carriers can get sick again and infect others.

Another disease common in developing countries is rotavirus. Babies and young children around the world are affected by this intestinal condition. Yet rotavirus is a leading killer of young children in the developing world. The severe diarrhea it causes can be deadly unless treated. Most of the estimated half-million deaths each year are in poor countries. But major studies show that two new vaccines called Rotarix and RotaTeq are safe and effective in preventing most cases of severe rotavirus in young children. Rotarix is already sold in some countries, but RotaTeq is not yet for sale. In 1991, the drug company Wyeth removed a rotavirus vaccine from the American market because it was blamed for some cases of an intestinal blockage. The studies of Rotarix and RotaTeq, however, show the two new vaccines did not show any increase in risk for that condition.

Section 2　Chinese Herbal Medicine

Chinese herbal medicine is well known throughout the world and in many places it's actually taken seriously! While Western medicine focuses on treating syndromes, Chinese medicine goes after the root of the problem, seeking to regulate the delicate vital balance in the body by compensating for certain deficiencies with elements found in mother nature.

If all that sounds a lot more complicated than simply popping a Quaalude, fear not! The people, ever solicitous foreign, is here to describe and prescribe some time-tested traditional Chinese medicinal remedies for many common ailments.

1. Diarrhea: One thing you can count on in China (besides an abacus) is diarrhea. Sooner or later, even those of us with great leap forward-forged cast-iron stomachs that can digest bowls of sawdust eventually wind up with it. As if having to spend half a day sitting on the toilet isn't bad enough, and you also have to listen to your friends and relatives giving you advice on how to rectify your sodden condition. It's enough to make you headache. A sure-fire cure for even the most persistent diarrhea is to simply soak some sour plums in liquor for a few mouths and cheers.

2. Constipation: If constipation is your problem, 5000 years of history and tradition dictates that a bar of soap up your butt is the cure. The people's personal panacea and prescription for pleasure is, of course, Beijing backyard moonshine (Erguotou). That is why people always carry a flask of it in one pocket and a jar of vinegar in the other. Just in case the people gets drunk, a couple of swigs are just what the doctor ordered to sober right up! (Speaking of vinegar, wash with it every day to keep your face looking white and beautiful.)

3. Sore throat: For a sore throat, just wet the tip of a chopstick, dab it in salt, and touch it to your uvula (the little thing that hangs down in the back of your throat). If you don't vomit, this is a guaranteed cure.

4. Fever: For relief from fever, try the following therapy that have someone rub a spoon vigorously up and down your back until your spine is nearly exposed. The excruciating pain will cause you to sweat until the fever breaks!

5. Backache: For simple chronic backaches, try cupping, a process by which someone smears black grease all over your back, lights a fire in a medicated glass jar and then slaps the burning contraption down onto your flesh, open-mouth side facing down. After the fire burns out they yank the jar off and it makes a popping sound like when you pull a plunger out of a toilet bowl. The bizarre procedure leaves your back, looking like a giant pepperoni pizza. It is good for the flu, too. Other antics include Dianxue, or pushing on pressure points to cure illness or paralysis and even improves eyesight.

While the above curative methods are practically cost-free, there are many Chinese herbal medicines that come with a hefty price tag. Ginseng sells for up to 500 dollars per gram. That is more expensive than cocaine. While Ginseng is basically an all-around restorative substance, one of its vital uses is to prolong the life of someone on their deathbed just long enough to give their relatives a chance to get to the hospital to say goodbye. There are also many other tonics and natural "cures" to be found in the animal world. To help heal a burn and prevent or heal a scar, try eating pigeons. Turtle is also known for its curative powers, as is the "dried oviduct fat of a Chinese forest frog". To boost vitality and keep up your overall resistance to illness, ground-up deer antlers are tops, as are shark bone power, snake power pills, dog kidney capsules and cow penis. Hugu Yaogao (tiger bone medicated patches) work great for sore muscles and joints. And then there is snake gall blander to improve your eyesight.

Some medicaments from the descriptions on the labels sounded too good to be true. The box of a certain product made from bear guts reads functions and indications: clearing away the heart fire, reducing fever, calming the liver, improving the eyesight and relieving spasm. It is suitable for treating hypertension, angina pectoris, coronary heart disease and arrhythmia, acute and chronic hepatitis, icterohepatitis and liver cirrhosis, cholecystitis, cholelithiasis, (among other things, various kinds of epilepsy), preventing and controlling attacks, affection after delivery, diabetes, sore throat, bronchitis, asthma, epidemic hemorrhagic conjunctivitis and nebula, hemorrhoid, injury, anti-fatigue and recovering physical strengthen. But what good is it, really, if it can't raise the dead?

The label on a bag of caterpillar fungus boasts it can build up the health and also has the special curative effect in treatment for asthma, tuberculosis and many other diseases. According to the label on a package containing the reproductive organs of a deer, its contents have the medical properties necessary to treat back or knee pain accompanied by cold sensation, limited movement of the joints, spermatorrhea, dizziness and tinnitus.

If all this sounds a little extraordinary to you, that's because it is. Chinese medicine, like the Chinese language and holding chopsticks, is too complicated and mysterious for you to possibly comprehend, but don't let that discourage you from trying!

A fun game: After boiling your pot of Chinese medicinal herbs, toss the gunk into the street for someone else to step on and subsequently get the illness which the medicine was intended to cure!

Section 3　Research Article

Anti-inflammatory effect of low molecular weight fucoidan from Saccharina japonica on atherosclerosis in apoE-knockout mice

1　Introduction

Atherosclerosis (AS) is the key cause of coronary heart disease (CHD), aortic aneurysm, cerebral infarction and peripheral arterial disease, and it is the pathological basis of a set of cardiovascular and cerebrovascular diseases. Currently, the morbidity and mortality rates of AS are sharply increasing worldwide. However, we still lack efficient prevention and treatment for stabilizing atherosclerotic plaques.

AS is a type of chronic inflammatory and metabolic disorder, mostly occurring in medium and large arteries. The inflammatory response and lipid metabolism disorders are both involved in the development and progression of AS. Local modifications in blood flow patterns and velocity alter the artery wall configuration; these areas of disturbed flow in vivo lead to the proliferation of endothelial cells and contribute to the apoptosis of endothelial cells. The permeability of aortic endothelial cells is elevated, and low-density lipoprotein (LDL) and many inflammatory and adhesion molecules can infiltrate into the intimal layer of arterial walls more easily. Infiltrating inflammatory cells, such as macrophages, monocytes and smooth muscle cells (SMCs) migrate into the intimal layer of arteries, which thicken and form plaques[1]. All the processes associated with the inflammatory response promote the development of AS.

Abundant data have linked dyslipidemia and chronic inflammation to AS. The oxidative modification of low density lipoproteins (ox-LDL) plays an important role in the formation of fatty plaques[2]. Following the internalization of ox-LDL, macrophages and SMCs becomes lipid-laden foam cells and ultimately initiate plaque formation around a necrotic core[3]. Studies have shown that almost all the cells involved in the pathogenesis of AS secrete various inflammatory cytokines, particularly macrophages, SMCs and lymphocytes. Scientists have broadly classified theses cytokines as pro-atherogenic or anti-atherogenic, depending on their effects. Interleukin 6 (IL-6), interleukin 1 (IL-1) and tumor necrosis factor-α (TNF-α) are considered pro-atherogenic cytokines, while interleukin 10 (IL-10) and interleukin 35 (IL-35) are anti-atherogenic[4]. The interplay between inflammatory cytokines and lipid metabolism aggravates the development of AS[5-7].

Traditional Chinese medicine has been extensively used in China for thousands of years and is considered a valuable asset for promoting health. Saccharina japonica, a kind of brown algae, is also a traditional Chinese medicine. Fucoidan is the main bioactive compound in Saccharina japonica. Fucoidan is a family of heteropolysaccharides composed of an α-L-fucose-enriched backbone that mostly contains fucose, galactose and sulfate and has a small amount of mannose, glucuronic acid, glucose, rhamnose, arabinose and xylose units. Because of its complicated and heterogeneous structures, fucoidan has various bioactivities. Studies have verified that the bioactivity of fucoidan is improved with a higher sulfate level and a lower molecular weight. Low molecular weight fucoidan (LMWF) is a highly sulfated fraction derived from fucoidan. Thus, LMWF has stronger bioactivity in some respects, such as anti-inflammatory, anticoagulant, antiangiogenic, antithrombosis, antioxidant and anti-adhesion effects[8-13].

Recent research has demonstrated that a purified fraction of fucoidan can effectively down-regulate the expression of major mediators of inflammation and can inhibit the expression of pro-inflammatory cytokines, including TNF-α, IL-1β, and IL-6 in lipopolysaccharide (LPS)-stimulated macrophages[4]. LMWF reduces IR-induced hepatic injury via JAK2/STAT1-mediated apoptosis and autophagy and attenuates liver enzymes in the serum and pathologic damage by inhibiting inflammatory reactions[14]. LMWF was also recommended as a natural and safe antibacterial and anti-adipogenic agent because of its marked effect in attenuating lipid accumulation[9]. An obvious regulating effect of LMWF was observed in hepatic glucose metabolism and antioxidant activities in db/db mice, and LMWF also decreased lipid metabolism in white adipose tissue[15].

Therefore, this study aimed to further investigate the preventive and therapeutic effects of LMWF on AS, and it focused on the regulatory function of LMWF on lipid metabolism and the inflammatory response in apoE-knockout mice. The bioactivity of LMWF may provide a new therapeutic application as well as its potential as an anti-atherogenic agent.

2　Materials and methods

2.1　Ethics statement

All the animal-related experiments were performed using the protocols approved by our institute (The Ethics Committee of Qingdao University Medical College, QUMC 2011-09).

2.2　Materials

LMWF was extracted from Saccharina japonica, molecular weight = 8177 Da. The LMWF was authenticated by high-performance liquid chromatography, capillary electrophoresis, monosaccharide composition analysis, methylation analysis, periodate oxidation, smith degradation, and many other tests[16]. The component analysis was composed as follows: fucose 35.07%, sulfate 36.85% and uronic acid 0.039%. LMWF was dissolved in distilled water.

2.3　Animals and treatment

Male KM mice (49 days old, SPF grade, strain: KM) and male apoE-knockout (-/-) mice (49 days old, SPF grade, strain: C57BL/6J-KO) were both purchased from the Institute of Laboratory Animal Science, Chinese Academy of Medical Sciences & Peking Union Medical College. All the mice were housed in standard environmental conditions at (22 ± 2) ℃, with (50 ± 5) % relative humidity and with natural illumination under natural light conditions. Food and water were given ad libitum.

After acclimation for one week, all the mice were randomly divided into 5 groups: (1) the normal group (n = 15): KM mice were fed a standard chow diet and received an identical volume of 0.9% saline; (2) the control group (n = 15): apoE (-/-) mice were fed a standard chow diet and received an identical volume of 0.9% saline; (3) the LF group (n = 15): apoE (-/-) mice were fed an atherogenic diet and received 200 mg/(kg·d) LMWF[17]; (4) the probucol group (n = 15): apoE (-/-) mice were fed an atherogenic diet and received 200 mg/(kg·d) of probucol[18]; (5) the model group (n = 15): apoE (-/-) mice were fed an atherogenic diet and received an identical volume of 0.9% saline.

The standard chow diet and the atherogenic diet (containing 21% fat and 0.15% cholesterol) were reserved in one batch throughout the experiment to avoid potential confounding effects[19]. All the treatments were administered by gavage between 8:00 and 10:00 for 11 weeks, and the mice were weighed twice a week. LMWF was dissolved in 0.9%

saline, and probucol was used as a positive drug and was dissolved in olive oil[18, 20]. The doses of LWMF and probucol were optimal according to previous studies[21-23].

At the end of the experiment, all the mice were anesthetized with 10% chloral hydrate. The blood sample as well as the aorta and liver were removed for subsequent tests.

2.4 Serum biochemical indexes

After anesthesia, the serums of all the mice were separated from the heart blood by centrifugation. The serums were sent to the clinical laboratory of the Affiliated Hospital of Qingdao University to ascertain serum biochemical indexes, such as total triglycerides (TRIG), cholesterol (CHOL), high-density lipoproteins (HDL), low-density lipoproteins (LDL), and apolipoprotein A and apolipoprotein B.

2.5 Histological studies

5 mice were randomly selected from each group. The aortas and heart were fixed in 4% paraformaldehyde. Several aortas from different groups were stained with en face Oil Red O to evaluate the gross atherosclerotic lesions. The other fixed aortas were embedded in optimum cutting temperature (OCT) compound (Sakura, USA) and quickly frozen using liquid nitrogen. Then, 10 μm thick sections were cut continuously at 500 μm intervals. Several sections of each group were stained with hematoxylin and eosin (HE) for analysis.

2.6 Tunel

The sections were stained to detect apoptotic cells in atherosclerotic plaques by labeling DNA strand breaks with the In Situ Cell Death Detection Kit, following the kit's guidelines. The apoptotic cells appeared as green fluorescence under a fluorescence microscope at 515 nm. The fluorescence intensity of five random non-overlapping views was measured using Image-Pro Plus 6.0 software.

2.7 Immunohistochemistry and immunofluorescence studies

Frozen sections were washed with Tris-HCl buffer solution (TBS), and endogenous peroxidases were inactivated by 3% H_2O_2. The washed sections were incubated with anti-p-SAPK/JNK antibody (1 : 200), anti-IL-6 antibody (1 : 200), anti-IL-10 antibody (1 : 50), and anti-cyclin D1 antibody (1 : 100), overnight at 4 °C. HRP-labeled secondary antibodies or fluorescence-labeled secondary antibodies (Alexa Fluor 488-conjugated goat anti-rabbit IgG, Alexa Fluor 594-conjugated goat anti-mouse IgG) were added onto the sections for 1 h at 37 °C.

A diaminobenzidine (DAB) specific reaction was performed for 5 min to detect positive immunohistochemistry expressions, with the positive cells appearing as brownish-yellow particles. Fluorescence intensity was detected using a fluorescence microscope, and positive cells appeared green (Alexa Fluor 488: A_{max} = 493 nm, E_{max} =519 nm) or red (Alexa Fluor 594: A_{max} = 493 nm, E_{max} = 519 nm). Five non-overlapping views of each section were randomly chosen to determine the positive expression level. The expression intensity of these proteins was measured using Image-Pro Plus 6.0 software.

2.8　Double immunofluorescence labeling

Frozen sections were also washed with Tris-HCl buffer solution (TBS), and endogenous peroxidases were inactivated by 3% H_2O_2. Anti-α-SMA antibody (1 ∶ 50) and anti-CD11b antibody (1 ∶ 200) were mixed in a 1.5 mL EP tube. The sections were incubated with the mixture overnight at 4 °C. Fluorescence-labeled secondary antibodies, Alexa Fluor 488 and Alexa Fluor 488, were mixed and added onto the sections for 1 h at 37 ℃ [24]. Fluorescence intensity was detected using a fluorescence microscope, and five non-overlapping views of each section were randomly chosen to determine the positive expression level. A-SMA-positive cells appeared red, and CD11b-positive cells appeared green. The expression intensity of these proteins was measured using Image-Pro Plus 6.0 software.

2.9　ELISA essay

5 mice were randomly selected from each group, and 20 mg aorta and liver tissues were separately lysed in RIPA buffer (with PMSF) on ice for 20 min. Then, the lysates were centrifuged at 12 000 r / min for 5 min, and the supernatants were collected. Concentrations of total protein were determined using SimpliNano microvolume spectrophotometer. All the proteins were stored in a −80 °C refrigerator. The supernatants were removed to Mouse IL-6, IL-10 and ox-LDL ELISA kit plates following the ELISA kits' protocols. The OD values were determined at 450 nm by an automatic microplate reader.

2.10　RT-qPCR essay

The total RNA was extracted from the aorta and liver tissues of all the mice by a Trizol kit. The RNA concentration was assessed using a SimpliNano microvolume spectrophotometer and was verified by 1% agarose gel electrophoresis. The RNA was reverse transcribed by a PrimeScript^{TM}RT kit. RT-qPCR was carried out in triplicate by the Light Cycler 480 system (Roche Molecular Systems, Inc, China). The reaction was performed in a 20 μL reaction volume containing 10 μL of SYBR Premix Ex Taq II, 1 μL of forward primers (final concentration 0.4 μmol/L), 1 μL of reverse primers (final concentration 0.4 μmol/L) and 50 ng of cDNA template. Relative expressions were normalized to GAPDH for an endogenous control. ΔCt was recorded, and the relative expression levels were calculated using the $2^{-\Delta\Delta Ct}$ method.

2.11 Western blotting

The proteins that were extracted from the aorta and liver tissues were separated by SDS-PAGE and then blotted onto polyvinylidene difluoride membranes (Solarbio Science & Technology Co., Ltd., China). The blotted membranes were incubated with anti-p-SAPK/JNK antibody (1 : 1000) and anti-cyclin D1 antibody (1 : 1000) at 4 °C overnight. After being washed with TBST, a peroxidase-conjugated secondary antibody (Solarbio Science & Technology Co., Ltd., China) was attached onto the immunoblotted membranes for 2 h at 37 °C. Blotted bands were revealed in accordance with the kit's protocol and were analyzed by ImageJ software. The relative values of the proteins were calculated as the gray value of the protein of interest/the gray value of the β-actin protein.

2.12 Statistical analysis

All the values were expressed as the means ± standard deviation (SD). SPSS 17.0 software was used for the statistical analyses. Multi-group comparisons were performed using a one-way analysis of variance (one-way ANOVA), and group-group comparisons were conducted using Bonferroni-corrected tests. Differences were considered statistically significant if P was less than 0.05.

3 Results

3.1 Effect of LMWF on the serum biochemical indexes

Several serum biochemical indexes were detected by an automatic biochemistry analyzer. Apolipoprotein A and apolipoprotein B of all the groups had no statistical significance, and LWMF had no obvious effect on apolipoprotein A and apolipoprotein B in atherosclerotic or non-atherosclerotic mice. The increases in TRIG, CHOL and LDL were the main characteristics in the progress of AS[25]. The TRIG, CHOL and LDL levels of the model group were obviously elevated, and HDL decreased, indicating that the apoE (-/-) mice had a lipid disorder after a long atherogenic diet. Compared with the model groups, the TRIG levels of the LF and the probucol group were down-regulated ($P < 0.05$), especially in the LF group ($P < 0.001$). In contrast, the HDL level of the LF group was increased compared with the model group ($P < 0.01$), even more than the control group ($P < 0.05$). But probucol did not have an obviously influence on the CHOL, TRIG and HDL levels; perhaps it's because of the medication time and physical exercise of mice[26-27]. The results showed that LMWF decreased the TRIG level and improved the HDL level in atherosclerotic mice but had no apparent effect on the CHOL and LDL levels.

3.2 Effect of LMWF on atherosclerotic plaques

To further illustrate the role of LMWF in AS, we examined its effect on AS development in apoE (-/-) mice by Oil-red O and HE stains. Figure 10-1 and Figure 10-2 showed that normal mice and the apoE (-/-) mice with a standard chow diet barely had any atherosclerotic plaques. In contrast, the model mice showed visible atherosclerotic lesion areas. Probucol evidently decreased the area of atherosclerotic plaques compared with the model group. The aorta of the LF group had inflammatory infiltration but no clear formed atherosclerotic plaques. The results showed LMWF inhibited the formation of atherosclerotic plaque and reduced the size of the plaque area. Therefore, LMWF treatment stabilized atherosclerotic lesions in apo (E-/-) mice.

3.3　LMWF inhibits ox-LDL levels in apoE (-/-) mice

Ox-LDL-induced macrophage apoptosis contributed to the formation of AS, and we further detected the effect of LMWF on lipid uptake in the livers and aortas of mice. Whether in the liver or the aorta, the ox-LDL of the model group was statistically increased. Figure 10-2 shows LMWF lowered the ox-LDL level to the normal standard of the control group, but the inhibitory effect of LMWF on ox-LDL was more significant in the aorta.

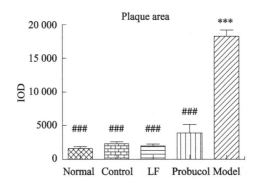

Figure 10-1　Effect of LMWF on the phenotype of the aorta and atherosclerotic plaques stained by Oil-red O

(a) Oil-red O staining of whole aortas and IOD quantification of the plaque area. (b) Oil-red O staining of cross section and IOD quantification. Data are expressed as the means ± SD. $n = 5$. $**P < 0.01$ and $***P < 0.001$ *vs* the normal group and $###P < 0.001$ *vs* the model group, scale bar = 100 μm in each panel.

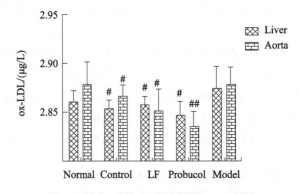

Figure 10-2　Effect of LMWF on ox-LDL

Data are expressed as the means ± SD. $#P < 0.05$ and $##P < 0.01$ *vs* the model group.

3.4   Effect of LMWF on cell apoptosis in the aorta

In AS, inflammation and excessively stimulated autophagy may cause cell death, such as in SMCs, vascular endothelial cells and macrophages. Figure 10-3 shows that there was much more apoptosis in the atherosclerotic aorta of the model group, notably in the intimal layer of the arterial wall. LMWF, like probucol, decreased the level of apoptosis in the arterial wall of apoE (-/-) mice compared with the model group ($P < 0.05$). Hence, LMWF stabilized established atherosclerotic lesions.

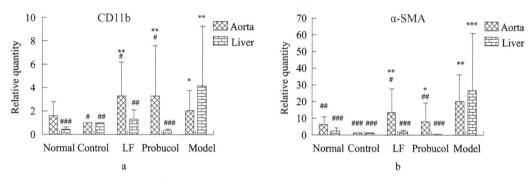

Figure 10-3   Effect of LMWF CD11b and α-SMA in the aorta

(a) Representative images of all the groups stained by double immunofluorescence labeling, scale bar = 100 μm in each panel. (b)The relative levels to GAPDH of CD11b and α-SMA from aorta and liver tissues by RT-qPCR. $^*P < 0.05$, $^{**}P < 0.01$ and $^{***}P < 0.001$ vs the normal group; $^\#P < 0.05$, $^{\#\#}P < 0.01$ and $^{\#\#\#}P < 0.001$ vs the model group.

3.5   Effect of LMWF on the inflammatory cytokines IL-6 and IL-10

IL-6 is one of the pro-atherogenic cytokines, and IL-10 functions as an anti-atherogenic cytokine in AS. Figure 10-4a reveals that LMWF did not influence the concentrations of IL-6 and IL-10 in the aorta and liver tissues. However, in the model group, the mRNA levels of IL-6 and IL-10 were both highly increased (Figure 10-4b). LMWF decreased the two inflammatory cytokines to normal levels, and the inhibition was more effective in the liver of apoE (-/-) mice.

3.6   Effect of LMWF on the inflammatory cytokines p–JNK and cyclin D1

P-JNK and cyclin D1 play essential roles in the inflammatory response. Figure 10-5a shows the elevated mRNA levels of p-JNK and cyclin D1 in the aorta and liver tissues of the model mice. LMWF decreased p-JNK levels in the aorta and returned liver p-JNK mRNA to normal levels. LMWF also decreased the mRNA levels of cyclin D1 in the aorta and liver tissues, but it didn't have noticeable effect on the protein expression levels of p-JNK and cyclin D1.

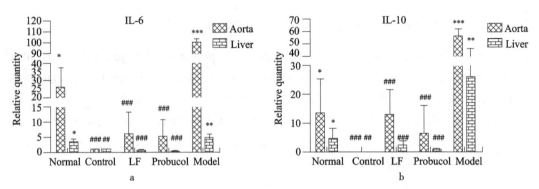

Figure 10-4　Effect of LMWF on the mRNA and protein levels of IL-6 and IL-10 in atherosclerotic mice

(a) Concentration of the secretion of IL-6 and IL-10 from aorta and liver tissues by ELISA. (b)The relative levels to GAPDH of IL-6 and IL-10 from aorta and liver tissues by RT-qPCR. $^*P < 0.05$, $^{**}P < 0.01$ and $^{***}P < 0.001$ vs the normal group; $^{###}P < 0.001$ vs the model group.

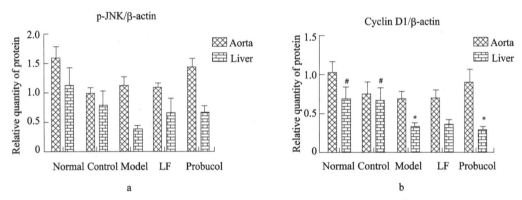

Figure 10-5　Effect of LMWF on the mRNA and protein levels of p-JNK and cyclin D1 in AS

(a) The relative levels to GAPDH of p-JNK and cyclin D1 from aorta and liver tissues by RT-qPCR. (b)Western blot analysis of the effects of LWMF on p-JNK and cyclin D1 levels. Representative images of p-JNK and cyclin D1 stained by immunofluorescence. $^*P < 0.05$, $^{**}P < 0.01$ and $^{***}P < 0.001$ vs the normal group; $^{###}P < 0.001$ vs the model group.

3.7　LMWF decreases the expression of CD11b and α-SMA in the aorta in apoE (-/-) mice

To observe the development of macrophages and SMCs in the formation of AS, we investigated the effect of LMWF on CD11b and α-SMA. Figure 10-3b shows that the mRNA levels of CD11b were up-regulated in the aorta but were down-regulated in the liver of apoE (-/-) mice after LMWF treatment. LMWF also decreased the mRNA levels of α-SMA, and this decrease was much stronger in the liver. CD11b and α-SMA both had visible expressions in the intimal layer of the aorta, and LMWF decreased these two-protein expression levels to normal levels (Figure 10-3a). The results show that LMWF ameliorated the occurrence and development of AS.

4   Discussion

It is becoming evident that AS is considered an inflammatory disease and that inflammatory processes are involved in different stages of plaque development. First, endothelial cells are activated, leading to the expression of adhesion molecules to attract inflammatory cells, such as neutrophils, T-cells and monocytes, to the early atherosclerotic lesion. After the plaque is formed, pro-inflammatory cytokines secreted by SMCs and endothelial cells stimulate the differentiation of monocytes into macrophages[3,28]. These macrophages develop into foam cells upon taking up ox-LDL and locally amplify the inflammatory response, attracting more immune cells and inducing the migration of SMCs into the plaque[29-30]; the migration and proliferation of SMCs are necessary for the formation of the fibrous cap. SMCs can be detected by the expression of α-SMA[31]. CD11b is a key integrin implicated in the inflammatory response; it is expressed on the surface of macrophages and monocytes. CD11b regulates the monocyte adhesion and migration processes and contributes to the formation of AS[32].

During the past few decades, LWMF has extensively been studied due to its broad spectrum of desirable biological functions[7, 14]. As a potential and novel inhibitor abstracted from traditional Chinese medicine, LMWF apparently has an anti-inflammatory effect. The results show that LMWF decreased the number of macrophages and ameliorated the inflammatory response through CD11b. The decrease in α-SMA by LMWF decreased the expression of SMCs in the intimal layer of the artery. Therefore, LMWF can decrease foam cells formed by inhibiting macrophages and can prevent SMCs from migrating to the intimal layer, thus decreasing the formation of atherosclerotic lesions.

Activated SMCs produce IL-6 by activating multiple intracellular pathways in AS[10]. However, IL-10 has been found to inhibit the SMC proliferation induced by TNF-α and basic fibroblast growth factor and to potently repress pro-inflammatory cytokine production in LPS-stimulated monocytes. LMWF distinctly down-regulated IL-6 transcriptional levels; meanwhile, the mRNA level of IL-10 was significantly increased with LMWF treatment. The JNK signaling pathway plays an important role in the development of AS, with multiple different transcription factors involved. MAPK pathway family members, such as Erk, JNK and p38, play crucial roles in many cell process, including cell proliferation, differentiation, apoptosis, migration and invasion. Activation of JNK pathways can induce tumor cell development, differentiation, proliferation and other cell processes. Previous studies also showed that JNK plays a critical role in VSMC proliferation and migration. Cyclin D1 forms cyclin-dependent kinases and controls the cell cycle transition from the G_1 to S phases, which results in increased cell proliferation. LMWF restored p-JNK and cyclin D1 to normal transcriptional levels and then alleviated the proliferation of SMCs and reduced the production of cytokines in response to inflammation, leading to cell proliferation, differentiation, apoptosis, migration and invasion. The results further showed that LMWF suppressed SMC proliferation and migration as well as atherosclerotic lesions and fibrous caps.

Proinflammatory cytokines increase the binding of LDL to SMCs and the endothelium; conversely, ox-LDL initiates a series of intracellular events that include the induction of proinflammatory cytokines and cellular apoptosis. Free CHOL and TRIG and ox-LDL are potent proinflammatory stimuli triggering the recruitment of more macrophages and are major components of plaque. Apoptosis may cause endothelial cell death resulting from local inflammatory mediators and is associated with macrophage infiltration. Our study showed that LMWF significantly decreased the levels of TRIG and ox-LDL and altered lipid metabolism and apoptosis.

In conclusion, our work demonstrated that LMWF modified lipid metabolism and reduced apoptosis. In addition, LMWF prevented macrophages from developing into foam cells and prevented SMC migration into the intimal layer of the aorta, thus inhibiting the formation of atherosclerotic plaques. LMWF regulated the production and expression of inflammatory cytokines, such as IL-6, IL-10, p-JNK and cyclin D1, and inhibited the inflammatory response in various stages of AS. Thus, LMWF can conclusively ameliorate the occurrence and development of AS.

References

[1] Goikuria H, Vandenbroeck K, Alloza I. Inflammation in human carotid atheroma plaques. Cytokine & Growth Factor Reviews, 2018.

[2] Xu J, Xia Z, Rong S, et al. Yirui capsules alleviate atherosclerosis by improving the lipid profile and reducing inflammation in apolipoprotein E-Deficient mice. Nutrients, 2018, 10(2): 142.

[3] Allahverdian S, Cheroudi A C, McManus B M, et al. Contribution of intimal smooth muscle cells to cholesterol accumulation and macrophage-like cells in human atherosclerosis. Circulation, 2014, 129(15) : 1551-1559.

[4] Faridi M H, Khan S Q, Zhao W, et al. CD11b activation suppresses TLR-dependent inflammation and autoimmunity in systemic lupus erythematosus. Journal of Clinical Investigation, 2017, 127(4): 1271-1283.

[5] Wong B W, Meredith A, Lin D, et al. The biological role of inflammation in atherosclerosis. Canadian Journal of Cardiology, 2012, 28(6): 631-641.

[6] Van Diepen J A, Berbée J F, Havekes L M, et al. Interactions between inflammation and lipid metabolism: relevance for efficacy of anti-inflammatory drugs in the treatment of atherosclerosis. Atherosclerosis, 2013, 228(2): 306-315.

[7] Ips F, Kka S, Samarakoon K W, et al. A fucoidan fraction purified from Chnoospora minima; a potential

inhibitor of LPS-induced inflammatory responses. International Journal of Biological Macromolecules, 2017, 104(Pt A): 1185-1193.

[8]　Kan J, Hood M, Burns C, et al. A novel combination of wheat peptides and fucoidan attenuates ethanol-induced gastric mucosal damage through anti-oxidant, anti-inflammatory, and pro-survival mechanisms. Nutrients, 2017, 9(9): 978.

[9]　Huang C Y, Kuo C H, Lee C H. Antibacterial and antioxidant capacities and attenuation of lipid accumulation in 3T3-L1 adipocytes by low-molecular-weight fucoidans prepared from compressional puffing pretreated sargassum crassifolium. Marine Drugs, 2018, 16(1).

[10]　Takahashi H, Kawaguchi M, Kitamura K, et al. An exploratory study on the anti-inflammatory effects of fucoidan in relation to quality of life in advanced cancer patients. Integrative Cancer Therapies, 2017, 17(2): 1534735417692097.

[11]　Juenet M, Aidlaunais R, Li B, et al. Thrombolytic therapy based on fucoidan-functionalized polymer nanoparticles targeting P-selectin. Biomaterials, 2018, 156: 204-216.

[12]　Fitton J H, Stringer D N, Karpiniec S S. Therapies from fucoidan: an update. Marine Drugs, 2015, 13(9): 5920-5946.

[13]　Wang X, Yi K, Zhao Y. Fucoidan inhibits amyloid-β-induced toxicity in transgenic Caenorhabditis elegans by reducing the accumulation of amyloid-β and decreasing the production of reactive oxygen species. Food & Function, 2017: 552-560.

[14]　Li J, Zhang Q, Li S, et al. The natural product fucoidan ameliorates hepatic ischemia-reperfusion injury in mice. Biomedicine & pharmacotherapy, 2017, 94: 687-696.

[15]　Lin H V, Tsou Y C, Chen Y T, et al. Effects of low-molecular-weight fucoidan and high stability fucoxanthin on glucose homeostasis, lipid metabolism, and liver function in a mouse model of type II diabetes. Marine Drugs, 2017, 15(4): 113.

[16]　Wang J, Zhang Q, Zhang Z, et al. Structural studies on a novel fucogalactan sulfate extracted from the brown seaweed Laminaria japonica. International Journal of Biological Macromolecules, 2010, 47(2): 126-131.

[17]　Xu Y, Zhang Q, Luo D, et al. Low molecular weight fucoidan ameliorates the inflammation and glomerular filtration function of diabetic nephropathy. Journal of Applied Phycology, 2016, 29(1): 1-12.

[18]　Li S, Liang J, Niimi M, et al. Probucol suppresses macrophage infiltration and MMP expression in atherosclerotic plaques of WHHL rabbits. Journal of Atherosclerosis & Thrombosis, 2014, 21(7): 648-658.

[19]　Peng N, Meng N, Wang S, et al. An activator of mTOR inhibits oxLDL-induced autophagy and apoptosis in vascular endothelial cells and restricts atherosclerosis in apolipoprotein E-/- mice. Sci Rep, 2014, 4(4): 5519.

[20]　Kim J H, Hong K W, Bae S S, et al. Probucol plus cilostazol attenuate hypercholesterolemia-induced exacerbation in ischemic brain injury via anti-inflammatory effects. International Journal of Molecular Medicine, 2014, 34(3): 687-694.

[21] Xu Y, Zhang Q, Luo D, et al. Low molecular weight fucoidan modulates P-selectin and alleviates diabetic nephropathy. International Journal of Biological Macromolecules, 2016, 91: 233-240.

[22] Pallebagegamarallage M M, Galloway S, Takechi R, et al. Probucol suppresses enterocytic accumulation of amyloid-β induced by saturated fat and cholesterol feeding. Lipids, 2012, 47(1): 27-34.

[23] Su X, Wang Y, Zhou G, et al. Probucol attenuates ethanol-induced liver fibrosis in rats by inhibiting oxidative stress, extracellular matrix protein accumulation and cytokine production. Clinical & Experimental Pharmacology & Physiology, 2014, 41(1): 73-80.

[24] Chudinova T V, Belekhova M G, Tostivint H, et al. Differences in parvalbumin and calbindin chemospecificity in the centers of the turtle ascending auditory pathway revealed by double immunofluorescence labeling. Brain Research, 2012, 1473(6): 87-103.

[25] Sacks F M, Jensen M K. From high-density lipoprotein cholesterol to measurements of function: prospects for the development of tests for high-density lipoprotein functionality in cardiovascular disease. Arteriosclerosis, thrombosis, and vascular biology, 2018, 38(3): 487-499.

[26] Moreira E L, Aguiar J A, De C C, et al. Effects of lifestyle modifications on cognitive impairments in a mouse model of hypercholesterolemia. Neuroscience Letters, 2013, 541(1): 193-198.

[27] Kasai T, Miyauchi K, Kubota N, et al. Probucol therapy improves long-term (>10-year) survival after complete revascularization: a propensity analysis. Atherosclerosis, 2012, 220(2): 463-469.

[28] Moon S M, Lee S A, Hong J H, et al. Oleamide suppresses inflammatory responses in LPS-induced RAW264.7 murine macrophages and alleviates paw edema in a carrageenan-induced inflammatory rat model. International Immunopharmacology, 2018, 56: 179-185.

[29] Hansson G K, Hermansson A. The immune system in atherosclerosis. Nature Immunology, 2011, 12(3): 204-212.

[30] Libby P. Inflammation in atherosclerosis. Nature. 2002, 420: 868.

[31] Roostalu U, Aldeiri B, Albertini A, et al. Distinct cellular mechanisms underlie smooth muscle turnover in vascular development and repair. Circulation Research, 2018, 122(2): 267-281.

[32] Subhi Y, Krogh Nielsen M, Molbech C R, et al. CD11b and CD200 on circulating monocytes differentiate two angiographic subtypes of polypoidal choroidal vasculopathy. Investigative Ophthalmology & Visual Science, 2017, 58(12) : 5242-5250.

Section 4　Words of TCM

1. 气为血帅 qi as the commander of blood
2. 血为气母 blood being the mother of qi
3. 离经之血 extravasation of blood
4. 气血之源 source of qi and blood
5. 血液亏虚 blood deficiency

6. 气滞血瘀 blood stasis due to qi stagnation

7. 寒凝气滞 qi stagnation due to cold

8. 腹痛拒按 unpalpable abdominal pain

9. 面色不华 lustreless comlexion

10. 脉细无力 thin and weak pulse

11. 强筋壮骨 body strengthening

12. 风热头痛 anemopyretic headache; headache due to pathogenic wind and cold

13. 肺虚咳嗽 pneumasthenic cough; cough because of asthenia of the lung

14. 外感风寒表证 exogenous exterior syndrome of wind-cold

15. 伤寒、肺炎 typhosis or typhoneumonia; pneumonia caused by typhoid

16. 伤寒毒素、毒血症、菌血症 typhotoxin, typhosepsis, typhemia

17. 骨度分寸 bone proportion cun; bone measurement

18. 手指同身寸 finger cun; finger measurement

19. 火针手法 needle-heated manipulation; manipulation of heating the needle

20. 通经活络 prescription for dredging meridians and activating collateral

21. 十八反 eighteen incompatible medicaments

22. 十九畏 nineteen medicaments of mutual antagonism

23. 十问 inquire about ten aspects of the patient

24. 十剂 ten kinds of prescription

25. 十二禁 twelve contraindications

26. 十二时 traditional twelve two-hour periods

27. 七方 seven prescriptions; seven formula

28. 七恶 the symptoms and signs indicating poor prognosis of suppurative infection of the exterior part

29. 七伤 seven kinds of impairments

30. 七冲门 seven important portals

31. 七日风 / 脐风 neonatal tetanus

32. 儿茶 catechu; black catechu; Catechu

33. 儿风 eclampsia

34. 儿枕痛 after-pains

35. 儿捧母心 breech presentation

36. 望神 spirit-inspecting

37. 望色 complexion-inspecting

38. 望形 build-inspecting

39. 望舌 tongue-inspecting

40. 望皮 skin-inspecting

(Xu Yingjie, Li Shan)

Chapter 11　Pain

Section 1　Pain and Aponia

Pain is a distressing feeling often caused by intense or damaging stimuli. The International Association for the Study of Pain's (IASP) widely used definition defines pain as an unpleasant sensory and emotional experience associated with actual or potential tissue damage, or described in terms of such damage; however, due to it being a complex, subjective phenomenon, defining pain has been a challenge. In medical diagnosis, pain is regarded as a symptom of an underlying condition.

Pain motivates the individual to withdraw from damaging situations, to protect a damaged body part while it heals, and to avoid similar experiences in the future. Most pain resolves once the noxious stimulus is removed and the body has healed, but it may persist despite removal of the stimulus and apparent healing of the body. Sometimes pain arises in the absence of any detectable stimulus, damage or disease.

Pain is the most common reason for physician consultation in most developed countries. It is a major symptom in many medical conditions, and can interfere with a person's quality of life and general functioning. Simple pain medications are useful in 20% ~ 70% of cases. Psychological factors such as social support, hypnotic suggestion, excitement, or distraction can significantly affect pain's intensity or unpleasantness. In some debates regarding physician assisted suicide or euthanasia, pain has been used as an argument to permit people who are terminally ill to end their lives.

Classification: In 1994, responding to the need for a more useful system for describing chronic pain, the IASP classified pain according to specific characteristics: (1) region of the body involved (e.g. abdomen, lower limbs), (2) system whose dysfunction may be causing the pain (e.g., nervous, gastrointestinal), (3) duration and pattern of occurrence, (4) intensity and time since onset, and (5) cause. However, this system has been criticized by Clifford J. Woolf and others as inadequate for guiding research and treatment. Woolf suggests three classes of pain: (1) nociceptive pain, (2) inflammatory pain which is associated with tissue damage and the infiltration of immune cells, and (3) pathological pain which is a disease state caused by damage to the nervous system or by its abnormal function (e.g. fibromyalgia, peripheral neuropathy, tension type headache, etc.).

Duration: Pain is usually transitory, lasting only until the noxious stimulus is removed or the underlying damage or pathology has healed, but some painful conditions, such as rheumatoid arthritis, peripheral neuropathy, cancer and idiopathic pain, may persist for years. Pain that lasts a long time is called chronic or persistent, and pain that resolves quickly is called acute. Traditionally, the distinction between acute and chronic pain has relied upon an arbitrary interval of time from onset; the two most commonly used markers being 3 months and 6 months since the onset of pain, though some theorists and researchers have placed the transition from acute to chronic pain at 12 months. Others apply acute to pain that lasts less than 30 days, chronic to pain of more than 6 months' duration, and subacute to pain that lasts 1 ~ 6 months. A popular alternative definition of chronic pain, involving no arbitrarily fixed duration, is pain that extends beyond the expected period of healing. Chronic pain may be classified as cancer pain or else as benign.

Nociceptive pain is caused by stimulation of sensory nerve fibers that respond to stimuli approaching or exceeding harmful intensity (nociceptors), and may be classified according to the mode of noxious stimulation. The most common categories are thermal (e.g. heat or cold), mechanical (e.g. crushing, tearing, shearing, etc.) and chemical (e.g. iodine in a cut or chemicals released during inflammation). Some nociceptors respond to more than one of these modalities and are consequently designated polymodal.

Nociceptive pain may also be divided into visceral, deep somatic and superficial somatic pain. Visceral structures are highly sensitive to stretch, ischemia and inflammation, but relatively insensitive to other stimuli that normally evoke pain in other structures, such as burning and cutting. Visceral pain is diffuse, difficult to locate and is often referred to a distant, usually superficial, structure. It may be accompanied by nausea and vomiting and may be described as sickening, deep, squeezing, and dull. Deep somatic pain is initiated by stimulation of nociceptors in ligaments, tendons, bones, blood vessels, fasciae and muscles, and is dull, aching, poorly-localized pain. Examples include sprains and broken bones. Superficial pain is initiated by activation of nociceptors in the skin or other superficial tissue, and is sharp, well-defined and clearly located. Examples of injuries that produce superficial somatic pain include minor wounds and minor (first degree) burns.

There are people in the world with an ability not feeling pain when they are hurting, breaking legs or giving birth. But a person unable to feel physical pain can be in danger and not know it. Last year, the magazine *Nature* published a report about 6 children with aponia, who have never suffered pain. The 6 children who apparently felt no pain come from three families from northern Pakistan. These children were 6 ~ 14 years of age. They sometimes burned themselves with hot liquids or steam. They sat on hot heating devices. They cut their lips with their teeth, but felt no pain. Two of the children bit off 1/3 of their tongue. Yet they could feel pressure and tell differences between hot and cold. A boy stood on burning coals and stabbed his arms with knives to earn money. Unfortunately, he died in a fall before the researchers could meet him.

Scientists studied deoxyribonucleic acid (DNA) from the children and the children's parents. They found that all had a gene with a mistake, or fault. Except of the genetic fault, the children had normal intelligence and health. The researchers found that each child received a faulty version of the gene from a parent. The gene is called SCN9A which gives orders to a protein that serves as a passageway for the chemical sodium. All nerve cells have such passages and this is how pain signals from a wound or injury are communicated to the myelon, or spinal cord, and brain. Two years ago, investigators discovered something important about SCN9A. They linked it to a rare condition in which patients suffered painful burning in their feet or hands. The problems of these patients were nearly opposite to those of the children who felt no pain. In patients with the burning hands and feet, SCN9A was too active. The findings may mean better medical help for pain and could happen if medicine can be developed to control the faulty gene. That would be welcome news to people whose pain resists current medicines.

Many American believe they are suffering more pain now than in earlier years. About 25% of American adults said they had a full day of pain in the month before they were questioned, 10% were more deeply affected and their pain continued for a year or more. Pain is rarely considered as a separate condition and the costs linked to pain overload the health care system.

Lower back pain was a big problem. More than 25% of adults who were asked said they had lower back pain in the past three months. Painful knees caused the most trouble of the body's joints. But some victims of knee pain did something about it. They had operations to replace the painful joint with man-made or artificial knees. Since 1992, rates of hospital stays for knee replacement rose almost 90% among older Americans of 65 years of age or older.

About 15% of adults suffered a migraine or other severe headache which affected young people three times as much as older adults in the past three months. Severe arthralgia, or joint pain, increased with age and women had painful joints more often than man.

The study showed that painful conditions caused use of narcotic drugs. Narcotics can be strong pain killers. The study compared 2 periods of which one lasted 6 years and ended in 1994, and the other began in 1999 and ended 4 years ago. Between those periods, the percentage of adults who said they used a narcotic for pain in the past month rose from 3% to 4%.

Opiates include morphine, codeine and methadone. Most of these drugs come from the poppy flower and have been used to treat pain for more than 2000 years. A new drug, oxycodone, called an opioid similar to an opiate has been used to control moderate to severe pain over a long period. For example, a woman with a painful back was in severe pain much of the time until the doctor ordered a form of oxycodone. She still has pain at some times of days now, but able to work at home and take part in at least some of the activities she loves.

Many doctors order, or prescribe, narcotic drugs for patients with continuing severe pain. Narcotic drugs may help to decrease pain, but can make many people sleepy. They also can be addictive and need increasing amounts to get the same effect. Some doctors have prescribed more narcotic drugs than are medically necessary. Doctors face possible arrest and jail sentences if they knowingly order narcotics for other than medical reasons.

Non-medical use of oxycodone and similar drugs has killed many Americans. Some people break them up and mix them with other drugs. Recently, the Centers for Disease Control and Prevention reported an increase in the number of accidental deaths from prescription drugs. The number increased more than 60% between 1999 and 2004. That made accidental drug poisoning the second largest cause of accidental death in the United States. Only traffic accidents rated higher. Clearly, strong painkillers can be dangerous, but many patients need them. To meet this need, some doctors and hospitals today provide special services for such patients. For example, some doctors offer advice and treatment for several kinds of pain.

The research into pain still continues around the world. Recently, a study suggested that women feel pain more than men. They found that women also feel pain in more body areas than men, and women suffer pain more often and for longer periods than men. In the study, several people at University of Bath held one arm in warm water and then put the arm in icy cold water. Both men and women were told to think about the physical nature of the pain. They did not think about their emotional reactions to it. Using this psychological trick, men said they felt less pain than women.

There are many explanations of these differences depend on genetic and hormonal influences. But the psychological and social reasons also are important. It is never fair to say someone is making too much of their pain, but no one can ever know what other people are feeling.

Section 2 Family and Friends

Sometimes family members are the first to learn of a loved one's cancer diagnosis. How does a family decide when or if to tell them? Should they be told? Are some people too emotionally fragile, too young, or too old? While most people can handle the news of a cancer diagnosis, each person takes a different amount of time to adjust and figure out what their diagnosis means to them.

If you are a family member trying to decide if you should tell a loved one they have cancer, consider this. You may think you are sparing them bad news, but they will sense something is wrong when they have many tests and/or don't feel well. Resentment can result when family members keep the diagnosis a secret from the person with cancer. Although you may think you are protecting the person with cancer, that person now might see this as dishonest. When people with cancer are not told about their diagnosis, they are unable to make important decisions about their treatment and their life. There may be things they want to do, personal matters they want to take care of, and legal papers that may need to be updated. Even when a person has a cancer with a good outlook, families need to discuss decisions about end-of-life care, including advance directives such as living wills and durable power of attorney for health care.

Often before one can express feelings, he or she must sort them out. Friends and family members may feel like scapegoats when their loved ones try to vent their feelings. If you are the target of anger and frustration, remember you are not the cause of this anger. The person is angry about the cancer and how it has affected his or her life. Even though family members and friends try to respond with love and friendship, it is natural to feel their own anger and frustration, and sometimes express it. Because they often have more responsibilities while handling many different emotions, families also have a difficult time adjusting to a diagnosis of cancer. Family members have to cope with their own emotions while also being sensitive to the needs of the person who has cancer. If the person with cancer feels the need to talk before others in the family are ready, you could say something such as "I am here when you are ready to talk". Your presence is also away to show your support for the person with cancer. Families and friends often try to raise a person's spirits by saying "Everything will be all right". But people with cancer and their families know everything is far from all right and might wonder if things will ever return to normal. Families and friends are also experiencing many different feelings, and they also need a way to share them. Being honest about these feelings can allow everyone to work through difficult times and enjoy the good days together.

Family and friends may struggle to find the right or proper words to say to someone who has been diagnosed with cancer. There is no right way to act or perfect words to say. Just listening to the person with cancer is often more helpful than talking. Reassuring them of your love and support is one of the most important things you can do for them. Most people with cancer do not want to face the experience alone and will need support from their family and friends. "I'm here for you" are the best words you can say to show your support for someone with cancer. But not everyone with cancer wants to talk about his or her feelings. They may have other ways to express their emotions, such as writing in a journal, or they may prefer to keep their feelings private. People with cancer might just want you to help them maintain their "normal" routine. Just be yourself and continue to do things with them just as you would if they didn't have cancer. Sometimes this isn't possible, but if you continue to spend time with them, they may change their mind and talk with you about their feelings.

For example, Sean, cancer survivor: I did not like to talk about my cancer with my friends or my family. I just wanted to get it over with. My oncologist had one of his patients who were diagnosed with testicular cancer a few years ago call me. He had the same treatment I received and was my age so we could easily communicate. He told me it would be a tough 6 months but I would get through it. Knowing that he made it through the same treatment was helpful.

The changes in the family: A diagnosis of cancer changes a family forever. Figuring out "what's for dinner" or "what your plans are for the weekend" is suddenly less important. Family and personal values are questioned and priorities are tested. Unsettled feelings and arguments may resurface during a family's struggle with cancer. Often a family must sort out and revisit old, unresolved feelings before they can start to battle with cancer as a family. Cancer can cause role changes in the family. The head of the household may now be more dependent on other family members. Others may need to work outside the home or work different hours to accommodate changes in the household. When family members take on new roles, the way they interact within the family can change. New responsibilities may overwhelm some family members. Parents might look to their children for support. If the children are old enough, they may be asked to take on more responsibilities within the household. These requests often come when children themselves need support. The behavior of younger children might regress in response to the stress on the family. This is their way of dealing with cancer and how it has changed their family. Adolescents who at this age are often rebelling and spending more time with friends may instead cling to their families for support. As a friend or family member helping to take care of the patient, you also have needs. Taking care of yourself will allow you to be able to care for others. When your needs are met the patient will also benefit. Overdoing is different from doing. Know your limits and rest when you need to. This rule applies to both caregivers and patients.

Often families find themselves treating the person like an invalid even when the person is fully capable of doing for himself or herself. Sometimes people will not want you to help them with activities such as bathing and dressing. These wishes should be respected if at all possible. While the patient may object to getting outside help, friends and family members should look at their own limits and get outside help when necessary. Certified nursing assistants, home health aides, and other resources can help with the care of the patient. Local churches may be able to help with cooking, shopping, transportation, and general housekeeping. Professional services may also be helpful although there usually is a fee involved.

Coping within the family: How a family handles cancer is greatly determined by how the family has dealt with crises in the past. Those who are used to communicating effectively and sharing feelings are usually able to discuss how cancer is affecting them. Families who solve their problems as individuals instead of a team might have greater difficulty coping with cancer. Cancer treatment includes care for the patient and the family not just the cancer. A mental health professional may already be a part of your cancer care team. If not, talk with your doctor or nurse to learn about additional resources that can help you cope with cancer in your family. Some family members have said they have avoided the family member with cancer because they felt as if they had nothing to offer, didn't know how to act, or felt they could do nothing to help make the situation better. Family and friends can find ways to relieve their stress by participating in activities outside the home. Resources outside the home, such as individual counseling or support groups, can serve as outlets for the frustrations you are facing within your family.

Section 3   Research Article

A new way: alleviating postembolization syndrome following transcatheter arterial chemoembolization

[Abstract] Background: Currently, most therapies of postembolization syndrome following transcatheter arterial chemoembolization (TACE) aim directly at a single symptom, thus leading to limitations. Objectives: To seek for a systematic approach to prevent and treat the syndrome, we carried out this study to observe the effect of ginsenosides (GS) and dexamethasone (Dex) in alleviating the postembolization syndrome following TACE. Methods: In the randomized, double-blinded and controlled trial, 120 patients with primary liver cancer were divided into 4 groups, with 30 patients in each group. The changes of clinical symptoms and laboratory tests before TACE and on the 3rd and 7th day respectively after TACE were observed. Results: The results indicated that Dex combined with GS not only markedly decreased the occurrence ratio and duration of such symptoms as nausea, vomiting, and fever, but also significantly reduced levels of total bilirubin, glutamic oxaloacetic transaminase, and glutamic-pyruvic transaminase (AST) and improved the Child-Pugh stage of liver function as compared with single use of GS or Dex. Conclusions: In conclusion, although single use of Dex or GS may improve some indices of adverse effects after TACE, the combination of Dex and GS can systematically prevent and treat the postembolization syndrome following TACE.

1   Introduction

Transcatheter arterial chemoembolization (TACE) is an effective treatment in advanced liver cancer and unresectable hepatocellular carcinoma[1-5]. However, the treatment usually leads to the occurrence of postembolization syndrome such as fever, nausea and vomiting, hepatalgia, and liver function impairment, which is mainly due to the toxicities of chemotherapeutic and embolic agents, the presence of stress responses, and underlying liver diseases. These symptoms often occur simultaneously and last for $1 \sim 2$ weeks. Patients do not need to be treated temporarily when the symptoms are mild, but in the setting of moderate to severe symptoms that have not been treated promptly, great effects on the prognosis and quality of life in patients will occur. Although antipyretic analgesics, antiemetics, and cytoprotection agents may relieve these symptoms[6], the combination of too many drugs will exacerbate the metabolic load of the liver. In addition, all these drugs aim directly at a single symptom after surgery and are single-targeted, thus not producing the systematic effects in preventing and treating the syndrome. To seek a systematic approach to preventing and treating the postembolization syndrome, we first proposed the combined drug strategy with ginsenosides (GS) and dexamethasone (Dex) in clinical practice, based on pharmacologic knowledge of traditional and Western medicine. Our study is a randomized, double-blinded, controlled trial to test the efficacy of GS combined with Dex in the treatment of post- embolization syndrome after TACE.

2 Patients and Methods

2.1 Enrollment criteria

According to clinical diagnostic criteria for primary liver cancer established in the Eighth National Liver Cancer Congress of the Society of Liver Cancer of the Chinese Anti-Cancer Association[7], patients with primary liver cancer were admitted to the Department of Traditional Medicine in Changhai Hospital in Shanghai between June 2004 and June 2007. According to the results of a preliminary test of this research, 28 patients were required for each study group. To compensate for nonevaluable patients, we planned to enroll 30 patients per group. The patients undergoing TACE were those in whom liver cancer had not been resected completely or recurred after surgery or was considered unresectable and those who were reluctant to receive surgery. In addition, they had to meet the following conditions: (1) suffused or multiple nodular liver cancer, (2) total bilirubin level < 50 mmol/L, (3) no tumor thrombi in portal vein, (4) ratio of liver tumor volume to entire volume < 70%, and (5) no upper gastrointestinal bleeding in the past 6 months. The exclusion criteria included the following: (1) not meeting the inclusion criteria above, (2) PT time exceeding normal control value beyond 5 seconds, (3) noncontrollable ascites, (4) leukocyte count < 3.0×10^9 and platelet count < 30×10^9, (5) Child-Pugh C stage, (6) extrahepatic metastasis, (7) arteriovenous fistula, (8) use of glucocorticoids (GCs) or GS in the past 3 months, (9) combined medication that affected the indices observed during the trial, and (10) patients who were not treated according to regulations in the setting of informed consent so that the efficacy was difficult to assess and patients whose information was not complete and the judgment of efficacy was affected. According to the inclusion and exclusion criteria, 120 patients were enrolled into this clinical trial eventually and completed the trial. The trial was given ethical approval by the Ethics Committee of Changhai Hospital in Shanghai according to the requirements of the country. At trial enrollment, informed consent was obtained from all patients prior to trial entry.

2.2   Randomization

The randomization code was prepared using computer generated random numbers by Dr. Zhai Xiaofeng. The trial code was held in the trial center. Every eligible participant obtained a code from the medical officer of the center before admission to the treatment groups, and the information was then given to the Pharmacy Department at Changhai Hospital. The details of the assignment and administration were unknown to any of the investigators or to the coordinator. All study personnel and participants were blinded to treatment assignment for the duration of the study. Only the study statisticians and the Data Monitoring Committee saw unblinded data, but none had any contact with study participants. To evaluate patient blinding, the questionnaire asked patients to evaluate which treatment they believed they had received (Dex, GS, Dex_GS, placebo, or don't know) at the 6th day. If patients answered either drugs or placebo, they were asked to indicate what led to that belief. At the end of the trial, 19% of the Dex recipients, 13% of the GS recipients, 21% of the Dex_GS recipients, and 11% of the placebo recipients correctly identified their group assignment ($P < 0.05$). The ability of participants to accurately guess their group assignment was no better than chance. Although insomnia and face flushing due to Dex may offer strong clues as to which intervention was received, the clinical outcome may also provide clues. The result means that blinding was successful.

2.3   Interventions

TACE. Chemoembolization procedures on all patients were performed by one group of doctors in the Department of Radiological Technology, at the Second Military Medicine University. The TACE procedure was modeled after the original HAE procedure of Chuang et al.[8] and modified by Coldwell et al.[9-10]. Via a transfemoral approach using the Seldinger technique[11], celiac and superior mesenteric arteriograms were performed with iohexol (Omnipaque; GE Healthcare, Princeton, NJ) 15 mL, to ascertain any variant arterial visceral anatomy and document portal vein patency. Coaxially through the selective catheter, a 16-F microcatheter was placed into the right or left hepatic artery trunk, where another arteriogram was performed to precisely delineate the distribution of all the vessels feeding the tumor and to determine optimal placement of the microcatheter tip for embolization. When the catheter was within the origin of the artery, 500 mg 5-fluorouracil, 20 mg epirubicin, 10 mg hydroxycamptothecin, and 10 ~ 20 mL ultrafluid lipiodol were infused slowly. The process lasted for about 20 minutes. Each patient was admitted to the hospital after the completion of the procedure.

Medication. Drugs were initially administered on 3 days before TACE and were withdrawn on 4 days after TACE in all groups. The course of treatment was 6 days. Group A: Patients were treated with oral placebo capsule (essential component was starch) twice a day. Group B: Patients were treated with one Dex capsule (2.25 mg Dex per pill) and one placebo capsule twice a day. Group C: Patients were treated with one GS capsule (200 mg GS per pill) and one placebo capsule twice a day. Group D: Patients were treated with one Dex capsule and one GS capsule twice a day. The drugs were given after breakfast and after supper, respectively. The Department of Chinese Drugs Preparation in Changhai Hospital of the Second Military Medical University supplied placebo capsule. Dex was purchased from Shanghai Shenyi Pharmaceuticals Company (Chongqing, China) and the batch number was 0707. GS capsules were purchased from Chongqing Dongya Medicine Co. Ltd. and the batch number was H50021734. The plant material was refluxed in 50% alcohol solution 3 times, 1.5 hour each time. The percentage of GS is about 90.3%. All these drugs bore the same appearance. In addition, the history of medication was identical in all patients. If adverse effects Ⅲ degree or higher occurred during the observation period, the same drugs were given to treat the symptoms routinely.

2.4   Clinical assessment

Such symptoms as nausea and vomiting, fever, and hepatalgia were observed from before surgery to one week after surgery. Liver function including total bilirubin (TB) level, the ratio of glutamic oxalacetic transaminase (ALT) to glutamic-pyruvic transaminase (AST), and alkaline phosphatase (AKP) level was performed before surgery, and on the 3rd and 7th day after surgery, respectively. The efficacy was assessed according to World Health Organization grading criteria on toxicities of anti-tumor drugs[12], and the Child-Pugh stages of liver function were achieved as well.

2.5   Statistical analysis

All data analysis was carried out according to a pre-established analysis plan. Analysis was performed using SPSS 11.0 (SPSS Inc., Chicago, IL). P values (0.05) were considered statistically significant for all tests. Enumeration data were analyzed through the analysis of variance; ranked data were analyzed through rank sum test. The comparison of numeration data was calculated using the analysis of variance test.

3 Results

All the participants completed the trial; the effect size was 30 per group. The baseline demographic and clinical characteristics are listed in Table 11-1. The results of the trial are summarized as follows.

Table 11-1 Demographic data of these patients

Group	n	Sex male	Sex female	Age / years	TNM Staging / % Ⅱ	TNM Staging / % Ⅲ
A	30	21	9	56.21 ± 12.42	22（73.3）	8（26.7）
B	30	25	5	51.45 ± 10.23	26（86.7）	4（13.3）
C	30	24	6	53.71 ± 11.92	25（83.3）	5（16.7）
D	30	22	8	57.67 ± 12.95	24（80.0）	6（20.0）

3.1 Degrees of adverse effects after TACE in each group

Different degrees of nausea and vomiting, fever, and hepatalgia occurred in 4 groups. The results of group comparison are as follows. Nausea and vomiting: The significant differences were observed between 4 groups ($P < 0.05$). The incidence of nausea and vomiting was 20% and 13.3% in group B and group D, respectively, which was markedly lower than that in group A (80%, $P < 0.01$). There were no significant differences between other groups (Figure 11-1). Fever: The incidence of fever was 26.7% and 20% in group B and group D, respectively, which was markedly lower than that in group A (70%, $P < 0.05$). No significant differences were seen between other groups, and fever of grade Ⅲ or higher did not occur in all groups (Figure 11-2). Pain: The incidence of pain was 40%, 30%, and 20% in group B, group C, and group D, respectively, which was markedly lower than that in group A (80%, $P < 0.01$). No significant differences were observed between group B, group C, and group D (Figure 11-3).

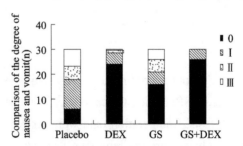

Figure 11-1　Comparison of nausea and vomiting degree between groups

The efficacy in Dex group and combined drug group is better than that in control group. 0 degree means no occurrence of nausea and vomiting; Ⅰ degree means the occurrence of nausea and vomiting; Ⅱ degree means transient vomiting and Ⅲ degree means vomiting that should be treated.

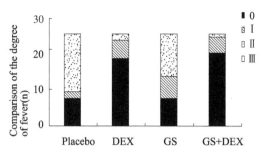

Figure 11-2 Comparison of fever degree between groups

The efficacy in Dex group and combined drug group is better than that in control group. 0 degree means no occurrence of fever; I degree means body temperature < 38 ℃ ; II degree means body temperature of 38 ~ 40 ℃ and III degree means body temperature > 40 ℃ .

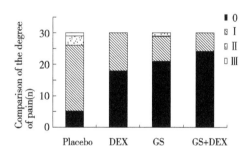

Figure 11-3 Comparison of hepatalgia degree between groups

The efficacy in single drug group and combined drug group are better than that in control group. 0 degree means no occurrence of hepatalgia; I degree is mild hepatalgia; II degree is moderate hepatalgia and III degree is severe hepatalgia.

3.2 Lasting time of clinical symptoms and signs after TACE in each group

The lasting time of nausea and vomiting was (1.29 ± 0.24) days and (1.02 ± 0.10) days in group B and group D, respectively, which was shorter than that in group A (2.56 ± 0.39) days. There were no significant differences between other groups.

The lasting time of fever was (1.78 ± 0.35) days and (1.13 ± 0.19) days in group B and group D, respectively, which was shorter than that in group A (4.40 ± 0.48) days. There were no significant differences between other groups.

The lasting time of pain was (1.58 ± 0.22) days, (1.86 ± 0.31) days, and (1.33 ± 0.20) days in group B, group C, and group D, respectively, which was lower than that in group A (5.15 ± 0.50) days. No significant differences were observed between group B, group C, and group D (Figure 11-4).

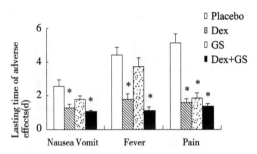

Figure 11-4　Lasting time of adverse effects after TACE in each group

3.3 Liver function before and after TACE in each group

TB level and ALT/AST ratio before and after TACE within each group: TB level and ALT/ AST ratio increased markedly after surgery compared with before surgery in group A, group B, and group C, and there were significant differences ($P < 0.05$). No significant change in the ratio was seen after surgery compared with before surgery in group D.

TB level and ALT/AST ratio before and after TACE between groups: On the 3rd day after surgery, the TB level in group D was markedly lower than that in group A, group B, and group C ($P < 0.05$). At the 7th day after surgery, the TB level in group D was still lower than that in other groups, but there were no significant differences.

There were no significant differences in AKP levels after surgery compared with before surgery in 4 groups ($P < 0.05$, Table 11-2).

Table 11-2　Comparison of liver function before and after the treatment in each group

Group	t/d	TB				AST / ALT				AKP			
		0	I	II	III	0	I	II	III	0	I	II	III
A	−3	27	2	1	0	26	3	1	0	27	3	0	0
	3	15	8	4	3	14	6	5	5	23	4	2	1
	7	20	8	2	0	21	7	1	1	24	4	2	0
B	−3	26	4	0	0	27	3	0	0	26	4	0	0
	3	16	6	6	2	15	7	4	4	24	3	3	0
	7	22	5	3	0	20	7	2	1	27	3	0	0
C	−3	29	1	0	0	29	1	0	0	28	2	0	0
	3	16	7	4	3	16	6	4	4	25	3	2	0
	7	23	5	2	0	21	6	3	0	25	4	1	0
D	−3	28	0	2	0	27	3	0	0	28	2	0	0
	3	25	4	1	0	26	3	1	0	27	1	1	1
	7	28	1	1	0	26	4	0	0	28	1	1	0

Combination of GS and Dex can reduce TB level and AST/ALT ratio after operation.

TB, AST/ALT, AKP: 0 degree $\leqslant 1.25 \times$ N; I degree $(1.26 \sim 2.5) \times$ N; II degree $(2.6 \sim 5) \times$ N; III degree $(5.1 \sim 10) \times$ N. N is the upline of the normal.

Stages of Child-Pugh before and after TACE within each group: There were significant differences in liver function stage in group A ($P < 0.05$). Although changes in stages of liver function were seen in group B, group C, and group D, there was no statistical significance ($P > 0.05$). Stages of Child-Pugh before and after TACE between groups: On the 3rd day after surgery, liver function impairment in group D was significantly milder than that in group A ($P < 0.05$). No significant differences were seen between other groups. There were no significant differences in the Child-Pugh stage on the 7th day after surgery compared with before surgery in each group. Pooled effects of GS and Dex are shown in Table 11-3.

Table 11-3   Pooled effects of GS and Dex

Index	Dex	GS	Dex + GS
Nausea/vomiting	√	—	√
Fever	√	—	√
Hepatalgia	√	√	√
TB	—	—	√
AST/ALT	—	—	√
Child-Pugh grade	—	—	√

Single use of Dex can alleviate such symptoms as nausea and vomiting, fever and pain, and decrease the occurrence of reduction of leucocyte and platelet. Single use of GS can alleviate the hepatalgia following intervention. Combination of Dex and GS can not only improve these symptoms above, but also prevent and treat the elevation of total bilirubin level and AST/ALT ratio effectively and protect liver function. √: effective; — : ineffective.

4　Discussion

In recent years, TACE has been generally applied as the first choice for treating liver cancer without surgical indications and preventing the recurrence of liver cancer after surgery[13-14]. The procedure is performed by selectively blocking the hepatic artery that supplies blood for tumor and infusing chemotherapeutics to achieve the goal of tumor necrosis and shrinkage. In clinical practice, postembolization syndrome is a common condition after TACE. The pathogenesis of the syndrome is complicated. The main aspects are as follows: (1) lipiodol-induced embolism may result in ischemia, hypoxia, and necrosis in some normal hepatic cells; (2) chemotherapeutic drugs have toxicities in themselves[15]; (3) the procedure itself can lead to considerable releasing of inflammatory factors[16]; (4) such stimuli as injury and drugs can contribute to stress responses in the human body. Up to now, there has not been a drug that can improve the postembolization syndrome effectively. Thus, it is of great importance to seek for an approach to improve the syndrome systematically.

The role that the typical GC Dex plays has been well known, with powerful antistress and anti-inflammatory actions. Dex can not only stabilize the lysosomal membrane and reduce cellular necrosis, but also inhibit the releasing of inflammatory mediators and participate in blood vessel endothelium inflammatory response and repair of injury[17-18]. Furthermore, Dex plays a role in the cerebral vomiting center and perceptual areas through cortical conduction[19].

Traditional Chinese Medicine ginseng has an effect of regulating qi, nourishing blood, and developing vital qi, with GS being the essential active component. It has been confirmed by modern pharmacologic studies that GS also has antistress and anti-inflammatory actions[20] as well as analgesic and sedative effects[21]. It can strengthen immunity, enhance T cell function[22-23] and protect cells from cisplatin (Platinol; Bristol Myers-Squibb, Princeton, NJ) intoxication[24]. These pharmacologic actions are in accordance with the pathogenesis of postembolization syndrome mainly following TACE. Therefore, we hypothesized that the combination of GS and Dex would prevent and treat postembolization syndrome more effectively.

Our study has shown that GS combined with Dex is equally effective with respect to controlling nausea, vomiting, and fever, shortening the lasting time of symptoms, and relieving myelosuppression. Single use of GS or Dex or their combination can bring about a better outcome than placebo with respect to improving hepatalgia degree and duration. However, combined use does not produce an obviously cumulative effect, suggesting there is a common pathway. These results indicate that the two drugs may produce analgesic effects by means of their own pathway. These results correspond completely with the pharmacological actions of Dex and GS mentioned above. Interestingly, GS combined with Dex can effectively prevent the elevation of TB level and ALT/AST ratio after TACE and improve the Child-Pugh stage, but single use does not result in a satisfactory outcome, suggesting that Dex and GS may produce synergistic effects in protecting liver function after surgery.

In view of the results above, single use of GS or Dex can prevent and treat some symptoms or improve some indices by means of their own pharmacologic effects after TACE. However, combination of GS and Dex can effectively improve the clinical symptom and protect liver function after TACE. Our study showed that the combination of GS and Dex can prevent and treat the postembolization syndrome more systematically.

Based on these results, we have preliminarily investigated the mechanisms of Dex combined with GS in preventing and treating postembolization syndrome. GC can play its biologic roles by binding with glucocorticoid receptor (GR) that resides in the cytoplasm. Then the GR and GC complex entered the cytoblast to initiate the GC-dependent gene network selectively[25]. Under the stress states, the secretion of corticosteroids increases while the GR level and its binding capacity decrease significantly[26-28]. Although the GC level is very high in vivo, the actual amount that can bind with GR to form ligand-receptor complex is very limited, thus leading to the fact that GCs cannot exhibit their biologic effects fully. If there is a drug that may up-regulate GR level or inhibit the down-regulation of GR induced by GC, can the combination of the two drugs produce synergistic effects to enhance the ability of anti-inflammation and anti-stress? Recent studies have demonstrated that GS is strongly associated with GR[29]. Although some GS monomers can down-regulate GR level[30-31] our research has discovered that GS may increase Dex-induced transcription of GR gene in the HL-7702 cell and partially reverse the inhibition of GR expression and binding capacity caused by Dex[32]. The experiments in vivo also have confirmed that GS can up-regulate GR level and combinative ability of GR in rats with heat injury. We supposed that GS increases the GR mRNA level and combinative ability of GR after stress stimuli, and that the synergistic effects of GS and GC are one of the mechanisms of their combination in preventing and treating the postembolization syndrome effectively. Unavoidably, we should take into account limitations of the study when analyzing the results. The experience of runners for TACE has particular importance to the results. In order to minimize the effect, all patients in 4 groups were accepted for TACE by the same group of doctors in the Department of Radiological Technology. In addition, the results in our study only refer to primary liver cancer. Many patients with metastasis in the liver underwent TACE that would have excluded them from the current study. Consequently, the results of this study do not address the occurrence of rare adverse events, nor can they be extrapolated to all patients seen in general clinical practice.

Because few studies about the treatment of postembolization syndrome have been published, it is difficult to compare these results with other relevant findings. In this trial, we have found that the combined drug strategy with GS and Dex can improve the postembolization syndrome markedly, but there is still a long way to go to draw the conclusion that GS could enhance the effect of GC. Further prospective studies should be performed to investigate several diseases that are treated with GC, such as systemic lupus erythematosus, dropsical nephritis, asthma, and so on. Only when all these trials present positive results could we more firmly say, "GS is a synergist of GC."

5   Conclusions

GS combined with Dex has an important role in the treatment of patients with post-embolization syndrome following TACE, based on this randomized controlled clinical trial.

Acknowledgement

This study was supported by E-institutes of Shanghai Municipal Education commission (E03008) and National Natural Science Foundation of China (30701132).

Disclosure Statement

No competing financial interests exist.

References

[1] Gay F. A comparison of lipiodol chemoembolization and conservative treatment for unresectable hepatocellular carcinoma. N Engl J Med, 1995, 332(19): 1256-1261.

[2] Vetter D, Wenger J J, Bergier J M, et al. Transcatheter oily chemoembolization in the management of advanced hepa-tocellular carcinoma in cirrhosis: results of a Western comparative study in 60 patients. Hepatology, 1991, 13: 427-433.

[3] Pelletier G, Roche A, Ink O, et al. A randomized trial of hepatic arterial chemoembolization in patients with unresectable hepatocellular carcinoma. Journal of Hepatology, 1990, 11(2): 181-184.

[4] Takayasu K, Arii S, Ikai I, et al. Prospective cohort study of transarterial chemoembolization for unresectable hepatocellular carcinoma in 8510 patients. Gastroenterology, 2006, 131(2): 461-469.

[5] Huang Y S, Chiang J H, Wu J C, et al. Risk of hepatic failure after transcatheter arterial chemoembolization for hepatocellular carcinoma: predictive value of the monoethylglycinexylidide test. American Journal of Gastroenterology, 2002, 97(5): 1223-1227.

[6] Miller A B, Hoogstraten B, Staquet M, et al. Reporting results of cancer treatment. Cancer, 1981, 47(1): 207-214.

[7] Society of Liver Cancer of Chinese Anti-Cancer Association. Clinical diagnosis and staging criteria for primary liver cancer. Chin J Hepatol, 2001, 9: 324.

[8] Chuang V P, Wallace S, Soo C S, et al. Therapeutic Ivalon embolization of hepatic tumors. Ajr Am J Roentgenol, 1982, 138(2): 289-294.

[9] Coldwell D M, Mortimer J E. Hepatic artery embolization in the treatment of hepatic malignancies. Researchgate, 1991, 3: 298-301.

[10] Coldwell DM, Mortimer J E. Transcatheter therapy for malignant neoplasms. West J Med, 1999, 151: 299-303.

[11] Seldinger S I. Catheter replacement of the needle in percutaneous arteriography. Acta Radiol Suppl, 2008, 434(5): 47-52.

[12] Zhou J C. Practice of Medical Oncology. Beijing: People's Medical Publishing House, 2003: 424.

[13] Mondazzi L, Bottelli R, Brambilla G, et al. Transarterial oily chemoembolization for the treatment of

hepatocellular carcinoma: a multivariate analysis of prognostic factors. Hepatology, 1994, 19(5): 1115-1123.

[14]   Jansen M C, Hillegersberg R V, Chamuleau R A F M, et al. Outcome of regional and local ablative therapies for hepatocellular carcinoma: a collective review. European Journal of Surgical Oncology, 2005, 31(4): 331-347.

[15]   Nagano M, Nakamura T, Niimi S, et al. Substitution of arginine for cysteine 643 of the glucocorticoid receptor reduces its steroid-binding affinity and transcriptional activity. Cancer Lett, 2002, 181: 109-114.

[16]   Distelhorst C W. Recent insights into the mechanism of glucocorticosteroid-induced apoptosis. Cell Death Differ, 2002, 9: 6-19.

[17]   Oberleithner H, Riethmuller C, Ludwig T, et al. Differential action of steroid hormones on human endothelium. Journal of Cell Science, 2006, 119(Pt 9): 1926-1932.

[18]   Tombrantink J, Lara N, Apricio S E, et al. Retinoic acid and dexamethasone regulate the expression of PEDF in retinal and endothelial cells. Experimental Eye Research, 2004, 78(5): 945-955.

[19]   Heron J F, Goedhals L, Jordaan J P, et al. Oral granisetron alone and in combination with dexamethasone: a double-blind randomized comparison against high-dose metoclopramide, plus dexamethasone in prevention of cisplatin-induced emesis. Annals of Oncology Official Journal of the European Society for Medical Oncology, 1994, 5(7): 579-574.

[20]   Junmo W. Pharmacy research progression of ginseng. Ginseng Res, 2001, 13: 2.

[21]   Yoon S R, Nah J J, Shin Y H, et al. Ginsenosides induce differential antinociception and inhibit substance P-induced nociceptive response in mice. Life Sci, 1998, 62: 319-325.

[22]   Jie Y H, Cammisuli S, Baggiolini M. Immunomodulatory effects of panax ginseng C.A. Meyer in the mouse. Agents & Actions, 1984, 15(3-4): 386-391.

[23]   C Cho J Y, Kim A R, Yoo E S, et al. Ginsenosides from Panax ginseng differentialy regulate lymphocyte proliferation. Planta Medica, 2002, 68(6): 497-500.

[24]   Liu S J, Zhou S W. Panax notoginseng saponins attenuated cisplatin-induced nephrotoxicity. Acta Pharmacol Sin, 2000, 21(3): 257-260.

[25]   Lu N Z, Cidlowski J A. Glucocorticoid receptor isoforms generate transcription specificity. Trends in Cell Biology, 2006, 16(6): 301-307.

[26]   Alexandrová M, Farkas P. Stress-induced changes of glucocorticoid receptor in rat liver. Journal of Steroid Biochemistry & Molecular Biology, 1992, 42(5): 493-498.

[27]   Herman J P, Watson S J, Spencer R L. Defense of adrenocorticosteroid receptor expression in rat hippocampus: effects of stress and strain. Endocrinology, 1999, 140: 3981-3991.

[28]   Liu D H, Su Y P, Zhang W, et al. Downregulation of glucocorticoid receptors of liver cytosols and the role of the inflammatory cytokines in pathological stress in scalded rats. Burns Journal of the International Society for Burn Injuries, 2002, 28(4): 315-320.

[29]   Li Y. Relationship between glucocorticoid receptor and deficiency syndrome and the regulation of traditional Chinese medicine. J Chin Integr Med, 2004, 2: 172-174.

[30]　Attele A S, Wu J A, Yuan C S. Ginseng pharmacology: multiple constituents and multiple actions. Biochemical Pharmacology, 1999, 58(11): 1685-1693.

[31]　Lee Y J, Chung E, Lee K Y, et al. Ginsenoside-Rg1, one of the major active molecules from Panax ginseng, is a functional ligand of glucocorticoid receptor. Molecular & Cellular Endocrinology, 1997, 133(2): 135-140.

[32]　Ling C, Li Y, Zhu X, et al. Ginsenosides may reverse the dexamethasone- induced down-regulation of glucocorticoid receptor. Gen Comp Endocr, 2006, 140(3): 302.

Section 4　Words of TCM

1. 经络之气 qi of meridians and collaterals
2. 经络辨证 meridian-collateral syndrome differentiation
3. 经络阻滞 obstruction of meridians and collaterals
4. 舒经活络 dredging meridians and collaterals
5. 孙络、浮络 minute collateral, superficial collateral
6. 十二正经 twelve main meridians; twelve regular channels
7. 十二经别 divergent branches of twelve meridians
8. 十二经筋 muscle along the twelve regular channels
9. 十二皮部 twelve skin areas
10. 十五别络 fifteen large collaterals
11. 奇经八脉 eight extra-ordinary meridians (channels)
12. 任脉 conception vessel; the ren channel; renmai
13. 督脉 the du channel; dumai
14. 冲脉 the chong channel; chongmai
15. 阴 / 阳跷脉 yin / yang heel vessel; yinqiao / yangqiao channel
16. 阴 / 阳维脉 yin / yang link vessel; yinwei / yangwei channel
17. 阴脉之海 sea of yin meridians (conception vessel)
18. 阳脉之海 sea of yang meridians (governor vessel)
19. 手太阴肺经 lung channel of hand taiyin (LU)
20. 手阳明大肠经 large intestine channel of hand yangming (LI)
21. 足阳明胃经 stomach channel of foot yangming (ST)
22. 足太阴脾经 spleen channel of foot taiyin (SP)
23. 手少阴心经 heart channel of hand shaoyin (HT)
24. 手太阳小肠经 small intestine channel of hand taiyang (SI)
25. 足太阳膀胱经 bladder channel of foot taiyang (BL)

26. 足少阴肾经 kidney channel of foot shaoyin (KI)

27. 手厥阴心包经 pericardium channel of hand jueyin (PC)

28. 手少阳三焦经 tri-energizer channel of hand shaoyang (TE)

29. 足少阳胆经 gallbladder channel of foot shaoyang (GB)

30. 足厥阴肝经 liver channel of foot jueyin (LR)

31. 奇穴 extra point; extra-ordinary point

32. 针灸穴 acupuncture point; acupoint

33. 十二井穴 twelve well-points

34. 十四经穴 accupuncture points on the fourteen regular channels

35. 十五络穴 fifteen main collaterals points

36. 十六郄穴 sixteen cleft points

37. 八脉交会穴 eight confluence points

38. 八会穴 eight hui-points; eight influential point

39. 八溪 eight joints

40. 七星针 / 梅芬针 seven star needle

(Ge Keli, Zhu Lin)

Chapter 12　Cancer

Section 1　About Cancer

Cancer is a group of diseases involving abnormal cell growth with the potential to invade or spread to other parts of the body. These contrast with benign tumors, which do not spread to other parts of the body. Possible signs and symptoms include a lump, abnormal bleeding, prolonged cough, unexplained weight loss, and a change in bowel movements. While these symptoms may indicate cancer, they may have other causes. Over 100 types of cancers affect humans.

People facing cancer often find themselves facing the possibility of their own death. At first, some focus on dying from cancer instead of living with cancer. As one woman explained, just after she was diagnosed with lung cancer she isolated herself from her family and spent a lot of time alone in her room. Soon, she realized her cancer wasn't going to disappear on its own. She realized that she could either keep pulling the covers over her head or she could tackle her cancer the way she did other challenges. This adjustment in thinking takes time.

Taking care of yourself: With the stress cancer causes, it is important that you take care of yourself — the person, and not just your cancer. Some people may want to become more "in tune" with themselves or participate in activities that take their mind off their disease. Do what you need to do. Physical activities such as walking and dance can improve your sense of well-being and make you more aware of your body. Poetry, music, drawing and reading are also creative ways to express yourself and keep your mind off cancer. Meditation and relaxation training can help with anxiety and symptom control. Taking on a new and challenging activity can provide a sense of accomplishment, as well as help reduce stress. There are many people selling herbs or treatments that claim to cure cancer. Some of these treatments are harmless in certain situations, while others have been shown to be clearly harmful. In addition, some of these treatments interact with other medications you may be taking and can cause unexpected effects.

Taking care of yourself also means accepting help from others. When people are diagnosed with cancer, many find they need to ask for and accept help for the first time. This can include help from friends and family or outside help. Asking for help does not mean you are a weak person. Arranging transportation to and from treatment, getting medical equipment such as a hospital bed, hiring a home health aide, or finding someone to watch the children while you are being treated are new tasks when people have cancer. Handling all of these changes in addition to your regular responsibilities can be stressful. In order to manage successfully, help is often necessary.

Adjusting to changes in your body and self-image: Cancer and its treatment can cause physical changes. Some people feel insecure about these changes in their body and self-image. Surgery can cause changes in physical appearance and other treatments can affect how a person feels. Side effects from cancer treatment such as weight loss or weight gain, fatigue, hair loss, and skin changes can alter a person's appearance. Partners, family members, and friends can help their loved ones work through their feelings about their different body image by offering their love, support, and understanding. It takes time for people with cancer to adjust to the way they feel about themselves and how they look.

The type of treatment as well as the dosage and schedule of medications and treatment helps determine the side effects a person may experience. The severity can vary from person to person and may occur in some and not in others. Let your doctor and nurse know which side effects you have, if any, and the severity of your symptoms. They can help you feel more comfortable when they know how treatment is affecting you physically and emotionally. Sometimes cancer treatments cause more illness or discomfort than the cancer itself. Ask your doctor what side effects you can expect and which side effects you need to report immediately. You will also want to know how to get in touch with your doctor after regular office hours if necessary.

Some find it hard to be optimistic when their treatment makes them feel bad. People with cancer can become frustrated when they do everything right but it does not help, or when treatment must be postponed because their body is unable to handle any more. It can be helpful to explain to friends and family that your treatment might cause mood swings. Sometimes these changes in your mood occur because of certain medications, while other times they occur because of the stress of coping with a cancer diagnosis.

Though hair loss resulting from some chemotherapy drugs is temporary and the loss of a limb after extensive surgery is permanent, they can both be difficult to handle because they are changes in physical appearance others can see. Many people who lose hair choose to wear scarves, wigs or hats. Some people choose prostheses and reconstructive surgery. These temporary or permanent solutions draw less attention to or hide a person's physical differences.

When making difficult decisions, talking with others who have had the same type of reconstructive surgery or wear the same type of prosthesis can be helpful. Ask your surgeon if he or she is able to share photographs that show actual results of reconstructive surgery. Check with your health insurance company about the details concerning coverage of reconstructive surgery or prostheses. If you do not have health insurance, your hospital social worker may be able to help you find resources. Insurance coverage can be limited either by dollar amount or the number of prostheses (that is, mastectomy bras and breast forms) you can purchase in a specified amount of time.

Sexuality and cancer: Personal qualities, such as a person's sense of humor, integrity, honesty, and spirit, are a large part of what makes someone attractive to their partner. Cancer treatment may seem to change these qualities, but the change is usually temporary. It is important to remember those qualities are still within but for the moment overshadowed by the cancer experience.

Some people fear physical intimacy because they think they will get cancer from their partner, or they are afraid they will hurt their partner. Cancer is not contagious and cannot pass the partner through sexual intercourse. In some cases, it may be necessary to abstain from sexual intercourse for a short period of time. For example, when a person is recovering from certain types of surgery and when they are more susceptible to infections. Ask your doctor if there are any precautions you need to take based on the treatment you or your partner will receive.

Issues such as fertility and birth control are important and should be discussed with your doctor before the treatment begins. Birth control should be used during cancer treatment because some treatments can have an adverse effect on a developing fetus. Even when sterility is a possible side effect of treatment, an effective method of birth control should be used.

Side effects of cancer treatment can also affect a person's sexuality. Some of these are lack of desire, feeling physically unattractive, vaginal dryness for women, and the inability to have or maintain an erection for men. Physical side effects, such as fatigue and nausea, can decrease a person's desire to have intimate contact with his or her partner. There are many reasons why these problems can exist, including fear, anxiety or depression. These side effects, like other physical and emotional side effects, can be managed or treated effectively. Although you may feel embarrassed, it is important to discuss them with your doctor.

Changes in your body image can affect your feelings about your sexual appeal. As a result, you may feel as if you are no longer sexually attractive. While sexual intimacy is a way to express love for someone, there are other ways to express this feeling. When physical intimacy becomes possible, let your partner know what is comfortable for you and when you feel up to it. Your partner may want to give you the space and time you need to adjust to changes in your body and self-image. Your partner may not want to rush you or appear insensitive, so it is helpful for you to communicate your desire for physical contact. Be specific about what you want. Physical contact other than sexual intercourse, such as hugging, kissing and touching may help you gradually feel more comfortable being intimate.

If you are single when you are diagnosed and recovering from cancer, you may be unsure about how and when to tell a new romantic partner. Only you can know if and when you trust someone enough to share this part of you. Whether someone is told early in a relationship or later on, it is up to you. You may find it helps to practice what you will say with a friend before sharing with your new partner.

Some people are afraid their partner will avoid physical with them. Others may fear the possibility of infidelity. If there were problems in the relationship before a cancer diagnosis, they will still be present after a cancer diagnosis. Likewise, if a couple works through problems well, chances are good and they will face this challenge in a similar way. When a couple communicates with one another, they can usually work toward resolving their feelings and the added stress that cancer places on a relationship.

Facing cancer as a couple can also strengthen a relationship. Cancer can help people realize what is really important to them. Priorities or problems they once viewed as important may now seem less important or smaller.

It is not unusual for people with cancer to withdraw from their partners when they experience changes in their body and self-image. People with cancer who are experiencing changes in their sexuality want to know their partners still care for them and are still attracted to them. As a partner of someone with cancer, there are several ways you can convey these feelings. Talk about your feelings and let the person with cancer talk about changes in their sexuality, body image and self-image.

People who are not able to gain support from their partners can find support elsewhere, such as counseling, a support group or friends. Counseling can help explore ways to improve communication and resolve problems in relationships. For those who are unable to work through these issues alone, professional counseling for individuals or couples is an option. Support groups that are offered by licensed or trained professionals may also be a source of practical advice and ideas about coping with changes in sexuality. Groups exist for people with cancer, for partners/spouses, and for couples.

Section 2　Tea: A Story of Serendipity

As legend has it, one day in 2737 BC, the Chinese Emperor Shennong was boiling drinking water over an open fire, believing that those who drank boiled water were healthier. Some leaves from a nearby Camellia sinensis plant floated into the pot. The emperor drank the mixture and declared it gave one vigor of body, contentment of mind, and determination of purpose. Perhaps as testament to the emperor's assessment, tea (the potion he unwittingly brewed that day) today is second only to water in worldwide consumption. The USA population drank its fair share of the brew, and drink 2.25 billion gallons of tea in one form or another (hot, iced, spiced, flavored, with or without sugar, honey, milk, cream, or lemon) in 1994. A serving of tea generally contains about 40 mg of caffeine (less than half as much caffeine as in coffee), but the actual levels vary depending on the specific blend and the strength of the brew, and the decaffeinated tea is also available. Many tea drinkers find the beverage soothing, and folk medicine has long valued it as a remedy for sore throats and unsettled stomachs. Recent studies have shown that certain chemicals in tea called polyphenols may help reduce the risk of far more serious illnesses, including atherosclerosis and some cancers, although the data are not conclusive.

The secret of fine tea picking is "two leaves and a bud at a time". The work is done chiefly by women to carry light bamboo baskets strapped to their backs. Tea comes in black, green and oolong varieties, all produced from the leaves of Camellia sinensis, a white-flowered evergreen. The method of processing the leaf distinguishes the three types. Herbal teas are made from leaves of other plants. Food and Drug Agency (FDA) requires that herbal tea labels carry the name of the plant the product derives from, such as chamomile.

The traditional method of producing black tea begins with withering. The plucked leaves are placed on shelves called withering racks, where excess moisture is removed. They are then rolled in special machines that release the leaves' enzymes and juices, which give tea its aroma and taste. Next, the leaves ferment in a room with controlled temperature and humidity; finally, they are dried in ovens. More recently some processors have forsaken the traditional method to speed production by using machines that finely chop the leaves, thereby cutting the time for withering and fermenting. Green tea is made by steaming or otherwise heating the leaves immediately after plucking to prevent the fermentation that makes black tea. Then the leaves are rolled and dried. Oolong tea is fermented only partially — to a point between black and green. While the leaves wilt naturally, enzymes begin to ferment them. Processors interrupt the fermentation by stirring the leaves in heated pans, then rolling and drying them.

Different varieties of Camellia sinensis grow in different geographic areas and produce leaves that vary from a very small Chinese leaf, perhaps 1/2 ~ 3/4 of an inch long, to the Assamese leaf, which may be 3 or 4 inches long. Certain varieties are better suited than others for a particular processing method. For example, the Chinese leaf from China produces the best oolongs.

Scented and spiced teas are made from black tea. Scented teas look just like any other tea because the scent is more or less sprayed on. They're flavored with just about anything — peach, vanilla, cherry. The spiced teas, on the other hand, usually contain pieces of spices — cinnamon or nutmeg or orange or lemon peel — so you can see there's something in there.

Orange pekoe refers to the size of the tea leaf. Processed tea leaves are sorted into sizes by passing them over screens with holes of different sizes. The largest leaves are orange pekoe, pekoe, and pekoe souchong. The smaller or broken leaves are classified as broken orange pekoe, broken pekoe souchong, broken orange pekoe fannings, and fines (also called "dust").

In brewing, flavor and color come out of the larger leaves more slowly than out of the broken and fine grades. The broken grades, which make up about 80% of the total black tea crop, produce a stronger, darker tea. The grades have nothing to do with the quality or flavor of tea; they simply refer to leaf size. Except for fanning and fine, the terms should apply only to black or fermented tea. But nowadays oolongs are often labeled orange pekoe, and even some green teas are labeled pekoe or flowery pekoe.

Tea tastes vary, and one aficionado who squirts lemon in his cup may cringe at the sight of another pouring milk or honey. But no matter how the tea may be doctored, the odds are overwhelming that it starts out black. Nearly 95% of all tea consumed here is black, 4% green, 1% oolong, and 1% flavored. The proclivity for drinking black tea over green or oolong may have been influenced by events in history. 60 years ago and more, the amount of black and green tea Americans drank was split fairly evenly — each accounting for about 40% of the market — with oolong constituting the rest. During World War II, however, the major sources of green tea — China and Japan — were cut off from the United States, leaving us with tea almost exclusively from British-controlled India, which produces black tea. Americans came out of the war drinking nearly 99% black tea.

With the Korean War in the 1950s, uncertainties about tea supplies resurfaced, and the United States began to look for other suppliers. Argentina filled the bill, because tea could grow very fast there. Although the country didn't produce an outstanding tea, it produced a good average tea.

Today, most of tea comes from Argentina, China (which got back into the USA market in 1978), and Java. 30 years ago most of it came from India and Ceylon (now Sri Lanka). Argentine black tea is the kind most used for iced tea, and that's another reason black tea dominates the US market.

What is green tea: What are different green teas made of exactly, and are they totally natural? Green, black and oolong teas come from the Camellia sinensis plant. Green tea consists of leaves that haven't been fermented so they contain the highest level of antioxidants. For example, flavonoid antioxidants account for about 30% of the dry weight of green tea leaves. Some of the antioxidants and healing compounds found in green tea include polyphenols, catechins and various other types of flavonoids — the same anti-aging compounds found in things like red wine, blueberries and dark chocolate. Despite that it does contain small amounts of caffeine, green tea consumption has been associated with more health benefits than even many of the healthiest foods available to us. Studies have found that the benefits of green tea are due to the fact green tea contains more healing compounds than many other herbs, spices, fruits and vegetables, truly making it a powerful super food.

Green tea nutrition facts: Flavan-3-ols, the type of flavonoids found in green tea and other teas, provide many of the anti-aging effects of green tea. Catechins in various types of teas are the polyphenols that seem to have the most potent antioxidant effects, according to Natural Standard, the leading and most respected reviewer of herbal compounds. Specific flavan-3-ols found in green tea include monomers (catechins) called: epicatechin, epigallocatechin, gallocatechin, and gallate derivatives.

A well-known compound found in green tea is called EGCG (which stands for epigallocatechin-3-gallate). EGCG is associated with enhanced metabolic activities that may prevent weight gain or assist with weight maintenance. Some of the ways that EGCG seems to work is by boosting thermogenesis (the body producing heat by using energy) and suppressing appetite, although not every study has found evidence that these effects are substantial.

Green tea also contains many other protective compounds, including: linoleic acid; quercetin; aginenin, methylxanthines, including caffeine, theobromine and theophylline; many different amino acids and enzymes (proteins make up about 15% ~ 20% of the leaves' dry weight); carbohydrate molecules, such as cellulose, pectins, glucose, fructose and sucrose; small amounts of minerals and trace elements like calcium, magnesium, chromium, manganese, iron, copper and zinc; small amounts of chlorophyll and carotenoids; volatile compounds like aldehydes, alcohols, esters, lactones and hydrocarbons.

Some of the benefits of green tea associated with the consumption of these compounds include reduced allergies, eye health and better vision, skin health, improved immune function, enhanced endurance, and protection from free radical damage and cancer.

How to use and steep green tea: Most experts recommend drinking about 3 ~ 4 cups per day for the most anti-aging benefits of green tea, but even drinking 1 ~ 2 cups is a step in the right direction. The standard way to brew green tea is: (1) Place your tea bag or high-quality tea leaves (purchase organic from a reputable company for the best tea) in your teapot. (2) Heat or boil water, but don't let it completely boil and become too hot, as this can destroy some of the delicate compounds found in green tea leaves. The "ideal" temperature for brewing green tea is 160 ~ 180 °F (traditionally standard Chinese green teas brew at a slightly higher temperature). Pour hot water into the teapot to steep the leaves for only about 1 ~ 3 minutes. Larger leaves need more time to steep than finer, smaller leaves. At this point you can also add any fresh herbs you plan on steeping. (3) Once brewed, pour a little tea at a time into each cup in order to have the tea's strength be evenly distributed. At this point, you can add some lemon juice or raw honey as the finishing touch.

Because it's used somewhat differently than regular green tea, directions for making matcha green tea are found below (note that directions can vary, so it's best to read the label of the product you purchase): (1) Fill kettle with fresh, filtered water and heat to just short of boiling. (2) Fill matcha bowl or cup with hot water and pour out (to warm the bowl/cup). (3) Add one teaspoon of matcha powder to bowl or cup and 2 ounces of nearly boiled water. (4) Whisk for a minute or two until it looks thick and frothy with tiny bubble, then add 3 ~ 4 more ounces of water before drinking.

Green tea recipes: A common practice around the world, such as in the Blue Zones, is to combine beneficial teas with fresh steeped herbs. Try steeping rosemary, ginger, wild sage, oregano, marjoram, mint or dandelion in tea for an extra antioxidant boost. You can also add fresh lemon juice or some orange to add a refreshing taste. Below are more recipe ideas for using green tea in smoothies or other interesting ways to get the benefits of green tea: (1) Make a mango green tea smoothie or one of 34 other green smoothie recipes. (2) Add matcha green tea powder to homemade berry muffins or pancakes. (3) Make homemade green tea coconut ice cream using chilled green tea and this ice cream recipe.

Section 3　Research Article

Up-regulation effect of ginsenosides on glucocorticoid receptor in rat liver

[Abstract]We have demonstrated earlier that ginsenosides (GSS) could partially reverse the dexamethasone (Dex)-induced down-regulation of glucocorticoid receptor (GR) and enhance Dex-induced transcription of GR reporter gene in HL 7702 cells, but whether it can play a similar role in vivo has not been studied. Male Sprague-Dawley rats were pretreated with saline (1 mL/ d) or GSS [50 mg/(kg·d)] for 5 days, and then subjected to GR down-regulation induced by polyvinyl alcohol containing hydrocortisone (F-PVA). The rats were killed by decapitation to determine liver GR and plasma corticosterone levels. Pretreatment with GSS resulted in up-regulation of GR with respect to binding capacity, cytoplasmic protein expression, and mRNA levels, but did not produce significant effects on GR binding affinity and serum corticosterone levels. Pretreatment with GSS also led to increase in GR translocation and TAT mRNA levels. Data obtained in the present study indicate that GSS may up-regulate GR levels in vivo and enhance glucocorticoid efficiency.

1　Introduction

Glucocorticoid (GC), a steroid hormone secreted by the adrenal gland, regulates many important physiological processes in the body, including growth, metabolism, and immunological reactivity. GC is also one of the most commonly used medicines in treating chronic asthma, rheumatoid arthritis, and systemic lupus erythematosus. It is generally believed that most of the GC functions are mediated by glucocorticoid receptors (GRs), a member of the nuclear receptor superfamily of ligand-dependent transcription factors. A number of studies have demonstrated that there is a direct correlation between the levels of GR and the responses to GC in steroid sensitive cell culture models[1-3], transfected cell studies[4-5], in vivo animal studies[6], and clinical studies[7]. Consequently, the level of GR is one of the principal determinants of GC sensitivity[4, 8-9].

However, some studies[8, 10-13] have also demonstrated that GC treatment decreased GR expression levels in a number of tissues and cell types and at multiple levels (transcriptional, post-transcriptional, and / or post-translational) in vitro and in vivo. It was also found that GC induced down-regulation of GR in vivo occurred rapidly while the recovery of GR was relatively slow[14-17]. It is therefore believed that homologous down-regulation plays an important role in the poor response to GC. If there was a medicine that may reverse the homologous down-regulation at least partially, it would enhance the efficacy of GC in patients with hormone dependent diseases.

Our laboratory has a continued interest in the regulation of GR by Chinese medicinal herbs[18-22]. Previously, we had demonstrated that compound prescriptions containing ginseng may up-regulate the GR level in stressed rats. We also found[23] that the main extracts of ginseng, GSS, which is one of the derivatives of triterpenoid dammarane consisting of 30 carbon atoms, could partially reverse dexamethasone (Dex)-induced down-regulation of GR and enhance the Dex-induced GR luciferase report gene expression in HL-7702 cells. Based on these findings, we made a further study to see whether GSS could reverse GC-induced GR down-regulation and enhance GC efficiency in vivo. Because liver is the prime target tissue for GC action, we determined cytosol GR in the liver in the present study by the method of exchange assay using ^{3}H-dexamethasone as the ligand, originally developed by Hubbard et al.[24] and modified by Tan et al.[25], and GR protein and GR mRNA expressions by Western blot and quantitative real-time RT-PCR.

2　Materials and methods

2.1　Chemicals

GSS was obtained from Professor Zheng Hanchen (Department of Natural Pharmacology, Second Military Medical University, Shanghai, China) with purity greater than 95%. The extract was dissolved in water at a water-bath temperature of 37 ℃. The concentrations of four major GSS were determined by reversed phase HPLC-MS/MS employing a quadrupole-ion trap mass spectrometer in samples (Rg1 = 20.88%, Re = 18.50%, Rb1 = 5.66%, and Rb2 = 2.38%). Other chemicals included Dex and dextran T-70 Sigma-Aldrich Chemicals, St. Louis, MO, USA); [1, 2, 4-3H]-Dex (^{34}Ci / mmol) (Amersham-Pharmacia Biotech, Buckinghamshire, UK); charcoal activated carbon (E-Merck, Darmstadt, Germany); and hydrocortisone (F) (Yangzhou

Pharmaceutical Co., Ltd., Yangzhou, China). All the other chemicals used were of analytical grade.

2.2 Animals and administration protocols

Sprague-Dawley male rats aged 6 ~ 8 weeks (200 ~ 250 g) were used. Male rats were used to avoid the variable steroid concentration during the normal estrous cycle of female animals. Animals were maintained on a 12-h light, 12-h dark cycle (7:00 – 19:00) at 22 ℃ with food and water available ad libitum. To avoid the influence of environmental changes, all the animals were housed for a week in a controlled environment before using in the experiment. The experiments were performed in accordance with the European Communities Council Directive of 24 November 1986 (86 / 609 EEC) and approved by the Ethics Committee of Changhai Hospital.

Thirty rats were equally assigned to five experimental groups: (1) the control group; (2) the sham group, where the animals were administered intragastrically with saline (1 mL/d) for five days, and then injected subcutaneously with polyvinyl alcohol (PVA) (0.5 mL, 120 mg/mL); (3) GSS group, where the animals were administered intragastrically with GSS [50 mg/(kg·d)] for five days, and then injected subcutaneously with PVA (0.5 mL, 120 mg/mL); (4) GC group, where the animals were administered intragastrically with saline (1 mL/d) for five days, and then injected subcutaneously with polyvinyl alcohol containing hydrocortisone (F-PVA) (0.5 mL, containing F 40 mg); and (5) GSS + GC group, where the animals were administered intragastrically with GSS [50 mg/(kg·d)] for five days, and then injected subcutaneously with F-PVA (0.5 mL, containing F 40 mg). Subcutaneous injection was done 12 h after the last intragastric drug administration, and the animals were killed by decapitation 12 h after the injection. To minimize the influence of diurnal variation, the intragastric administrations, injection of F-PVA, and decapitation were performed at 8:00 – 9:00, 18:00 –20:00, and 6:00 – 8:00 respectively.

Approximately 1 mL of trunk blood was collected into centrifuge tubes containing 100 μL of 0.3 mol/L EDTA for radioimmunoassay. Collected blood was immediately centrifuged by using a Sorvall RC-3 centrifuge at 3000 g for 15 min. The supernatant was stored at − 70 ℃ .

2.3 Radioligand binding analysis for GR in liver

After the rats were killed, the blood in the liver was washed out immediately from the portal vein with precooled saline. Then, a portion of the liver was removed, weighed, minced, and homogenized in 50 mmol/L Tris buffer (pH 7.5; 1 : 3, w/v) containing 0.25 mol/L sucrose, 25 mmol/L KCl, 1 mmol/L MgCl$_2$, 1 mmol/L CaCl$_2$, 10 mmol/L sodium molybdate and 0.1% β-mercaptoethanol. The homogenate was centrifuged at 4 ℃ for 30 min at 175 000 g, and then the upper fatty layer was discarded and the supernatant (cytosol) was collected. The cytosol was treated with 5% dextran-coated charcoal (DCC) (5 g charcoal and 0.5 g dextran T-70 dissolved in 10 mmol/L Tris, pH 7.5) for 3 min at 0 ℃ . The supernatant was then centrifuged at 12 000 g for 5 min at 4 ℃ . The resulting clear supernatant was used as the cytosol fraction for exchange assays.

The protein concentration was determined by the method of Bradford with BSA as the standard. The liver cytosol was incubated with ^{3}H-dexamethasone at a final concentration of 5 ~ 40 nmol/L (with or without 1000-fold unlabelled Dex) at 25 ℃ for 30 min. Later, they were incubated at 0 ℃ for 2 h and treated with 5% DCC again to determine the bound ^{3}H-dexamethasone. The radioactivity was assayed by scintillation counting with scintillation cocktail. The results were standardized as femtomoles of ^{3}H-dexamethasone bound per milligram of protein. Maximum binding (B max) and Kd were deprived by Scatchard analysis.

2.4 Western blot

Cytoplasmic and nuclear proteins were extracted with an NEPER Nuclear and Cytoplasmic Extract kit (Pierce, Rockford, USA) according to the manufacturer's instructions. Briefly, 100 mg of liver was homogenized in CER I Reagent using a glass Teflon homogenizer. Then the CER II Reagent was added to the homogenates. After incubation on ice for 1 min, the homogenates were centrifuged at 12 000 g for 5 min at 4 ℃ . The resulting supernatant was collected (Cytoplasmic extraction) and the pellet was resuspended in ice-cold NER, respectively. The nuclear suspension was placed on ice, continued with vortexing for 15 s every 10 min for a total of 40 min, and then centrifuged at 12 000 g for 10 min at 4 ℃ . The supernatant (nuclear extraction) was collected and stored at − 70 ℃ until use.

Total protein concentrations in cytoplasmic and nuclear extractions were measured using a BCA protein assay kit. The supernatants were mixed 1 : 4 with SDS reducing buffer containing 50 mmol/L DTT. The samples then were heated at 100 ℃ for 5 min. SDS-PAGE was performed by the method of Laemmli[26]. Samples containing the same amount of proteins (80 μg for cytoplasmic protein and 40 μg for nuclear protein) were then loaded onto 8% discontinuous gels with a 5% stacking gel, and run at 110 mV for 120 min. After electrophoresis, gels were allowed to equilibrate in 20% methanol blotting buffer. Blotting was performed for 90 min at 100 V. After completion of the protein transfer, the ready membranes were incubated for 2 h at room temperature in TBS buffer (50 mmol/L Tris-HCl, 150 mmol/L NaCl, 0.05% Tween-20, pH 8.0), containing 5% nonfat dry milk powder to saturate the nonspecific protein binding sites and then incubated with specific primary antibodies diluted in 1% nonfat dry milk-TBST (anti-GR polyclonal antibody, Santa Cruz, CA, USA) overnight at 4 ℃ with mild agitation. Membranes were then washed with TBST three times for 10 min and incubated for 2 h with secondary antibodies (goat-anti-rabbit, Bio-Rad, CA, USA) in 1% nonfat milk-TBST with gentle agitation. Final detection was performed by ECL detection reagents according to the manufacturer's instructions. The computer-assisted densitometry program was used to determine optical density reading for the single GR band.

2.5 RNA extraction and real-time quantitative RT-PCR

Total RNA was isolated from the liver with Trizol Reagent (Invitrogen, Paisley, UK) according to the manufacturer's instructions. The concentration and purity of total RNA were determined by a spectrophotometer (Eppendorf, Hamburg, Germany) and the integrity of total RNA was determined by formaldehyde-agarose gel electrophoresis. cDNA synthesis was performed using oligo dT primers RT mixtures with AMV (Promega, Madison, WI, USA) reverse transcriptase 15 U / 20 μL, total RNA 1 μg / 20 μL. cDNA was stored at −20 ℃ . Primers for real time PCR were as follows: GR primers, sense: 5'-AGC AGA GAA TGT CTC TAC-3', antisense: 5'-GGA ATT CAA TAC TCA TGG TC-3' (365 bp); tyrosine aminotransferase (TAT) primers, sense: 5'-GCA TTT CCC GGA ATT CGA-3' , antisense: 5'-GAC AGC CTG CTC CGC AAT-3' (63 bp); β-actin primers, sense: 5'-CCT CTA TGC CAA CAC AGT GC-3', antisense: 5'-GTA CTC CTG CTT GCT GAT CC-3' (211 bp). Real-time quantitative PCR reaction was performed in a Light Cycler® (Roche Diagnostic, Mannheim, Germany) using Toyobo SYBR Green PCR mastermixed (TOYOBO, Osaka, Japan) according to the manufacturer's instructions. PCR condition was 3 min at 95 ℃ , 40 cycles of 20 s at 95 ℃ , 20 s at 54 ℃ , and 25 s at 72 ℃ . Amplification of the single product in PCR was confirmed by monitoring the melting curve from 65 ℃ to 95 ℃ . Each real-time PCR was done in duplicate. The relative expression level of GR mRNA in each sample was normalized to its β-actin content. The relative expression levels of GR mRNA were calculated as $2^{-\Delta\Delta Ct}$.

2.6 Radioimmunoassay of corticosterone

The plasma samples were thawed. The corticosterone concentration was determined with a rat corticosterone RIA DSL-80100 kit supplied by Diagnostics System Laboratories (Webster, TX, USA) according to the manufacturer' s instructions.

2.7 Statistical analysis

Data are expressed as means ± SD (SEM), unless otherwise indicated. One-way analysis of variance (ANOVA) followed by Student-Newman-Keuls tests were used for statistical analysis. Statistical significance was established at $P < 0.05$.

3 Results

3.1 GR concentrations and apparent dissociation constants in liver

In this study, GR binding capacity was determined by the method of exchange assay. GR binding capacity in the control and sham groups was (673 ± 54) fmol/mg and (577 ± 36) fmol / mg protein, respectively. Single GSS treatment resulted in a general increase of GR binding capacity. GR binding capacity in GSS group was (734 ± 76) fmol / mg protein and administration of GC induced a significant decrease of GR level. The results were consistent with results of previous reports. F-PVA injection resulted in a significant down-regulation of GR, which decreased to (413 ± 14) fmol / mg protein in GC group and (521 ± 33) fmol / mg protein in GSS + GC group. However, the administration of GSS did not produce significant effect on apparent dissociation constants (Kd).

3.2 GR protein expression in liver

A single prominent band was detected at approximate 95 kD in liver cytoplasmic and nuclear preparations. Figure 12-1 indicates the change in GR protein expression in the liver after F-PVA and / or GSS treatment. Cytoplasmic GR expression decreased in animals treated with F-PVA as compared with that of sham animals (Figure 12-1a). GR expression in cytoplasmic extraction elevated slightly in animals treated with GSS alone as compared with that in control animals. GR expression in cytoplasmic extraction elevated significantly in GSS + GC group animals as compared with that in GC group animals. There was no significant difference of GR expression in cytoplasmic extraction between GSS + GC group animals and GC group animals.

Although cytoplasmic protein decreased in GC group, nuclear protein increased (Figure 12-1b), indicating that the increase of GC level could promote GR protein translocation from the cytoplasma to the nucleus. There was a roughly equivalent increase of nuclear GR protein in rats treated with GSS alone as in GC group rats. The combined use of GSS and F-PVA produced a significant increase of nuclear GR protein compared with F-PVA used alone.

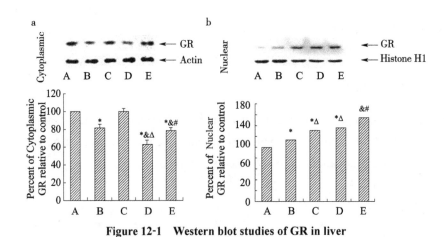

Figure 12-1   Western blot studies of GR in liver

Cytoplasmic and nuclear proteins were prepared as described in Section Materials and Methods. The samples were electrophorsed and analyzed by Western blot with monoclonal GR antibody. A: cytoplasmic protein; B: nuclear protein. Upper panel A = control, B = sham, C = single GSS treatment, D = GC treatment, E = GSS + GC treatment. Lower panel: quantities for densitometric analysis of GR. Each bar represents the means ± SEM of three rats assayed in triplicate. $^*P < 0.01$, *vs* control; $^#P < 0.01$, *vs* GC group; $^&P < 0.01$, *vs* single GSS treatment; $^\Delta P < 0.01$, *vs* sham.

3.3   GR mRNA in liver

Real time RT-PCR was used to determine the change of GR mRNA after the administration of GSS or F-PVA. Previous reports[8, 17] showed that GR mRNA decreased significantly after administration of GC. The same phenomenon was observed after injection of F-PVA in this study (Figure 12-2). Compared with the control group, GR mRNA decreased significantly in GC group. Although GR mRNA also decreases in the sham, GSS and GSS+GC groups, the significant difference between GC group and GSS+GC group indicates that the 5-day pretreatment with GSS attenuated the down-regulation of GR mRNA induced by F-PVA.

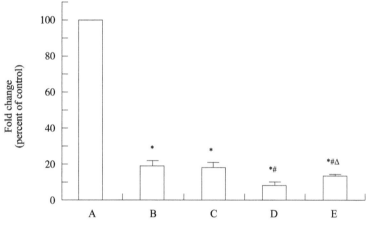

Figure 12-2   Change of GR mRNA in rat liver

GR mRNA level was determined by real-time RT-PCR. The fold change in GR mRNA expression was calculated using the $2^{-\Delta\Delta Ct}$ method [$\Delta\Delta$ Ct = (Ct$_{GR}$ – Ct$_{\beta\text{-actin}}$) Experimental groups – (Ct$_{GR}$ –Ct$_{\beta\text{-actin}}$) Control]. The results are expressed as fold change relative to control. Values are shown as fold-change $\pm$ SEM (n = 6). A, B, C, D, and E represent control, sham, GSS, GC, and GSS + GC, respectively. $^{*}P < 0.01$, vs control; $^{\#}P < 0.01$, vs sham; $^{\Delta}P < 0.01$, vs GC control.

3.4   Corticosterone in plasma

The administration of GC would lead to a secondary increase of total GC and consequently will suppress the hypothalamic-pituitary-adrenal (HPA) axis. Since a rat corticosterone RIA kit was used during this study, the plasma corticosterone level was determined but the exogenous cortisol was not detectable (Figure 12-3). The plasma corticosterone concentration in the control, sham, and GSS groups was (66.4 $\pm$ 13.8) ng / mL, (178.1 $\pm$ 12.5) ng / mL and (186.7 $\pm$ 12.8) ng / mL, respectively. F-PVA injection caused a significant decrease of the corticosterone levels in GC and GSS + GC groups though the difference between the two groups was not significant.

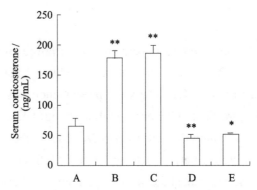

Figure 12-3　Change of serum corticosterone

Serum corticosterone was determined with radioimmunoassay. Each bar represents the means ± SD ($n = 6$). A, B, C, D, and E represent control, sham, GSS, GC, and GSS + GC, respectively. $^*P < 0.05$, *vs* control; $^{**}P < 0.01$, *vs* control.

3.5　TAT mRNA in liver

Although GSS showed little effect on the corticosterone levels, it increased both cytoplasmic and nuclear GR protein levels as indicated above in the GSS and GSS + GC groups. To demonstrate whether GSS could enhance the GC effect in the liver, we examined the tyrosine aminotransferase (TAT) mRNA level in the liver. Figure 12-4 shows that TAT mRNA level increased significantly in GSS, GC, and GSS + GC groups compared with that in the control and sham groups. GSS pretreatment and later F-PVA injection significantly increased TAT mRNA level in the liver compared with F-PVA injection alone.

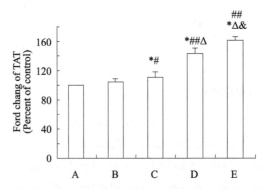

Figure 12-4　Change of TAT mRNA in rat liver

TAT mRNA level was determined by real-time RT-PCR. The fold change in TAT mRNA expression was calculated using the $2^{-\Delta\Delta Ct}$ method [$\Delta\Delta$ Ct = (Ct_{GR} − $Ct_{\beta\text{-actin}}$) experimental groups −(Ct_{GR} − $Ct_{\beta\text{-actin}}$) control]. The results are expressed as fold change relative to control. Values are shown as fold-change ± SEM ($n = 6$). A, B, C, D, and E represent control, sham, GSS, GC, and GSS + GC, respectively. $^*P < 0.01$, *vs* control; $^{\#} P < 0.05$, *vs* sham; $^{\#\#} P < 0.01$, *vs* sham; $^{\triangle}P < 0.01$, *vs* GSS; $^{\&}P < 0.01$, *vs* GC control.

4 Discussion

In the present study, we have investigated the effect of GSS on GR in rat liver. It was found that cytoplasmic GR protein, activity, and GR mRNA decreased significantly after hormone treatment, which is consistent with previous studies. GSS pretreatment attenuated the down-regulation of cytoplasmic GR and GR mRNA induced by GC and increased the nuclear GR protein level. However, GSS treatment did not alter the ligand-affinity of GR, and had little effect on endogenous secretion of corticosterone with or without GC treatment. The treatment with GSS also induced a higher TAT mRNA level with or without GC treatment.

Glucocorticoid therapy is one of the most effective medications in the acute and chronic management of many diseases such as allergic diseases and autoimmune diseases. However, many patients respond poorly to GC therapy due to GR down-regulation induced by GC, especially in chronic and prolonged courses of treatment[8-9]. In the present study, we simulated a GC therapy process in rats by F-PVA injection as described by Xu and Tan[15]. Combination use of F and PVA could delay the release of F.

GSS pretreatment increased cytoplasmic and nuclear GR levels in both GSS and GSS + GC groups as compared with the sham and GC groups respectively, indicating that GSS could not only increase the GR activity and cytoplasmic protein but promote GR translocation from cytoplasma to nucleus, thus improving tissues sensitivity to GC and enhancing the efficacy of GC. To evaluate whether GSS could really enhance the efficacy of GC in the liver, we examined TAT mRNA levels in the liver for previous studies indicating that the induction of TAT by GC was mainly on the transcriptional level[27-28]. We found that TAT mRNA level increased more significantly in GSS + GC group than that in GC group, indicating that GSS did enhance the GC effect in the liver. There are two possibilities accounting for the increase in GR binding capacity, the number of GR protein molecules and the hormone binding activities.

However, our results showed that the apparent dissociation constants (Kd) did not change with or without GSS and / or F-PVA administration. So the increase of GR protein may be the main reason for the up-regulation of GR binding capacity. Moreover, our data showed that GC treatment led to more serious decrease of mRNA than that of protein, indicating that besides the increase of GR protein expression, the increase of protein stabilization may also contribute to the increase of GR protein. Our results suggested that both the transcriptional and post-transcriptional mechanisms are involved in the up-regulation of GR.

Kim et al.[29] reported that GSS could inhibit stress-induced increase of plasma corticosterone levels in mice. But data from our study showed that GSS had no effect on corticosterone levels with or without GC treatment, indicating that GSS may not activate the suppressed HPA axis.

Ginseng is one of the most effective herbs in traditional Chinese medicine (TCM). It has been reported that ginseng has a wide range of pharmacological activities in cardiovascular, endocrine, immune, and central nervous systems. Ginseng and its constituents have been used for their tonic, immunomodulatory adaptogenic, anticancer, antistress, anti-inflammatory, and anti-aging activities. Our results also suggest that elevating GR level and promoting GR translocation by increasing the GC effect may be the common mechanism of GSS effects.

In the treatment of GC-dependent diseases, GR would be down-regulated after the exogenous GC administration[3, 13]. Since almost all the GC functions are mediated by GR[8], the down-regulation of GR may limit the efficiency of GC[9]. Our data suggests that the pretreatment of GSS may antagonize the down-regulation of GR. Our results indicate that GSS may be a potential drug for enhancing GC efficiency. We will further investigate the efficiency of GC in combination with GSS in the treatment of glucocorticoid-dependent and glucocorticoid-resistant diseases.

Acknowledgement

The work was supported by grants from the National Natural Science Foundation of China (90709024, 30472271, and 30701132). The authors thank Prof. Zheng Hanchen for the supply of ginsenosides. The authors declare that there is no conflict of interest that would prejudice the impartiality of this scientific work.

References

[1]   Bourgeois S, Newby R F. Correlation between glucocorticoid receptor and cytolytic response of murine lymphoid cell lines. Cancer Research, 1979, 39(11): 4749-4753.

[2]   Dong Y, Aronsson M, Gustafsson J A, et al. The mechanism of cAMP-induced glucocorticoid receptor expression: correlation to cellular glucocorticoid response. Journal of Biological Chemistry, 1989, 264(23): 13679-13683.

[3]   Oakley R H, Cidlowski J A. Homologous down regulation of the glucocorticoid receptor: the molecular machinery. Crit Rev Eukaryot Gene Expr, 1993, 3(2): 63-88.

[4]   Vanderbilt J N, Miesfeld R, Maler B A, et al. Intracellular receptor concentration limits glucocorticoid-dependent enhancer activity. Molecular Endocrinology, 1987, 1(1): 68-74.

[5]   Bellingham D L, Sar M, Cidlowski J A. Ligand-dependent down-regulation of stably transfected human glucocorticoid receptors is associated with the loss of functional glucocorticoid responsiveness. Molecular Endocrinology, 1992, 6(12): 2090-2102.

[6]   Yang Y L, Tan J X, Xu R B. Down-regulation of glucocorticoid receptor and its relationship to the induction of rat liver tyrosine aminotransferase. Journal of Steroid Biochemistry, 1989, 32(1A): 99-104.

[7]   Bloomfield C D, Smith K A, Peterson B A, et al. Glucocorticoid receptors in adult acute lymphoblastic

leukemia. Cancer Research, 1981, 41(11 Pt 2): 4857-4860.

[8]　Schaaf M J, Cidlowski J A. Molecular mechanisms of glucocorticoid action and resistance. Journal of Steroid Biochemistry & Molecular Biology, 2002, 83(1-5): 37-48.

[9]　Bamberger C M, Schulte H M, Chrousos G P. Molecular determinants of glucocorticoid receptor function and tissue sensitivity to glucocorticoids. Endocrine Reviews, 1996, 17(3): 245-261.

[10]　Burnstein K L, Bellingham D L, Jewell C M, et al. Autoregulation of glucocorticoid receptor gene expression. Steroids, 1991, 56(2): 52-58.

[11]　Burnstein K L, Cidlowski J A. The down side of glucocorticoid receptor regulation. Molecular & Cellular Endocrinology, 1992, 83(1): 1-8.

[12]　Burnstein K L, Jewell C M, Sar M, et al. Intragenic sequences of the human glucocorticoid receptor complementary DNA mediate hormone-inducible receptor messenger RNA down-regulation through multiple mechanisms. Molecular Endocrinology, 1994, 8(12): 1764-1773.

[13]　Silva C M, Powelloliver F E, Jewell C M, et al. Regulation of the human glucocorticoid receptor by long-term and chronic treatment with glucocorticoid. Steroids, 1994, 59(7): 436-442.

[14]　Shipman G F, Bloomfield C D, Gajlpeczalska K J, et al. Glucocorticoids and lymphocytes Ⅲ: effects of glucocorticoid administration on lymphocyte glucocorticoid receptors. Blood, 1983, 61(6): 1086-1090.

[15]　Xu R B, Tan J X. Regulation of glucocorticoid receptor by glucocorticoids (Ⅱ): the studies on rat liver, brain and spleen. Science China Chemistry, 1990, 33(3): 288-293.

[16]　Alexandrová M, Farkas P. Stress-induced changes of glucocorticoid receptor in rat liver. Journal of Steroid Biochemistry & Molecular Biology, 1992, 42(5): 493-498.

[17]　DuBois D C, Xu Z X, MacKay L, et al. Differential dynamics of receptor down-regulation and tyrosine aminotransferase induction following glucocorticoid treatment. J Steroid Biochem Mol Biol, 1995, 54: 237-243.

[18]　Li M, Zhao F J, Guo J S. Effects of Jawei Shengmai San on the glucocorticoid and its receptor in heat-stressed rats. Acad J Sec Military Med Univ, 1996, 17: 284-286.

[19]　Lu J H, Ling C Q, Tan J X. Effects of Gu Tuo Tang on the glucocorticoid receptors in rats during hemorrhagic shock. Chin J Pathophysiol, 1998,14 : 136-139.

[20]　Ling C Q, Li M, Tan J. Experimental study on protective effect of Chinese herbal medicine on glucocorticoid receptor . Chin J Int Tradit Western Med, 1999, 19 : 302-303.

[21]　Li Y. Relationship between glucocorticoid receptor and deficiency syndrome and the regulation of traditional Chinese medicine. Journal of Chinese Integrative Medicine, 2004, 2(3): 172-174.

[22]　Li M, Ling C Q, Huang X Q, et al. Effects of ginsenosides extracted from ginseng stem and leaves on glucocorticoid receptor in different viscera in heat-damaged rats. J Chin Int Med, 2006, 4: 156-159.

[23]　Ling C Q, Li Y, Zhu X Y, et al. Ginsenosides may reverse the dexamethasone-induced down-regulation of glucocorticoid receptor. Gen Compar Endocrinol, 2006, 140(3): 302.

[24]　Hubbard J R, Tanvir A S, Kalimi M. Rapid high temperature exchange assay for the hepatic glucocorticiod receptor. Mol Cell Biochem, 1984, 65: 95-99.

[25] Tan J X, Xu R B. An improved method for the exchange assay of glucocorticoid receptor. Prog Biochem Biophy, 1987, 4: 56-58.

[26] Laemmli U. Cleavage of structural proteins during the assembly of the head of bacteriophage T4. Nature, 1970, 227: 680-684.

[27] Baki L, Alexis M N. Regulation of tyrosine aminotransferase gene expression by glucocorticoids in quiescent and regenerating liver. Biochemical Journal, 1996, 320 (Pt 3)(3): 745-753.

[28] Nickol J M, Lee K L, Kenney F T. Changes in hepatic levels of tyrosine aminotransferase messenger RNA during induction by hydrocortisone. Journal of Biological Chemistry, 1978, 253(11): 4009-4015.

[29] Kim D H, Jung J S, Suh H W, et al. Inhibition of stress-induced plasma corticosterone levels by ginsenosides in mice: involvement of nitric oxide. Neuroreport, 1998, 9(10): 2261-2264.

Section 4　Words of TCM

1. 病位病性 location and nature of disease
2. 表里同病 simultaneous exterior-interior disease
3. 真寒假热 real cold with false heat
4. 真热假寒 real heat with false cold
5. 热证转寒证 heat syndrome transforming into cold syndrome
6. 气有余便是火 excessive qi causing fire
7. 卫气营血传变 transmission of wei, qi, ying and xue
8. 主色与客色 normal individual complexion and varied normal colors
9. 精神不振 dispiritedness
10. 精气充足 sufficiency of essence and qi
11. 气机调畅 harmonious functional activities of qi
12. 气郁化热 qi stagnation transforming heat
13. 气不摄血 qi failing to keep blood circulation within vessels
14. 气不固精 qi failing to consolidate essence
15. 元气虚衰 decline of primordial qi
16. 四诊结合 synthesis of the four diagnostic methods
17. 未病先防 preventing measures taken before occurrence of disease
18. 表情淡漠 indifferent expression
19. 水气凌心 water attacking the heart
20. 和血止痛 regulating blood to alleviate pain
21. 大肠热结 retention of heat in the large intestine
22. 轻宣润燥 dispersing lung qi and moistening dryness

23. 心脉瘀阻 blood stasis in the heart vessels
24. 四肢抽搐 convulsion of the limbs
25. 饥不欲食 hunger without desire for food
26. 脉有胃气 pulse with stomach qi
27. 清里泄热 clearing away heat in the interior
28. 表邪入里 invasion of the exterior pathogenic factors into the interior
29. 祛风解痉 expelling wind to relieve convulsion
30. 恶寒 / 恶热 aversion to cold / heat
31. 潮热盗汗 tidal fever and night sweating
32. 口干唇裂 dry mouth with cracked lips
33. 高热谵妄 high fever with delirium
34. 脉数无力 rapid and weak pulse
35. 补气健脾 invigorating qi and strengthening the spleen
36. 外感胃脘痛 stomachache due to exogenous pathogenic factors
37. 寒因寒用 treating pseudo-cold syndrome with herbs of cold nature
38. 塞因塞用 treating obstructive syndrome with tonifying therapy
39. 寒邪郁而化热 stagnation of pathogenic cold changing into heat
40. 舌淡苔白而润滑 light-colored tongue with white and slippery coating

(Ge Keli, Zhu Lin)

Chapter 13　Nails

Section 1　Nails and Overall Health

Healthy nails are an important part of overall health. When nails are in good physical shape, people are not only aesthetically pleasing, but they make it easier to perform everyday tasks. However, not many of us put a lot of thought into our nails, either finger or toe, until there appears to be something wrong. The nails can be windows to a patient's overall health. While the nail itself is dead tissue, the areas under the cuticle and beneath the nail are alive and these areas are particularly vulnerable to infection and damage, which is why it is important to see a dermatologist with any nail changes, so that the problem can be diagnosed and treated.

Cosmetics: Keeping the nails healthy and neat looking has become an important grooming ritual for both men and women as the number of consumers that frequent nail salons and use nail cosmetics at home has increased. Nail cosmetics and salon services are generally quite safe, but there are potential problem areas associated with the use of nail cosmetics and salon services: infection, allergic reactions and mechanical damage to the nail. While these are fairly rare occurrences, they can be serious and consumers should take some simple measures to guard against these potential health concerns.

Contracting an infection is the most serious health risk related to nail cosmetics, particularly from manicure and pedicure tools and implements that have not been properly sterilized. Viral, bacterial and fungal infections may be transmitted to unsuspecting consumers from improperly sterilized implements.

Allergic reactions occur when a nail cosmetic ingredient sensitizes the skin which may result in itching, redness, blisters and pain every time the ingredient is used. Some of the more common ingredients that can create an allergic reaction are the acrylic materials found in a wide variety of nail products. Another potential allergen is tosylamide formaldehyde resin, an ingredient found in some nail polishes. If you experience itching or burning of the skin following a nail salon service or the application of nail cosmetics at home, you are recommend to remove the product as soon as possible and to visit a dermatologist to determine which ingredient is responsible for the allergic reaction.

Fungus: Fungal infections, known as onchomycosis or tinea unguium, make up approximately 50% of all nail disorders and since the infection occurs under the nail plate or in the nail bed, it can be difficult to treat. Fungal infections often cause the end of the nail to separate from the nail bed, the skin on which the nail rests. Fungus — colored white, green, yellow or black — may build up under the nail plate and discolor the nail bed. Toenails are more susceptible to fungal infections because they are confined in a warm, moist, weight-bearing environment. Candida or yeast infections are common in fingernails especially if the hands are always in water, as they are in profession such as fishermen, dishwashers or those who work at aquariums or aquatic theme parks.

Fungal infections are contagious and organisms can sometimes spread from one person to another especially where the air is often moist and people's feet are bare. This can happen both at home and in public places like shower stalls, bathrooms or locker rooms or they can be passed around by sharing a nail file or emery board. A recent study noted an increase in athletes' feet, a fungal infection that can grow and multiply on human skin, at boarding schools where students share the same living spaces. One way to reduce the risk of contracting toenail fungus is to always wear shower slippers in public showers, lockers rooms and around swimming pools.

The psoriatic nail: Approximately 50% of patients with psoriasis, a disease of the immune system which causes skin lesions that range from patches of mild scaling to extensive thick, red, scaling plaques, have psoriatic changes in their finger and toenails. Nail changes in psoriasis fall into general categories that may occur singly or all together. These changes can include a deeply pitted nail plate, yellow or yellow-pink discoloration of the nail, white areas under the nail plate or a nail plate that flakes off in yellow patches. In some cases, the nail is entirely lost due to psoriatic involvement of the nail matrix, where the nail and cuticle meet, and the nail bed. Psoriasis of the fingernails also can resemble other conditions such as chronic infection or inflammation of the nail bed or nail fold, the hard skin overlapping the base and sides of the nails.

Psoriasis of the toenails can resemble a chronic fungal infection. Psoriatic nails can be treated by the dermatologist as part of the overall treatment of the disease and dermatologists are beginning to study the use of biologic treatments. Therapies for the psoriatic nail have been limited because topical treatments do not penetrate down into the nail fold where the psoriasis is actually disfiguring the nail plate. The introduction of biologic therapies to control skin psoriasis also may be beneficial for patients with psoriatic nails since these treatments work with the body's immune system to prevent the body from triggering a psoriasis flare.

Nail malignancies: Subungal, or under the nail, melanoma appears as a brown to black colored streak underneath the nail, which is often mistaken for a bruise or the nail streaks that frequently occur in people with dark skin. Subungal melanoma accounts for approximately 2% of melanomas in Caucasians, and 30% ~ 40% of melanomas in patients with skin of color. Subungal melanoma occurs with equal frequency in males and females, appears most often in people over 50 years of age, but can develop at any age and is seen most often under the nail of the thumb or the big toe. Subungal melanoma should be suspected whenever a nail streak appears without known injury to the nail, the nail discoloration does not gradually disappear and a bruise or the size of the nail streak increases over time. It's important to see a dermatologist immediately if any changes are noticed on the nail since treatment for this condition should begin as soon as possible.

Overall, it's important when caring for the nails at home or having a service in a salon to make sure that the nails are being treated gently and safely. Paying careful attention to the nails can help ensure that any infections or diseases are identified early and that treatment begins as soon as possible.

As the nation's 375 000 nail technicians buff, polish and file our fingers and toes, the workplace exposure to chemicals in the polish and glue can pose a real threat. But it's not just the amount of those substances that can turn them toxic; it is also the way they get into workers' bodies. Workplace conditions in certain nail salons, expertly laid out last week in an investigation by The New York Times's Sarah Maslin Nir, can alleviate or exacerbate these issues. Chemicals inside of the glues, removers, polishes and salon products, which technicians are often exposed to at close proximity and in poorly ventilated spaces, can be hazardous individually. When combined, however, they could potentially cause even greater harm. Yet it is difficult to know how these chemicals affect the body because current evaluations do not look at these substances comprehensively. There are also few reports looking at how each compound individually affects nail workers.

The risks are many: Dust shavings from filed nails can settle on the skin like pollen and cause irritation or can be inhaled (and those small particles could contain chemicals from the polishes or acrylics). Technicians could also inhale harmful vapors or mists from the chemicals in the shop. The compounds could also settle into workers' eyes. Moreover, these substances could be swallowed while eating, drinking or puffing on a cigarette during a break.

The US Occupational Safety and Health Administration (OSHA), which sets workplace safety standards, cites a laundry list of chemicals that nail salon workers encounter daily. For the typical nail salon client these chemicals may not pose a large threat, but for workers who are exposed to this potentially toxic brew day after day there's an elevated level of risk. Studies documenting the health problems of nail technicians often describe respiratory, skin and musculoskeletal issues. Respiratory problems, unsurprisingly, were typically associated with the reporting of workplace exposures such as poor air quality. Some of these chemicals are also linked with birth defects. Yet, as with many environmental exposures, it can be difficult to prove that an adverse health effect was the direct result of workplace exposures instead of those encountered elsewhere in life.

Nail salons could help protect workers by providing certain safety equipment. Public health officials say wearing nitrile gloves (not latex or vinyl) could help shield workers from chemical exposures. Using a proper mask to protect workers from chemicals or nail-filing dust would also help. Paper dust masks (like those most often seen in a salon), however, only protect the wearer from some dusts but not chemicals. Good ventilation in a nail salon would also typically eliminate the need for workers to wear heavy-duty respirator masks with organic vapor cartridges.

Section 2   Angong Niuhuang Wan

Angong Niuhuang Wan (ANW) or AnGongNiuHuang Wan is a composite prescription of traditional Chinese medicine (TCM) composed of Calculus Bovis, Cornu Bubali, Moschus, Margarita, Cinnabaris, Realgar, Rhizoma Coptidis, Radix Scutellariae Baicalensis, Fructus Gradeniae, Radix Curcumae and Borneolum Synthcticum. In China, ANW is generally prescribed for patients suffering from acute and chronic cerebral diseases, such as hypoxic-ischemic encephalopathy, viral encephalitis, cerebral paralysis, hypertensive cerebral hemorrhage, severe craniocerebral trauma and diffuse axonal injury. However, the clinical application of ANW is limited by the existence of two known hepatorenal toxic metalloids, mercury (Hg) and arsenic (As) found in cinnabar (contains 96% HgS) and realgar (contains 90% As_2S_2), respectively .

In recent years, it was reported that cinnabar and realgar, as well as ANW, protected dopaminergic neurons against lipopolysaccharide-induced neurotoxicity by inhibiting the microglia activation and pro-inflammatory factor production. Moreover, cinnabar and realgar exerted similar effects as ANW on changes in levels of cortical catecholamine and its metabolites in endotoxin-induced intracerebral hemorrhage in rats. Evidence from in vitro and in vivo studies suggest that both cinnabar and realgar are probably the main contributors to the neuroprotective effect of ANW.

Because cinnabar and realgar are relatively poorly water-soluble in the form of sulfides and have long history of safe use at therapeutic doses, they are considered to be less poisonous than common mercurials (mercuric chloride and methylmercury) and arsenicals (arsenite and arsenate). In addition, both the cinnabar and realgar almost cannot cross this blood-brain barrier because they cannot pass through slit junctions and have difficulty traversing the lipid cell membrane. However, in the liver and kindey tissues, a large part of the basement membrane is exposed due to large discontinuous capillaries, through which most small molecule drugs can pass into the hepatic and renal interstitium. Thus, the liver and kidneys have been suggested as the main target organs of cinnabar and realgar-induced toxicity. Long-term use or overdose of cinnabar or cinnabar-containing preparations could induce hepatic and renal dysfunction due to the accumulation of mercury being present as non-sulfur bound species. When animals were exposed continuously and chronically to cinnabar at clinical dosage, free mercury could be released and absorbed, causing a pronounced depletion of sulfur groups of enzymes, oxidizing intramitochondrial NADH and NADPH, and enhancing depolarization of the mitochondrial inner membrane, hence leading to reactive oxygen species (ROS) generation and lipid peroxidation (LPO). On the other hand, soluble arsenic contents of realgar were measured (0.6% of the total arsenic content) under simulated gastric fluid. If realgar-containing medicines were taken for long periods of time or in excessive dosages, soluble forms of arsenic could also be absorbed from the gastrointestinal tract into blood circulation, freely crossing cell membrane and finding distribution in target organs, especially the liver and kidneys. Similar to mercury, the soluble arsenic in realgar could accelerate production of oxygen-derived free radicals (such as H_2O_2 and superoxide) by binding to biological ligands containing sulfhydryl groups especially vicinal thiols, leading to oxidation of DNA and proteins and oxidative damage to the liver and kidneys. Hence, oxidative stress plays a seminal role in the pathogenesis of chronic liver and kidney injury elicited by mercury-containing cinnabar and arsenic-containing realgar.

Chronic inflammation is also an important pathological mechanism underlying the progression of mercury and arsenic-induced hepatic and renal lesions. Studies in the past decades have demonstrated that mercury and arsenic generate ROS that trigger activation of pro-inflammatory signals, including mitogen-activated protein kinase superfamily members (MAPK), phosphatidylinositol 3 kinase (PI3K), Akt and nuclear factor-kappa B (NFκB). It has been reported that mercury and arsenic-activated MAPK/NFκB and PI3K/Akt/NFκB signal pathways play critical roles in the multiple steps of inflammatory responses by regulating the transcription of a chain of pro-inflammatory mediators. Considering the pro-oxidative and pro-inflammatory properties of cinnabar and realgar, antioxidant and/or anti-inflammatory intervention might represent an effective strategy to ameliorate cinnabar and realgar-induced hepatorenal toxicity.

As noted previously, cinnabar and realgar are not used alone in ANW; they are combined with other herbs as adjuvants in the form of a composite formula. Previously published studies described that multiple constituents of four combined herbs in ANW, including Radix Scutellariae Baicalensis flavones, Rhizoma Coptidis alkaloids, Fructus Gradeniae iridoids and Radix Curcumae curcuminoids, contributed to protective effects against both liver and kidney injury owing to their anti-oxidative and anti-inflammatory properties. However, the ameliorative effects of the above mentioned herbs in ANW to cinnabar and realgar-induced hepatorenal toxicity were still not investigated.

According to modern toxicology principles, metal-containing traditional preparations are extremely toxic and hazardous even in therapeutic doses. However, it is noted that the heavy metals in these formulae are not used alone, but rather combined with different kinds of medicinal herbs and/or animal-based products. In spite of the wide use of polyherb-metallic formulae in modern pharmaceuticals and in ethnopharmacology, the rationale of including metals and herb-metal interactions in traditional remedies still needs to be addressed. As a representative example, ANW formula contains cinnabar and realgar as principal elements, along with several types of medicinal herbs and animal products. Thus, studies on ANW may be considered as a pilot model exploring how herbal medicines in the formula exert potential protective effects against hepatorenal toxicity induced by heavy metals.

In ANW, mercury and arsenic interact with herbal constituents, which might serve as adjuvants to potentiate therapeutic effects or to reduce mercury and arsenic-induced toxicity. The main herbal components of ANW are Rhizoma Coptidis, Radix Scutellariae Baicalensis, Fructus Gradeniae, and Radix Curcumae with berberine, baicalin, geniposide and curcumin as major active constituents, respectively. Intriguingly, there has been growing body of literature reporting the aforementioned herbal components in ANW and their constituents as having hepatorenal protective potentials. For example, berberine has shown protective effects against hepatic damage induced by lead acetate. Oral administration of baicalin apparently inhibited acetaminophen-induced hepatotoxicity. Moreover, it was previously demonstrated that geniposide and crocetin derivatives might be responsible for the hepatoprotective effect of gardenia fruits against carbon tetrachloride-induced hepatic damage in mice. Also, Sankar et al. treated rats with sodium arsenite and curcumin and they found that curcumin significantly protected the liver and kidneys from arsenic-induced injury. Thus, it is plausible to assume that the herbal components in ANW and their constituents, including berberine, baicalin, geniposide and curcumin, act synergistically to combat damage induced by cinnabar and realgar. This hypothesis was confirmed by the histological examination of liver and kidney sections of mice. Co-administration of other herbs with cinnabar and realgar in ANW revealed no abnormality in the architecture of the liver and kidneys, and reversed cinnabar and realgar-induced histopathological changes.

Although the mechanisms by which cinnabar and realgar cause hepatorenal damage are not fully defined, recent studies have shown that cinnabar and realgar exert their toxic effects by inducing oxidative stress in mice or rats, by consumption of GSH, by interacting with sulfhydryl groups of proteins or by generating ROS such as superoxide anion $[O_2 \cdot]^-$, hydroxyl radical $[HO \cdot]^-$ and hydrogen peroxide (H_2O_2). As a non-enzymatic antioxidant, GSH, conjugates directly with mercury and arsenic through its sulfhydryl group and preserves functional integrity of cell membranes. Furthermore, CAT is generally considered as an enzymatic antioxidant and provides protection against the deleterious effects of H_2O_2-mediated oxidative injury.

Nowadays, naturally occurring antioxidants are recognized as important compounds in combating heavy metal-induced toxicity. In ANW, a variety of herbal compounds, including berberine, baicalin, geniposide and curcumin, have strong anti-oxidative and detoxifying activities in a wide range of diseases. Thus, the potential protective effects of herbal constituents in ANW against cinnabar and realgar-induced hepatorenal toxicity could be associated with the reestablishment of the sulfhydryl groups and redox homeostasis.

Innate immune-mediated inflammatory response is another critical pathological mechanism amplifying cinnabar and realgar-induced hepatorenal injury. It is generally reported that if the binding capacity of GSH becomes saturated, the elevated accessibility of unbound mercury and arsenic triggers a series of events causing severe necrosis of hepatocytes and renal cells. Subsequently, macrophages infiltrate into sites of initial injury and release pro-inflammatory cytokines such as IL1 β and TNFα and chemokines to recruit more monocytes and neutrophils into regions of necrosis. The macrophages and neutrophils produce a great quantity of cytotoxic agents and superoxide radical anions, which further exacerbate the local injury to the liver and kidney tissues in the later stage. Numerous pro-inflammatory enzymes are involved in local tissue lesion during the chronic inflammatory process. Among them, the inducible isoform of cyclooxygenase (COX-2) and nitric oxide synthase (iNOS) have been identified with the pathogenesis of inflammatory diseases. Elevation of COX-2 activity is responsible for the biosynthesis of pro-inflammatory prostaglandins (PGs) at the inflammatory site, including PGE2. It has been found that arsenite or mercuric chloride exposure induces COX-2 overexpression accompanied by an increased level of PGE2 production in endothelial cells. Many studies have also shown that development and propagation of inflammation are highly correlated with enhancement of enzyme activity of iNOS. Under inflammatory conditions, iNOS in infiltrated macrophages, renal cells and hepatocytes is activated to produce biologically active NO. High concentrations of NO react with superoxide anion to generate a cytotoxic prooxidant, peroxynitrite anion $[ONOO \cdot]^-$. It has been demonstrated that acetaminophen-induced hepatorenal injury is positively correlated with the overproduction of NO and intracellular GSH depletion. Also, inhibition of iNOS-mediated NO production has been shown to protect against acute tubular necrosis induced by mercuric chloride.

It has been reported that berberine significantly reduced the lipopolysaccharide-induced procoagulant activity and expression of tissue factors through the concomitant inactivation of the ERK/JNK/P38 MAPK, Akt and NFκB pathways in human monoblastic leukemia THP-1 cells. Recently, Liao et al. have also demonstrated that baicalin treatment can effectively attenuate acetaminophen-induced liver injury by down-regulating hepatic phosphorylated ERK1/2 expression in a mice model. Recent studies have also revealed geniposide inhibits lipopolysaccharide-induced release of inflammation-associated mediators, mainly through suppression of phosphorylation of ERK1/2, p38 MAPK and IκBα in murine microglia and peritoneal macrophages. Furthermore, curcumin shows protective effects against coxsackievirus B3-induced myocarditis through suppressing the local myocardial expression of pro-inflammatory cytokines (TNFα, IL1β, and IL6) in a PI3K/Akt/NFκB pathway dependent manner.

Section 3　Research Article

Astragalus injection

[Abstract] Background: Astragalus is a widely used traditional Chinese medicine and has been proven beneficial for many aspects of human health. It is important to explore the neuroprotective effect and mechanism of astragalus injection in cerebral ischemia reperfusion injury. Methods: The focal cerebral ischemic model with middle cerebral artery occlusion (MCAO) reperfusion was established by Longa's method in healthy adult male Wistar rats, and treated by injecting intraperitoneally astragalus injection (3 mL/kg). The neurobehavioral function of rats was evaluated by Longa's test. The cerebral blood flow (CBF) was measured by laser Doppler flowmetry and the cerebral infarct volume was calculated by tetrazolium chloride (TTC) stain. The shape and structure of neurons in parietal cortex was observed by HE stain and the neuronal apoptosis was detected by terminal deoxynucleotidyl transferase mediated dUTP nick end labeling (TUNEL) and flow cytometry. The expressions of c-jun N-terminal kinase 3 (JNK3) mRNA and protein were determined by RT-PCR and immunohistochemical assay and Western blotting respectively. Results: After treatment with astragalus injection, the expressions of JNK3 mRNA and protein reduced significantly, the number of neuronal apoptosis decreased, the cerebral infarct volume shrank, CBF increased, and the neuronal shape-structure and animal neurobehavioral function improved significantly compared with those in model rats. Conclusions: It is suggested that astragalus injection could inhibit neuronal apoptosis, reduce infarct volume and improve neurobehavioral function by down-regulating the expression of JNK3 gene after cerebral ischemia reperfusion injury in rats.

Keywords: astragalus injection; cerebral ischemia; reperfusion injury; apoptosis; JNK3; rats

1　Background

Astragalus (Astragalus membranaceus) has long been known in traditional Chinese medicine as an immune-modulating herb. In clinical practice, administration of astragalus has achieved widespread use in the treatment of diabetes, and in the treatment of kidney abnormalities caused by diabetes. Polysaccharoses, astragaloside, isoflavones and saponin glycosides are the primary astragalus extracts. Recent studies have demonstrated that astragalus has an antifibrotic effect in a rat model, and can inhibit the expression of transforming growth factor β1 (TGFβ1), reduce extracellular matrix component (ECM) synthesis, and block tubular epithelial to mesenchymal transition (EMT) processes. Results of a meta-analysis revealed that astragalus injection had therapeutic effects in diabetic nephropathy (DN) patients, including reduced urine protein and improved renal function. Astragaloside Ⅳ, one of the main active ingredients of astragalus, was shown to ameliorate podocyte apoptosis, prevent acute kidney injury, and attenuate glycated albumin-induced EMT in renal proximal tubular cells.

Neuronal apoptosis in ischemic penumbra is one of the mechanisms of neuronal damage in ischemic cerebrovascular disease[1]. The c-jun amino terminal kinase (c-Jun N-terminal kinase, JNK) signaling is an important pathway of mitogen-activated protein kinase (MAPK)[2] and plays an important regulatory role in programmed cell death[3]. The encoding JNK genes found presently in mammalian cells included jnk1, jnk2 and jnk3, and their corresponding coding product JNK1 and JNK2 expressed widely, while JNK3 expressed only in brain, heart and testicular tissues[4]. JNK3 is the key signal in neuronal apoptosis during brain ischemia[5], and the JNK3 gene knockout not only reduces the c-jun phosphorylation but also protects the brain injury caused by cerebral ischemia/hypoxia[6], so that inhibiting JNK3 expression and neuronal apoptosis may be one of important methods to prevent and treat cerebral ischemic injury[7]. Lijima et al.[8] reported that propofol could get rid of free radicals in the body, improve cerebral blood microcirculation, and inhibit neuronal apoptosis in hippocampus caused by ischemia in rats[9]. Previous experiments shown some ingredients of traditional Chinese medicine have neuroprotctive role[10-11]. Qu et al.[12-13] reported that astragaloside, a main ingredient of astragalus injection, could decrease leukocyte infusion in cerebral ischemia reperfusion tissue, and reduce inflammatory reaction and brain edema. The research results of Ye et al.[14-15] indicated that astragalus injection could inhibit the apoptosis-associated gene JNK3 expression, but its neuroprotective mechanism is not very clear now[16-17]. This study aims further to study the influence of astragalus injection on the expression of JNK3 and neuronal apoptosis following cerebral ischemia reperfusion injury, as well as its neuroprotective mechanism.

2 Methods

2.1 Establishment of animal models

Total of 70 healthy adult male Wistar rats (SPF grade with 4 months age and 203 ~ 250 g body weight) were supplied by the Laboratory Animal Center of Qingdao Drug Inspection, the license number is SCXK (Lu) 20090007. The disposition on animals in the experiments are in accordance with the relevant provisions of the guidance to take care of the experimental animals issued by the Science and Technology Department of the People's Republic of

China[18]. Of them 20 rats ($n = 20$) were randomly selected as control group and the rest 50 rats were established focal cerebral ischemic models by inserting intraluminally a monofilament suture into middle cerebral artery from external-internal carotid artery according to Longa's methods[19]. After ischemia 2 h, the monofilament thread was withdrawn to reperfuse blood flow, and the rats in the control group was subjected the same surgical operation without inserting a monofilament suture. Core body temperature was maintained at 36 ~ 37 ℃ using an electric homeothermic blanket during and after the operation, and the cerebral blood flow (CBF) in parietal cortex was continuously monitoring with laser Doppler flowmetry (PeriFlux 5000, Sweden). The rat was considered as a successful model when its CBF reduced to 30% and appeared Horner's sign with right forelimb flexing and circling rightward as running. 10 died or unsuccessful rats were except of and 40 successful models were internalized into the experiment and then subdivided randomly into model group ($n = 20$) and treatment group ($n = 20$).

2.2   Treatment

Astragalus injection (No. Z31020084) is provided by Chengdu Diao Jiuhong Pharmacy Co., Ltd.. Each milliliter (mL) astragalus injection contains 1 mg astragaloside (molecular weight: 784.97, molecular formula: $C_{41}H_{68}O_{14}$). According to the treatment dose reported by Liu et al.[20], the rats in the treatment group were intraperitoneally injected 3 mL/kg (3 mg/kg) of astragalus injection at ischemia 2 h and before reperfusion, while equal normal saline for rats in the control and model groups.

2.3   Evaluating indexes

Neurobehavioral function: After treatment 24 h with astragalus injection, the neurobehavioral function was evaluated according to Longa's test[19]. Score 0: no behavioral deficiency. Score 1: forelimb reflexing (the tail lifting-suspension test positive). Score 2: lateral thrust resistance decreased (lateral thrust test positive) and forelimb reflexing, no circling. Score 3: the same as midrange behavior and circling spontaneously. The higher score, the severe neurological function deficiency.

Cerebral blood flow (CBF): CBF of the lateral hemisphere (parietal cortex) was continuously monitored with laser Doppler flowmetry. The head of laser fiber was placed stereotactically (SN-3, Narishige, Tokyo, Japan) in the area known to be ischemia after MCAO by a stainless cannula (the right caudate anterior 18.0 mm, right 8.0 mm, and height 18.0 mm) according to an atlas. The rat CBF was recorded by Perisoft ware and calculated by CBF index (CBFI %) = (CBF of ischemic side / CBF of contralateral side) × 100.

Cerebral infarct volume (CIV): After treatment 24 h with astragalus injection, 5 rats in each group were randomly selected and anesthetized with 10% chloral hydrate 0.3 mL

(300 mg/kg) to be sacrificed by cutting the neck. The brain was removed rapidly and taken out completely to be cut into five coronal sections of 2 mm thickness backward from optic chiasma. Then the sections were immersed in 2% 2, 3, 5-triphenyltetrazolium chloride (TTC) at 37 ℃ for 10 min. The normal brain tissue showed red and infarct tissue white. The CIV is determined by Adobe PhotoShop CS after taking a photograph and presented as the percentage (%) of (cerebral infarct area / contralateral hemisphere area)×100.

Histopathology: After treatment 24 h with astragalus injection, 5 rats in each group were anesthetized with 10% chloral hydrate and perfused from heart with 200 mL of normal saline and 200 mL of 4% paraformaldehyde solution. The brain was taken out of and dehydrated by gradient ethanol, cleared by xylene, embedded in paraffin and cut coronally backward from optic chiasma into pieces of thickness 5 μm, then adhered to the glass slices, and finally stored at 4 °C. Four paraffin sections from each rat were selected to stain with hematoxylin for 5 min, differentiated by 75% hydrochloric acid ethanol for 30 s, and stained by acidification eosin for 1 min. The neuron morphology in parietal cortex was observed in four non-overlapping visual fields under light microscope and presented as degenerative cell index (DCI): the number of degenerative cells / total cells in the visual field (Mean ± SD).

Neuronal apoptosis: According to the instruction of TUNEL apoptosis detection kit (Wuhan Boster Biotech. Co. Ltd., China), four paraffin sections from each group were conventionally de-waxed and hydrated to dispose with 3% H_2O_2 for 10 min at room temperature, and then digested by proteinase K (1 ∶ 200) for 10 min at 37 ℃ . Mixing TdT (1 μL) and Dig-dUTP (1 μL) into labeling buffer (18 μL) and add on each paraffin slice to react for 2 h at 37 °C. Add biotin anti-digoxin antibody (1 ∶ 100) and react for 30 min at 37 °C, then add SABC (1 ∶ 100) to react for 30 min at 37 ℃ and colored with HRP-DAB reagent kit (Beijing Tiangen Biotech. Co. Ltd.). The TUNEL positive cells showed orange-brown nuclei under light microscope (Olympus CK2, Japan). Under high magnification (400 times), four non-overlapping visual fields in hippocampus were randomly selected from each section to calculate the neuronal apoptosis index (NAI). NAI = the number of TUNEL-positive cells / the number of total cells in the field (Mean ± SD).

Immunohistochemical assay: The rabbit anti-rat antibody and immunohistochemical SP kit (Wuhan Boster Biotech. Co. Ltd.) were used to detect the expression JNK3 in parietal cortex. Referring to the instructions of kit, four sections from each group were de-waxed and hydrated to dispose 3% H_2O_2 for 10 min at room temperature, adding antibody (1 ∶ 100) to react for 2 h at 37 ℃ and SP (1 ∶ 100) to incubate at 37 ℃ for 30 min, and colored with HRP-DAB. The JNK3 positive cells appeared brown cytoplasm and measured by UV spectrophotometer (Beckmann USA) in four non-overlapping visual fields in each section. The JNK3 expression intensity was presented by relative absorbance (A) index (RAI): the A value of JNK3 positive cells minus the background A value, Mean ± SD.

Flow cytometry: After treatment 24 h with astragalus injection, 5 rats in each group were anesthetized with 10% chloral hydrate and perfused from heart with 200 mL of normal saline. Then take out off the whole brain and put in the distilled cool water, peel off the vessel and membranous tissues and cut 100 mg of left hippocampal tissue. According to the instruction of annexin V-FITC apoptosis detection kit (Nanjing Biotech. Co. Ltd.), flow cytometry analysis was operated by FACScan Calibur (BD Company, USA) within 1 h and the result of neuronal apoptotic ratio (NAR %) was calculated by CELL Quest program analysis.

Western blotting: After treatment 24 h with astragalus injection, 5 rats from each group were deeply anesthetized and perfused with normal saline. The whole brain was frozen in liquid nitrogen at −80 ℃ and separated 100 mg of left hippocampus to grind with equal RIPA lysate at 4 ℃. After ultrasonic slurry and centrifuged with 12 000 r/min for 10 min at 4 ℃ (Eppendorf 5801, Germany), the supernatant was collected to determine the total protein concentration by BCA-100 kit. Take protein sample 50 μg to subject to electrophoresis on 10% SDS-polyacrylamide gels (SDS-PAGE) and transfer onto PVDF membrane (Millipore, Bedford, MA, USA) using a semi-dry electrophoretic transfer system. The PVDF membrane were blocked for 1 h at room temperature and then incubated with the primary goal anti-rat JNK3 antibody (1 : 300) overnight at 4 °C. Finally the membrane was exposed 2 ~ 4 min in X-ray box, developed an image for 40 s, fixed 2 min, washed 5 min and dried. The absorbance (A) value was determined by Quantity One software. In the same specimen, the value of 3-glyceraldehyde-phosphate dehydrogenase (GAPDH) was also detected to calibrate the concentration of each target protein. The relative A value (RAV) was calculated as follows: the A value of JNK3 / the A value of GAPDH.

RT-PCR: The above frozen sample was homogenized in Trizol reagent (Life Tech, USA) using 1 mL of Trizol per 50 mg of tissue. Total RNA was extracted from the tissue according to the manufacturer's protocol and calculated the content by $A_{260\,nm\,/\,280\,nm}$ spectrophotometer. Using RT-PCR kit (Invitrogen, USA, USA), cDNA was synthesized from total RNA (5 μg). JNK3 sense primer: 5'-CTG ATG CAG TGC ACG ATC TAC-3', anti-sense primer: 5'-AGC GTC GTA CTA GAC GTT GCG AT-3', the product: 197 bp. GAPDH sense primer: 5'-TAG TCT ACA TGC TGC AGT ACT ACT-3', anti-sense primer: 5'-CGA CTT GAT GTT AGC GAG ATA TC-3', the product: 225 bp. PCR cycling conditions with reference to the use of JNK3 mRNA kit (Santa Cruz, USA), 95 ℃ predegeneration for 3 min; at 94 ℃ modified for 30 s; 56 ℃ for 30 s; 72 ℃ for 40 s, for 30 cycle. Finally extension at 72 ℃ for 3 min. The experiment is repeated 3 times with a 2% agarose gel electrophoresis of PCR products, and visualized under ultraviolet illumination by ethidium bromide (EB) staining. The A value of each mRNA band in the same gel was captured and determined through Scion analysis software. The relative A value (RAV) of JNK3 mRNA were presented as: the A value of JNK3 / the A value of GAPDH.

2.4 Statistical analysis

The experimental results were adopted to the analysis of SPSS15.0 software (SPSS, Chicago, IL, USA). The experimental data was showed in (means ± SD), and we use single factor for analysis of variance between groups, LSD-t test for comparing in pairs.

3 Results

3.1 Neurobehavioral function

The neurobehavioral function of rats in the control group was normal and Longa's test was 0 scales. The Longa's test scales of rats in the model group was significantly higher than those in the control group ($t = 30.82$, $P < 0.01$), while in the treatment group decreased more significantly than that in the model group ($t = 7.57$, $P < 0.01$) and also higher than that in the control group ($t = 27.30$, $P < 0.01$)(Table 13-1).

3.2 Cerebral blood flow

The cerebral blood flow index (CBFI %) of rats in the control group was 100, which in the model group (73.25 ± 5.45) reduced significantly ($t = 30.26$, $P < 0.01$), while in the treatment group (81.60 ± 6.30) was significantly higher than that in model group ($t = 6.11$, $P < 0.01$) and also lower than that in the control group ($t = 18.10$, $P < 0.01$) (Table 13-1).

Table 13-1 Longa's test scales and CBFI of rats (Mean ± SD)

Groups	n	Longa's test scales	CBFI / %
Control group	20	0.00 ± 0.00	3.53 ± 1.13
Model group	20	$2.25 \pm 0.45^*$	$73.25 \pm 5.45^*$
Treatment group	20	$1.553 \pm 0.35^{\triangle \#}$	$81.50 \pm 6.30^{\triangle \#}$

Compared with control group, $^*t = 30.26 \sim 30.82$, $P < 0.01$; $^\triangle t = 18.10 \sim 27.30$, $P < 0.01$; $^\#$Compared with the model group, $t = 7.57 \sim 6.11$, $P < 0.01$.

3.3 Cerebral infarct Volume

The normal brain tissues showed red and infarct tissue white. No cerebral infarct area was found in the brain tissue of the control group rats (CIV = 0), while a large infarct volume (CIV = 70.50 ± 6.75) existed in model group, which reduced to (CIV = 45.35 ± 5.62) in the treatment group significantly ($t = 8.11$, $P < 0.01$).

3.4 The pathology in parietal cortex

Hematoxylin-eosin (HE) staining showed that the neurons in parietal cortex arranged neatly, the cellular structure was completed and chromatin shade evenly, and the degenerative cell index (DCI) was 022 ± 0.07. In the model group, the neurons degenerated seriously, triangular or irregular shape, the cytoplasm and nucleus concentrated, and the DCI (0.56 ± 0.20) was higher than that in the control group ($t = 4.54$, $P < 0.01$). In treatment group, the DCI (0.33 ± 0.14) was significantly lower than that in the model group ($t = 2.43$, $P < 0.05$) and also higher than that in the control group ($t = 2.35$, $P < 0.05$).

3.5 Neuronal apoptosis in hippocampus

TUNEL staining showed that a few apoptotic neurons existed in the control group (NAI = 0.12 ± 0.02). The number of apoptotic neurons in the model group (NAI = 0.33 ± 0.07) increased significantly than that of the control group ($t = 8.16$, $P < 0.01$), while decreased more significantly in the treatment group (NAI = 0.26 ± 0.04) than that of the model group ($t = 2.46$, $P < 0.05$) and also higher than that in the control group ($t = 8.86$, $P < 0.01$).

Flow cytometry indicated that neuronal apoptotic ratio (NAR) in model group (6.56 ± 1.65) increased more significantly than that in the control group (1.67 ± 0.35) ($t = 8.20$, $P < 0.01$). In the treatment group, the NAR (4.35 ± 1.12) decreased more significantly than that in the model group ($t = 3.13$, $P < 0.01$) and also higher than that in the control group ($t = 6.46$, $P < 0.01$).

3.6 The expression of JNK3

Immunohistochemical staining showed that the expression of JNK3 in parietal cortex of the control group (RAI = 0.14 ± 0.05) was weakly, which increased more significantly in the model group (RAI = 0.37 ± 0.12) than that of the control group ($t = 5.00$, $P < 0.01$), while reduced more obviously in the treatment group (RAI = 0.26 ± 0.08) than that of the model group ($t = 2.15$, $P < 0.05$) and also higher than that in the control group ($t = 3.59$, $P < 0.01$).

Western blotting of quantitative analysis (Figure 13-1) indicated that JNK3 (11kD) expressed weakly in the control group (RAV = 0.33 ± 0.08), and increased significantly in the model group (RAV = 0.87 ± 0.21), higher than that in the control group ($t = 6.84$, $P < 0.01$), while reduced more obviously in the treatment group (RAV = 0.56 ± 0.14) than that in the model group ($t = 3.54$, $P < 0.01$) and also higher than that in the control group ($t = 4.04$, $P < 0.01$).

3.7 The expression of JNK3 mRNA

The relative A values of JNK3 and GAPDH present the relative content of PCR products. The JNK3 mRNA in the control group (RAV = 0.33 ± 0.07) expressed weakly, which expressed significantly in the model group (RAV = 0.93 ± 0.21) stronger than that in the control group (t = 7.67, P < 0.01), while decreased more in the treatment group (RAV = 0.67 ± 0.17) than that in the model group (t = 2.72, P < 0.01) and also higher than that in the control group (t = 6.26, P < 0.01).

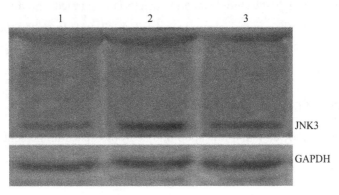

Figure 13-1   The fragmentation formed by JNK3 protein detected by Western blotting

Line 1: a weaker fragment was formed by JNK3 protein in the control group. Line 2: a strong fragment was formed by JNK3 protein in the model group. Line 3: a middle fragment was formed by JNK3 protein in the treatment group.

4   Discussion

Diabetic nephropathy (DN) is a major microvascular complication of diabetes mellitus, as well as the leading cause of end-stage renal disease. A pathological change associated with DN is the accumulation of normal and abnormal extracellular matrix components (ECM) in renal glomeruli and interstitium. TGFβ is a secreted protein that plays a critical role in renal fibrosis and the accumulation of ECM, and intraperitoneal injections of TGFβ alone were sufficient to initiate a prominent renal fibrotic response. Further, TGFβ isoforms and their receptors were upregulated in both experimental models of DN, as well as in human DN. We chose to focus on TGFβ1 because it is the most abundantly expressed isoform in the kidney, and has been most closely linked to the pathophysiology of DN. Additionally, it was reported that TGFβ1 was stimulated by high glucose levels, and was chiefly expressed in renal tubular epithelial cells in diabetic mice.

Cerebral ischemia and reperfusion can induce neuronal apoptosis which related very closely to the expression of apoptosis related genes c-jun N-terminal kinase 3 (JNK3)[21]. Recanalizing the occluded artery as early as possible to restore the regional blood supply in ischemic penumbra and trying to save neurons to restore their functions are the main purpose of the treatment[22]. How to prevent delayed neuronal death to rescue ischemic penumbra becomes the main direction of the current treatment[23]. JNK3 is located in the cytoplasm of neurons, which is stimulated in emergency by cerebral ischemia reperfusion injury before the activation transfers into the nucleus, activated transcription factors c-Jun and Jun D. The activating transcription factors combined with cis function components to cause a large number of apoptosis related gene expression, which associated closely to delayed cell death[24-26].

Ren et al.[27] reported that astragalus could: (1) eliminate free radicals and avoid lipid peroxidation to improve cerebral function, (2) reduce the content of excitatory amino acid and restrain the expression of heat shock protein 70 and alleviated the cerebral ischemic injury, (3) reduce the permeability of blood vessel and improve of hemorrheology after ischemia, and (4) restrain the hypernormal expression of glial fibril acidic protein in early period of cerebral ischemia and inhibit neuronal apoptosis effectively. Ye et al.[14] reported that astragalus injection could inhibit neuronal apoptosis and expression of JNK3 after hypoxia/hypoglycemia and re-oxygenation in hippocampal neurons.

In this experiment, the results show that the expressions of JNK3 mRNA and protein increased significantly after cerebral ischemia reperfusion to induce neuronal apoptosis, neuronal degeneration and cerebral infarction, which caused neurobehavioral function disorderly. In the model group, RT-PCR results indicated that JNK3 mRNA expressed significantly, immuno-histochemical staining and quantitative Western blotting showed JNK3 protein expressed higher than those in the control group, at the same time, TUNEL assay and flow cytometry also showed neuronal apoptosis highly, and hematoxylin-eosin staining showed neuronal degeneration seriously with large ischemic infarction and neurobehavioral dysfunction of rats. These results further indicated that cerebral ischemia caused JNKS expression to inducing neuronal apoptosis and nervous dysfunction. After the treatment with astragalus injection, the expressions of JNK3 mRNA and JNK3 protein in hippocampus decreased more significantly than those in the model group, so reduced the JNK3 protein activity and inhabit neuronal apoptosis, and as a result, reduced the cerebral infarction volume and improved the neuronal structure and neurobehavioral function of rats. Our research results were coincident with the previous reports[28-29], which further suggested that astragalus injection could recover the cerebral blood flow to the ischemic area, reduce the cerebral infarct volume and improve the neurobehavioral function of rats. It might be the molecular mechanism of astragalus reducing JNK3 expression and inhibiting neuronal apoptosis to recover neuronal structure and function of rats after cerebral ischemia reperfusion injury.

5   Conclusions

Astragalus injection could reduce infarction volume and improve neurobehavioral function by reducing the expression of JNK3 to inhibit neuronal apoptosis following cerebral ischemia in rats.

References

[1] Blomgren K, Zhu C, Hallin U, et al. Mitochondria and ischemic reperfusion damage in the adult and in the developing brain. Biochemical & Biophysical Research Communications, 2003, 304(3): 551-559.

[2] Davis R J. Signal transduction by the JNK group of MAP kinases. Cell, 2000, 103(2): 239-252.

[3] Ginet V, Puyal J, Magnin G, et al. Limited role of the c-Jun N-terminal kinase pathway in a neonatal rat model of cerebral hypoxia-ischemia. Journal of Neurochemistry, 2010, 108(3): 552-562.

[4] Bogoyevitch M A, Kobe B. Uses for JNK: the many and varied substrates of the c-Jun N-terminal kinases. Microbiol Mol Biol Rev, 2006, 70(4): 1061-1095.

[5] Kuan C Y, Whitmarsh A J, Yang D D, et al. A critical role of nalml-specific JNK3 for ischemic apoptosis. Prog Nail Acad Sci USA, 2003, 100: 15184-15189.

[6] Pirianov G, Brywe K G, Mallard C, et al. Deletion of the c-Jun N-terminal kinase 3 gene protects neonatal mice against cerebral hypoxic-ischaemic injury. J Cereb Blood Flow Metab, 2007, 27(5): 1022-1032.

[7] O'Collins V E, Macleod M R, Donnan G A, et al. 1026 experimental treatments in acute stroke. Annals of Neurology, 2006, 59(3): 467-477.

[8] Lijima T, Mishima T, Akagawa K, et al. Neuroprotective effect of propofol on necrosis and apoptosis following oxygen-glucose deprivation-relationship between mitochondrial membrane potential and mode of death. Brain Res, 2006, 1099: 25-32.

[9] Lai Z, Yao C K, Cheng S B. Study of radix astragali on neuronal apoptosis in reperfusion local cerebral ischemia rats brains. Journal of Emergency in Traditional Chinese Medicine, 2008, 17: 1565-1569.

[10] Guo Y, Xu X, Li Q, et al. Anti-inflammation effects of picroside 2 in cerebral ischemic injury rats. Behavioral & Brain Functions, 2010, 6(1): 43-53.

[11] Li Q, Li Z, Xu X Y, et al. Neuroprotective properties of picroside II in a rat model of focal cerebral ischemia. International Journal of Molecular Sciences, 2010, 11(11): 4580-4590.

[12] Qu Y Z, Zhao Y L, Gao G D. Effects of combined use of tetramethylpyrazine and astragalus on neuronal apoptosis and expression of Fos protein following cerebral ischemia/reperfusion. Chinese Journal of Integrated Traditional & Western Medicine in Intensive & Critical Care, 2006, 13: 123-125.

[13] Zhuo M, Chen H L, Cai N L, et al. A study on clinical effects and immunological mechanism of intravenous astragalus injection therapy in neonates with hypoxic ischemic encephalopathy. Chinese Journal of Integrated Traditional & Western Medicine in Intensive & Critical Care, 2008, 15: 13-15.

[14] Dong-Qing Y E, Gao W J, Qian T, et al. Astragalus injection inhibits the expression of JNK3 after hypoxia/hypoglycemia and reoxygenation in hippocampal neurons of rats. Chinese Journal of Pathophysiology, 2010, 26(1): 77-82.

[15] Li W Z, Ming L, He T, et al. Effects of extract of astragalus on hippocampal delayed neuronal death in rats. Chin Pharmacol Bull, 2005, 21(5): 584-587.

[16] Liang S L, Xu B, Zhang Y Y. The effect of astragalus injection on neuronal apoptosis in cerebral ischemic injury in rats. Zhejiang J Integr Tradit Chin West Med, 2011, 21: 159-161.

[17] Qu Y Z, Li M, Gao G D. Protective effects of astragalus injection on blood-brain barrier and expressions of occludin and zonula occludens protein-1 after cerebral ischemia and reperfusion in rats. Chinese Journal of Integrated Traditional & Western Medicine in Intensive & Critical Care, 2011, 18: 263-265.

[18] The Ministry of Science and Technology of the People's Republic of China. Guidance Suggestions for the Care and Use of Laboratory Animals. (2006-09-30)[2018-01-20]. http://www.most.gov.cn.

[19] Longa E Z, Weinstein P R, Carlson S, et al. Reversible middle cerebral artery occlusion without craniectomy in rats. Stroke, 1989, 20(1): 84-91.

[20] Liu S S, Gao W J, Qian T, et al. Effect of astragalus on expression of JNK3 in hippocampus of cerebral ischemia reperfusion rats. Chin Pharmacol Bull, 2012, 28: 665-670.

[21] Sun W, Gould T W, Newbern J, et al. Phosphorylation of c-Jun in avian and mammalian motoneurons in vivo during programmed cell death: an early reversible event in the apoptotic cascade. Journal of Neuroscience, 2005, 25(23): 5595-5603.

[22] Ma K F. Vascular endothelial growth factor on acute cerebral infarction and experimental cure. Foreign Medical Sciences Section on Neurology & Neurosurgery, 2001, 28: 377-379.

[23] Kaushal V, Schlichter L C. Mechanisms of microglia-mediated neurotoxicity in a new model of the stroke penumbra. Journal of Neuroscience, 2008, 28(9): 2221-2230.

[24] Johnson G L, Lapadat R. Mitogen-activated protein kinase pathways mediated by ERK, JNK, and p38 protein kinases. Science, 2002, 298(5600): 1911-1912.

[25] Lv J R, Ma H Z, Xue R L. The expression of c-Jun in hippocampus of rats global cerebral ischemia reperfusion and the effect of heat shock precondition on it. J Xi'an Commun Univ (Med Sci), 2007, 27: 337-340.

[26] Wang N, Xue R L, Yao F Z. Effects of JNK signal passway on brain ischemia reperfusion in rats. J Xi'an Commun Univ (Med Sci), 2007, 28: 617-618.

[27] Ren F, Gong S Y, Zhi L M, et al. Effectiveness of astragulus for cerebral ischemic injury. Chinese Journal of Clinical Rehabilitation, 2006, 10(3): 149-151.

[28] Zhang Y L, Gao W J, Yan F X. Study on the inhibitory action of astragalus injection on apoptosis of hippocamal neurons induced by hypoxia hypoglycemia and reoxygenation. Chinese Journal of Gerontology, 2009, 29(7): 793-796.

[29] Yan F X, Gao W J, Qian T. The effect of astragalus injection on the expression of caspase-3 after hypoxia/hypoglycemia and reoxygenation in hippocampal neurons of rats. Chinese Pharmacological Bulletin, 2010, 42(1): 14-21.

Section 4　Words of TCM

1. 水液代谢 water metabolism, body fluid metabolism
2. 排泄糟粕 excreting the waste
3. 小肠实热 asthenic heat of small intestine
4. 大肠主传导 large intestine controlling transportation
5. 久痢脱肛 proctoptosis due to prolonged dysentery
6. 地道不通 menopause
7. 肾阳式微 declination of kidney yang
8. 脾阳不振 inactivation of spleen yang
9. 脾胃虚弱 hypofunction/weakness of the spleen and stomach
10. 温肾健脾 warming the kidney and strengthening the spleen
11. 平肝和胃 soothing the liver and harmonizing the stomach
12. 肝旺脾虚 hyperfunction of the liver and weakness of the spleen
13. 大肉陷下 obvious emaciation and muscular atrophy; extreme emaciation
14. 脘腹胀闷 epigastric distension and depression
15. 嗳气酸腐 eructation with fetid odor
16. 消导积滞 promoting digestion and removing food retention
17. 养阴清热 nourishing yin and clearing away heat
18. 湿邪犯肺 pathogenic dampness invading the lung
19. 祛风散寒 expelling/eliminating wind to disperse cold
20. 潜阳息风 suppressing yang to quench wind
21. 阴盛则阳病 predominance of yin leading to disorder of yang
22. 阴盛则阳病 an excess of yin leads to deficiency of yang
23. 阳盛生外热 exuberance of yang leading to exterior heat
24. 阴阳胜复 alternative predominance of yin and yang
25. 扶阳退阴 strengthening yang to reduce yin
26. 阴阳离绝 separation of yin and yang
27. 阴中求阳 obtaining yang from yin
28. 绝对偏盛 absolute predominance
29. 阳虚则寒 yang deficiency leading to cold
30. 阳虚发热 fever due to yang deficiency
31. 止咳散 cough-checking powder
32. 生脉散 pulsation-promoting powder
33. 鸡鸣 / 苏散 cock-crowing / cock-waking powder
34. 百合固金汤 lily lung-strengthening decoction

35. 温经汤 meridian-warming decoction

36. 定喘汤 asthma-relieving decoction

37. 健脾丸 spleen-enhancing pill

38. 四逆汤 sini decoction

39. 拳参 red legs; sweet-dock

40. 乌鸡白凤丸 wuji baifeng pill; black cock and white phoenix pill

(Li Hongguo, Ji Yaqing)

Chapter 14   Hypertension

Section 1   High Blood Pressure

Definitions of normal, borderline and high blood pressure are far from arbitrary. Pressures higher than 120/80 mmHg mean that the heart must pump unnaturally hard to circulate blood. Over time, the muscle may fail from the added strain. High pressures encourage fatty plaques to build up abnormally fast in the coronary arteries. This may clog the arteries completely, starving the heart of its supply of blood. High blood pressure injures and weakens blood vessels in the brain, the kidneys and the eyes which can lead in turn to strokes, kidney failure and blindness.

Although high blood pressure affects different people in various ways, its ravages are matters of medical fact. For example, one study showed that risks of death or disability from stroke, coronary disease or kidney failure rose sharply as soon as blood pressure exceeded 120/80 mmHg. Insurance companies' actuarial tables make an even more convincing case for matters of medical fact. One table stated that a 35-year-old man with a blood pressure of 120/80 mmHg can expect to live additional 41.5 years, but that a man of the same age with a blood pressure of 140/95 mmHg can expect to live only 37.5 years more. Raise the numbers only slightly and the stakes go up significantly. The 35-year-old man who has a blood pressure of 150/100 mmHg has a life expectancy of only 25 more years.

Clearly, then, there is no safe level above normal. If you are told you have high blood pressure, follow your doctor's instructions for lowering it. In contrast to the situation of the 1930s, doctors today know how to reduce blood pressure to nonthreatening levels in about 85% of the cases. Sometimes the treatment is remarkably simple steps that you take on your own. If you are overweight, the first step in your treatment will probably be to reduce. Obesity imposes an added burden on the heart because blood volume increases with body weight. To circulate the extra blood through an extra-large body, the heart must pump at higher pressure.

Smoking is harmful to the body because the nicotine in tobacco smoke is widely believed to constrict blood vessels and boost blood pressure. The sodium contained in salt makes the body retain fluid. Increased fluid retention raises the total volume of blood flowing through the circulatory system and hence raises the blood pressure. In about one out of every three cases of hypertension, a diet that stringently restricts sodium intake leads to some lowering of blood pressure. This means eliminating or sharply curbing your consumption of such salty food as dill pickles, luncheon meats, corned beef, bacon, ham, canned soups, cheeses (except dry cottage cheese), bakery goods and many commercially canned or frozen vegetables. Many seasonings — ketchup, relishes, soy sauce and, of course, table salt — should be avoided altogether.

Medically supervised exercise programs can help reduce blood pressure, too, so can learning to relax for short periods of time during the working day, at night and on weekends. Blood pressure drops as you relax, and it reaches a daily low when you sleep. There are many specific relaxation techniques as a means of treating high blood pressure, such as yoga and meditation, which have their roots in ancient religious rituals. Others, such as biofeedback, employ the latest technology. One noted experiment showed that relaxation techniques, including biofeedback, can help borderline hypertension reach normal blood pressure levels.

For many other hypertensives, however, it is not enough to lose weight, stop smoking, eliminate salt from the diet, exercise or learn to relax. These people need active medical treatment includes anti-hypertensive drugs. For years, medical science struggled to discover compounds that lowered blood pressure. Doctors in many cases prescribed sedatives such as phenobarbital for hypertensive patients, but the results were disappointing. Then, in the 1950s, a variety of potent pressure-reducing drugs became available. At first, doctors were somewhat reluctant to prescribe these new medications — particularly for mild or borderline hypertension. They were afraid that drug therapy was not worth the bother, the expense and possible side effects. These can include weakness, sleepiness, digestive upsets, lethargy and sexual problems. Some anti-hypertensive medicines have produced fainting episodes in their users, caused by sudden drops in blood pressure to very low levels when posture changed abruptly. But the evidence favoring drug therapy has come to outweigh most such reservations. Results of studies published in 1967 and 1970s showed that for 500 middle-aged American men who had moderate or severe hypertension, drug therapy reduced significantly the incidence of other forms of cardiovascular disease and death.

Still, many physicians remained hesitant to prescribe drugs for patients with mild or borderline hypertension. Then, at the end of the 1970s came overwhelming scientific evidence that aggressive drug therapy could prove a lifesaver ever for mild hypertensives. In a five-year study called the Hypertension Detection and Follow-up Program, the National Heart, Lung, and Blood Institute screened almost 159 000 Americans between the age of 30 and 69. Using an arbitrary diving line — diastolic pressure above 90 mmHg — the researchers selected almost 11 000 subjects as having some degree of hypertension, and divided that group into three categories: those with diastolic pressures between 90 mmHg and 104 mmHg, between 105 mmHg and 114 mmHg, and above 115 mmHg. About half of the patients in each group then were referred to their physicians or local clinics for care. The remaining half of the patients in each group were treated with drugs designed to bring diastolic pressure below 90 mmHg. If one drug failed to work, another was added, until some patients received as many as four drugs simultaneously. The results were persuasive for every high blood pressure group designated in the study. There were almost 45% fewer deaths from stroke and 26% fewer from heart attack.

The extra evidence, reported in 1980, came from a six-year study conducted by the National Heart Foundation of Australian. The researcher screened about 3400 residents who suffered from mild high blood pressure, which the Australian team defined as a diastolic reading between 95 mmHg and 110 mmHg. The subjects were then divided into two groups: one group was given active pressure-reducing drugs; the other, placebo tables — medically inactive tablets. At the end of the study, Australians in the actively treated group had suffered 50% fewer strokes — and of those who suffered strokes 50% fewer died — than those given placebos. The overall death rate from cardiovascular disease was 2/3 lower in the drug-treated half than in the placebo half. Projected nationwide, the results of the study indicated that drug treatment of mild hypertension could reduce cardiovascular disease in Australia by 7000 cases per year and stroke deaths by 2000.

Thus, the case is strong for using drugs when simpler means of reducing high blood pressure fail. Luckily, half of all hypertensives can be helped by the least objectionable of the drugs — diuretics. These force the body to excrete more water and sodium than usual, reducing the total blood volume — and thus the blood pressure. Diuretics such as chlorothiazide and furosemide sometimes can lower high blood pressure by themselves. Quite often, however, diuretics are used in combination with other medications. The choice of additional drugs depends on the degree of hypertension. It also depends on how the patient reacts to the drugs. A doctor treating a hypertensive patient may start with a low dose of one drug, increase the dose somewhat if it is ineffective, then step up to a second drug, and so on, continuing up a ladder of higher doses and different drugs until effective control is achieved.

One category of drugs often used in combination with diuretics is made up of vasodilators, such as hydralazine and diazoxide. These medications act directly on the muscle walls of blood vessels, relaxing them and causing them to enlarge. This reduces resistance to the flow of blood, and thus lowers the blood pressure. The other major group of antihypertensive drugs, the sympatholytics, acts on the nervous system, interfering with the chemical nerve messengers that help control blood pressure. One of the oldest such drugs is the tranquilizer reserpine, which inhibits nerve messages to the adrenal glands, making them secrete less of their pressure-raising hormones.

If your doctor prescribes any of these drugs to lower blood pressure, you should resist a common temptation — to stop taking the medicine once pressure has been brought under control. That is almost always a grievous error on two counts. Stopping some of these drugs may produce harmful side effects. For example, if clonidine is discontinued suddenly, blood pressure may zoom above the original high reading. But in addition, most people who need a blood pressure drug require lifelong treatment. If you stop taking the drug, you give up the protection it provides against a trio of cardiovascular diseases that hypertension can bring on: congestive heart failure, coronary heart disease and, perhaps most demonstrably, stroke.

Section 2   Hypertension in Chinese Medicine

The patients manifest as increasingly high blood pressure, accompanied with general symptoms like vertigo and headache. Some senile patients have high blood pressure, but are free from marked subjective symptoms. In this case, diagnosis should be made on the basis of the lab examinations.

Hyperactive yang due to yin deficiency: Headache, dizziness, tinnitus, blurred vision, insomnia, dream-disturbed sleep, soreness and flaccidity of the waist and knees, occasional flushed face, numbness of limbs, red tongue with thin fur or without fur, taut, thready and rapid pulse. It is advisable to nourish yin and suppress yang. The prescription used is the modified Tianma Gouteng Decoction (Decoction of Gastrodia and Uncaria). As for the traditional Chinese patent medicine, select Zhibai Dihuang Pill (Pill of Anemarrhena, Phellodendrono and Rehmannia).

Yin deficiency of the liver and kidney: Light-headedness, unsmooth and dry eyes, tinnitus, deafness, lumbar soreness, flaccidity of legs, pain of heels, red tongue without fur, deep, thready and slow pulse. It is suitable to nourish and tonify the liver and kidney. The prescription used is the modified Qiju Dihuang Bolus (Bolus of Six Drugs, Rehmannia with Wolfberry and Chrysanthemum). It is also advisable to select the medicine of the same name.

Deficiency of both yin and yang: Light-headedness with the sensation of walking like sitting in a boat, lusterless complexion, occasional fever, palpitation, short breath, soreness and flaccidity of the waist and knees, frequent and profuse nocturnal urine, or edema, pale and tender tongue, deep and thready or tense pulse. It is advisable to regulate and strengthen yin and yang. The prescription used is the modified Er-xian Decoction. As for the traditional Chinese patent medicine, select Jingui Shenqi Pill.

There are many other rehabilitation methods.

1. Regulating emotions: Emotional dissatisfaction, excessive joy and anger often affect the hepatic function of regulating qi and blood, the renal function of nourishment, giving rise to continuous high blood pressure. Therefore, regulating emotions is of great importance for the rehabilitation of the disease.

(1) Enlightening method: Adopt the methods of interpretation, consolation, encouragement and assurance to lessen and eliminate abnormal emotional reactions and pathogenic emotional factors.

(2) The behavior therapy: Adopt more biofeedback therapies, and apply the continuous value-displaying electronic manometer, dermothermometer and electromyography to instruct patients in judging the effect of lowering blood pressure from the readings of these instruments or other visible and audible signals. Besides, train the patients to practice muscular relaxation and normal respiration. Synthesize the results displayed in the instruments to adjust the training methods constantly. Maintain the self control over blood pressure by means of repeated self somatopsychic training.

2. The recreation therapy: Participate in recreational activities like gardening, fishing, practicing calligraphy and painting, playing a musical instrument and appreciating music. As for the musical therapy, select the type of music of expressing emotions and removing depression alternatively.

3. Physical training: Physical training can lower blood pressure to a certain extent. Practicing Taijiquan is very suitable. The patients with good constitution may play the whole set of simplified Taijiquan while the patients with poor constitution may play half, or several postures of it. Besides, the patients can have other activities like jogging to increase the amount of exercise, extend the distance and quicken the speed gradually. The patients should not have the activities with the movement of the head below the horizontal position so as to avoid aggravating the symptom of discomfort of the head due to the gravitational influence no matter whatever sports events are selected. It is not advisable to have competitive activities to prevent emotional excitement. Do not have weight-carrying activities to avoid breath holding which conversely and reflexively elevates blood pressure.

4. Acumox and massage

(1) Acumox: The commonly-used acupoints include Fengchi, Baihui, Quchi, Zusanli, Sanyinjiao, etc.. In case of relative hyperactive hepatic yang, add Xingjian, Xiaxi and Taichong; in case of hepatorenal yin deficiency, Ganshu and Shenshu; in case of excessive phlegm, Fenglong, Zhongwan and Jiexi. Puncture the acupoints once every other day and 7 days constitute one course of treatment. Besides, the acupoint injection may be alternatively applied on the above-mentioned acupoints. Select two acupoints each time with the acupoint injection of 1 mL of 0.25% procaine hydrochloride for each acupoint, once a day; or select Chimai with the acupoint injection of 1 mL of vitamin B_{12}, once a day and 7 days constitute

one course of treatment. The commonly-used auricular acupoints include Pizhixia, Jiangyagou, Naogan, Neifenmi, Shenmen, Xin, etc.. Select one or two acupoints every day or every other day and retain the needle for 30 minutes. Besides, the needle-embedding therapy may be adopted, or apply Wangbuliuxing (Semen Vaccariae) on the auricular acupoints instead of the needle-embedding therapy.

(2) The cupping therapy: Select the acupoints of the first lateral line of the dorsal gallbladder meridian and Jianyu, Quchi, Shousanli, Weizhong, Chengjin, Zusanli, Fenglong, Fengchi, etc.. Cup ten acupoints or so each time for 10 ~ 15 minutes.

(3) Massage: Apply self massage mainly. The commonly-used methods include kneading Zanzhu, scrubbing the nose, beating the Heavenly drum (Tiangu), combing the hair with the hand, kneading Taiyang, wiping the forehead, pressing-kneading Naohu, rubbing the hands to bath the face, kneading Yanyan and scrubbing Yongquan. Simultaneously, pat the relevant regions with the fist and palm.

5. The dietary therapy: In case of hepatorenal yin deficiency, select Haizhe Biqi Soup (Soup of Cavum Rhopilemae and Bulbus Heleocharis Dulcis). If the conditions permit, select Fengru (Lac Apis Melliferum) to eat. In case of hyperactive yang due to yin deficiency, select cold celery in sauce. Meanwhile, it is also advisable to decoct 5 ~ 10 g of Juhua (Flos Chrysanthemi) or Yejuhua (Flos Chrysanthenmi Indici) in water until the water boils for 3 ~ 5 minutes. Drink the decoction like tea. In case of deficiency of yin and yang, select 20 g of Heizhima (Semen Sesami), Goujizi (Fructus Lycii) and Hutaorou (Semen Juglandis) respectively to be decocted in water. Take the dregs and the decoction simultaneously, once a day. The commonly-used dietary prescriptions for lowering blood pressure are as follow:

(1) Stewed Sea Cucumber: Stew 30 g of sea cucumber (soaked in water) in a proper amount of water with slow fire until it is thoroughly cooked. Then, add a proper quantity of crystal sugar to be dissolved for eating.

(2) Stewed Edible Fungus: Soak 10 g of tremella or black fungus in water. Then, wash it clean and add a proper amount of water to it. Next, stew it with slow fire until it is thoroughly cooked. Finally, add a proper quantity of crystal sugar to it. Take it in the evening.

(3) Shelled Peanut Pickled in Vinegar: Soak 250 g of shelled peanut (with the red coating) in a proper amount of vinegar for 5 ~ 7 days. Eat it three times a day, a proper amount each time.

(4) Fermented Juhua (Flos Chrysanthemi): Cook 10 g of Flos Chrysanthemi and a proper amount of glutinous rice wine in a pot until the wine boils. Take it at a draught, twice a day.

(5) Egg Stewed with Tianma (Rhizoma Gastrodiae): Decoct 9 g of Tianma in water for one hour. Then, remove the dregs and stew two eggs in the decoction. Take it orally.

The patients should eat more melon, fruit and vegetable usually, of which celery, water melon, etc. have the action of lowering blood pressure to a certain extent. Do not over-eat fat meat and fine grain and do not eat the vegetarian diet all the time, either. They should eat the low salt diet with a daily intake of less than 5 g of salt.

6. Drugs for external treatment

(1) Mix a proper amount of the minced Wuzhuyu (Folium Evodiae) with vinegar. Then, apply the drug on Yongquan on the sole. Conduct the dressing change once a day.

(2) Decoct 6 g Cishi (Magnetitum), Shijueming (Semen Cassiae), Dangshen (Radix Angelicae Sinensis), Huangqi (Radix Astragali seu Hedysari), Danggui (Radix Angelicae Sinensis), Sangzhi (Ramulus Mori), Zhike (Fructus Aurantii), Wuyao (Radix Linderae), Manjingzi (Fructus Viticis), Baijili (Fructus Tribuli), Baishao (Radix Paeoniae Alba), Chaoduzhong (parched Cortex Eucommiae) and Niuxi (Radix Achyranthis Bidentatae) respectively and 18 g of Duhuo (Radox Angelicae Pubescentis). Soak the feet in the decoction for an hour once a day.

(3) Make a medicinal pillow with Yejuhua (Flos Chrysanthemi Indici), Danzhuye (Herba Lophatheri), Dongsangye (Folium Mori collected in winter), Shengshigao (Gypsum Fibrosum), Baishao (Radix Paedoniae Alba), Chuanxiong (Rhizoma Ligustici Chuanxiong), Cishi (Magnetitum), Manjingzi (Fructus Viticis) and Cansha (Excrementa Bombycum). Use it for more than 6 hours a day. It is applicable to the patients with hyperactive yang due to yin deficiency. Besides, Lüdouke (Testa Phaseoli Radiati) can be used to make the medicinal pillow as well.

Section 3　Research Article

Hypertension

Hypertension (HTN or HT), also known as high blood pressure (HBP), is a long-term medical condition in which the blood pressure in the arteries is persistently elevated. High blood pressure usually does not cause symptoms. Long-term high blood pressure, however, is a major risk factor for coronary artery disease, stroke, heart failure, atrial fibrillation, peripheral vascular disease, vision loss, chronic kidney disease, and dementia.

High blood pressure is classified as either primary (essential) high blood pressure or secondary high blood pressure. 90% ~ 95% of cases are primary, defined as high blood pressure due to nonspecific lifestyle and genetic factors. Lifestyle factors that increase the risk include excess salt in the diet, excess body weight, smoking, and alcohol use. The remaining 5% ~ 10% of cases are categorized as secondary high blood pressure, defined as high blood pressure due to an identifiable cause, such as chronic kidney disease, narrowing of the kidney arteries, an endocrine disorder, or the use of birth control pills.

Blood pressure is expressed by two measurements, the systolic and diastolic pressures, which are the maximum and minimum pressures, respectively. For most adults, normal blood pressure at rest is within the range of 100 ~ 130 mmHg systolic and 60 ~ 80 mmHg diastolic. For most adults, high blood pressure is present if the resting blood pressure is persistently at or above 130/90 or 140/90 mmHg. Different numbers apply to children. Ambulatory blood pressure monitoring over a 24 h period appears more accurate than office-based blood pressure measurement.

Lifestyle changes and medications can lower blood pressure and decrease the risk of health complications. Lifestyle changes include weight loss, decreased salt intake, physical exercise, and a healthy diet. If lifestyle changes are not sufficient then blood pressure medications are used. Up to three medications can control blood pressure in 90% of people. The treatment of moderately high arterial blood pressure (defined as >160/100 mmHg) with medications is associated with an improved life expectancy. The effect of treatment of blood pressure between 130/80 mmHg and 160/100 mmHg is less clear, with some reviews finding benefit and others finding unclear benefit. High blood pressure affects between 16% and 37% of the population globally. In 2010, hypertension was believed to have been a factor in 18% of all deaths (9.4 million globally).

1   Signs and symptoms

Hypertension is rarely accompanied by symptoms, and its identification is usually through screening, or when seeking health-care for an unrelated problem. Some with high blood pressure report headaches (particularly at the back of the head and in the morning), as well as lightheadedness, vertigo, tinnitus (buzzing or hissing in the ears), altered vision or fainting episodes. These symptoms, however, might be related to associated anxiety rather than the high blood pressure itself.

On physical examination, hypertension may be associated with the presence of changes in the optic fundus seen by ophthalmoscopy. The severity of the changes typical of hypertensive retinopathy is graded from I to IV; grades I and II may be difficult to differentiate. The severity of the retinopathy correlates roughly with the duration or the severity of the hypertension.

Secondary hypertension: Hypertension with certain specific additional signs and symptoms may suggest secondary hypertension, i.e. hypertension due to an identifiable cause. For example, Cushing's syndrome frequently causes truncal obesity, glucose intolerance, moon face, a hump of fat behind the neck / shoulder (referred to as a buffalo hump), and purple abdominal stretch marks. Hyperthyroidism frequently causes weight loss with increased appetite, fast heart rate, bulging eyes, and tremor. Renal artery stenosis (RAS) may be associated with a localized abdominal bruit to the left or right of the midline (unilateral RAS), or in both locations (bilateral RAS). Coarctation of the aorta frequently causes a decreased blood pressure in the lower extremities relative to the arms, or delayed or absent femoral arterial pulses. Pheochromocytoma may cause abrupt (paroxysmal) episodes of hypertension accompanied by headache, palpitations, pale appearance, and excessive sweating.

Hypertensive crisis: Severely elevated blood pressure (equal to or greater than a systolic 180 mmHg or diastolic of 110 mmHg) is referred to as a hypertensive crisis. Hypertensive crisis is categorized as either hypertensive urgency or hypertensive emergency, according to the absence or presence of end organ damage, respectively.

In hypertensive urgency, there is no evidence of end organ damage resulting from the elevated blood pressure. In these cases, oral medications are used to lower the BP gradually over 24 to 48 hours.

In hypertensive emergency, there is evidence of direct damage to one or more organs. The most affected organs include the brain, kidney, heart and lungs, producing symptoms which may include confusion, drowsiness, chest pain and breathlessness. In hypertensive emergency, the blood pressure must be reduced more rapidly to stop ongoing organ damage; however, there is a lack of randomized controlled trial evidence for this approach.

Pregnancy: Hypertension occurs in 8% ~ 10% of pregnancies. If two blood pressure measurements apart of six hours were greater than 140/90 mmHg hypertension in pregnancy could be diagnosed. High blood pressure in pregnancy can be classified as pre-existing hypertension, gestational hypertension, or pre-eclampsia.

Pre-eclampsia is a serious condition of the second half of pregnancy and following delivery characterized by increased blood pressure and the presence of protein in the urine. It occurs in about 5% of pregnancies and is responsible for approximately 16% of all maternal deaths globally. Pre-eclampsia also doubles the risk of death of the baby around the time of birth. Usually there are no symptoms in pre-eclampsia and it is detected by routine screening. When symptoms of pre-eclampsia occur, the most common are headache, visual disturbance (often flashing lights), vomiting, pain over the stomach, and swelling. Pre-eclampsia can occasionally progress to a life-threatening condition called eclampsia, which is a hypertensive emergency and has several serious complications including vision loss, brain swelling, seizures, kidney failure, pulmonary edema, and disseminated intravascular coagulation (a blood clotting disorder). In contrast, gestational hypertension is defined as new-onset hypertension during pregnancy without protein in the urine.

Children: Failure to thrive, seizures, irritability, lack of energy, and difficulty in breathing can be associated with hypertension in newborns and young infants. In older infants and children, hypertension can cause headache, unexplained irritability, fatigue, failure to thrive, blurred vision, nosebleeds, and facial paralysis.

2　Causes

Primary hypertension: Hypertension results from a complex interaction of genes and environmental factors. Numerous common genetic variants with small effects on blood pressure have been identified as well as some rare genetic variants with large effects on blood pressure. Also, genome-wide association studies (GWAS) have identified 35 genetic loci related to blood pressure; 12 of these genetic loci influencing blood pressure were newly found. Sentinel SNP for each new genetic loci identified has shown an association with DNA methylation at multiple nearby CpG sites. These sentinel SNP are located within genes related to vascular smooth muscle and renal function. DNA methylation might affect in some way linking common genetic variation to multiple phenotypes even though mechanisms underlying these associations are not understood. Single variant test performed in this study for the 35 sentinel SNP (known and new) showed that genetic variants singly or in aggregate contribute to the risk of clinical phenotypes related to high blood pressure.

Blood pressure rises with aging and the risk of becoming hypertensive in later life is considerable. Several environmental factors influence blood pressure. High salt intake raises the blood pressure in salt sensitive individuals; lack of exercise, obesity, and depression can play a role in individual cases. The possible role of other factors such as caffeine consumption, and vitamin D deficiency are less clear. Insulin resistance, which is common in obesity and is a component of syndrome X (or the metabolic syndrome), is also thought to contribute to hypertension. One review suggests that sugar may play an important role in hypertension and salt is just an innocent bystander.

Events in early life, such as low birth weight, maternal smoking, and lack of breastfeeding may be risk factors for adult essential hypertension, although the mechanisms linking these exposures to adult hypertension remain unclear. An increased rate of high blood urea has been found in untreated people with hypertensive in comparison with people with normal blood pressure, although it is uncertain whether the former plays a causal role or is subsidiary to poor kidney function. Average blood pressure may be higher in the winter than in the summer.

Secondary hypertension: Secondary hypertension results from an identifiable cause. Kidney disease is the most common secondary cause of hypertension. Hypertension can also be caused by endocrine conditions, such as Cushing's syndrome, hyperthyroidism, hypothyroidism, acromegaly, Conn's syndrome or hyperaldosteronism, renal artery stenosis (from atherosclerosis or fibromuscular dysplasia), hyperparathyroidism, and pheochromocytoma. Other causes of secondary hypertension include obesity, sleep apnea, pregnancy, coarctation of the aorta, excessive eating of liquorice, excessive drinking of alcohol, and certain prescription medicines, herbal remedies, and illegal drugs such as cocaine and methamphetamine. Arsenic exposure through drinking water has been shown to correlate with elevated blood pressure.

3　Pathophysiology

In most people with established essential hypertension, increased resistance to blood flow (total peripheral resistance) accounts for the high pressure while cardiac output remains normal. There is evidence that some younger people with prehypertension or borderline hypertension have high cardiac output, an elevated heart rate and normal peripheral resistance, and termed hyperkinetic borderline hypertension. These individuals develop the typical features of established essential hypertension in later life as their cardiac output falls and peripheral resistance rises with age. Whether this pattern is typical of all people who ultimately develop hypertension is disputed. The increased peripheral resistance in established hypertension is mainly attributable to structural narrowing of small arteries and arterioles, although a reduction in the number or density of capillaries may also contribute.

It is not clear whether or not the vasoconstriction of arteriolar blood vessels plays a role in hypertension. Hypertension is also associated with decreased peripheral venous compliance which may increase venous return, increase cardiac preload and, ultimately, cause diastolic dysfunction.

Pulse pressure (the difference between systolic and diastolic blood pressure) is frequently increased in older people with hypertension. This can mean that systolic pressure is abnormally high, but diastolic pressure may be normal or low. The high pulse pressure in elderly people with hypertension or isolated systolic hypertension is explained by increased arterial stiffness, which typically accompanies aging and may be exacerbated by high blood pressure.

Many mechanisms have been proposed to account for the rise in peripheral resistance in hypertension. Most evidence implicates either disturbances in the kidneys' salt and water handling (particularly abnormalities in the intrarenal renin-angiotensin system) or abnormalities of the sympathetic nervous system. These mechanisms are not mutually exclusive and it is likely that both contribute to some extent in most cases of essential hypertension. It has also been suggested that endothelial dysfunction and vascular inflammation may also contribute to increased peripheral resistance and vascular damage in hypertension. Interleukin 17 has garnered interest for its role in increasing the production of several other immune system chemical signals thought to be involved in hypertension such as tumor necrosis factor alpha, interleukin 1, interleukin 6, and interleukin 8.

Consumption of excessive sodium and / or insufficient potassium leads to excessive intracellular sodium, which contracts vascular smooth muscle, restricting blood flow and so increases blood pressure.

4 Diagnosis

Hypertension is diagnosed on the basis of a persistently high resting blood pressure. Traditionally, the National Institute of Clinical Excellence recommends three separate resting sphygmomanometer measurements at monthly intervals. The American Heart Association recommends at least three resting measurements on at least two separate health care visits.

For an accurate diagnosis of hypertension to be made, it is essential for proper blood pressure measurement technique to be used. Improper measurement of blood pressure is common and can change the blood pressure reading by up to 10 mmHg, which can lead to misdiagnosis and misclassification of hypertension. Correct blood pressure measurement technique involves several steps. Proper blood pressure measurement requires the person whose blood pressure is being measured to sit quietly for at least five minutes which is then followed by application of a properly fitted blood pressure cuff to a bare upper arm. The people should be seated with their back supported, feet flat on the floor, and with their legs uncrossed. The person whose blood pressure is being measured should avoid talking or moving during this process. The arm being measured should be supported on a flat surface at the level of the heart. Blood pressure measurement should be done in a quiet room so the medical professional checking the blood pressure can hear the Korotkoff sounds while listening to the brachial artery with a stethoscope for accurate blood pressure measurements. The blood pressure cuff should be deflated slowly (2 ~ 3 mmHg per second) while listening for the Korotkoff sounds. The bladder should be emptied before a person's blood pressure is measured since this can increase blood pressure by up to 15/10 mmHg. Multiple blood pressure readings (at least two) spaced 1 ~ 2 minutes apart should be obtained to ensure accuracy. Ambulatory blood pressure monitoring over 12 to 24 hours is the most accurate method to confirm the diagnosis.

An exception to this is those with very high blood pressure readings especially when there is poor organ function. Initial assessment of the hypertensive people should include a complete history and physical examination. With the availability of 24-hour ambulatory blood pressure monitors and home blood pressure machines, the importance of not wrongly diagnosing those who have white coat hypertension has led to a change in protocols. In the United Kingdom, current best practice is to follow up a single raised clinic reading with ambulatory measurement, or less ideally with home blood pressure monitoring over the course of 7 days. The United States Preventive Services Task Force also recommends getting measurements outside of the healthcare environment. Pseudohypertension in the elderly or noncompressibility artery syndrome may also require consideration. This condition is believed to be due to calcification of the arteries resulting in abnormally high blood pressure readings with a blood pressure cuff while intra arterial measurements of blood pressure are normal. Orthostatic hypertension is when blood pressure increases upon standing.

Once the diagnosis of hypertension has been made, healthcare providers should attempt to identify the underlying cause based on risk factors and other symptoms, if present. Secondary hypertension is more common in preadolescent children, with most cases caused by kidney disease. Primary or essential hypertension is more common in adolescents and has multiple risk factors, including obesity and a family history of hypertension. Laboratory tests can also be performed to identify possible causes of secondary hypertension, and to determine whether hypertension has caused damage to the heart, eyes, and kidneys. Additional tests for diabetes and high cholesterol levels are usually performed because these conditions are additional risk factors for the development of heart disease and may require treatment.

Serum creatinine is measured to assess for the presence of kidney disease, which can be either the cause or the result of hypertension. Serum creatinine alone may overestimate glomerular filtration rate and recent guidelines advocate the use of predictive equations such as the Modification of Diet in Renal Disease (MDRD) formula to estimate glomerular filtration rate (eGFR). eGFR can also provide a baseline measurement of kidney function that can be used to monitor for side effects of certain anti-hypertensive drugs on kidney function. Additionally, testing of urine samples for protein is used as a secondary indicator of kidney disease. Electrocardiogram (ECG) testing is done to check for evidence that the heart is under strain from high blood pressure. It may also show whether there is thickening of the heart muscle (left ventricular hypertrophy) or whether the heart has experienced a prior minor disturbance such as a silent heart attack. A chest X-ray or an echocardiogram may also be performed to look for signs of heart enlargement or damage to the heart.

Adults: In people aged 18 years or older hypertension is defined as either a systolic or a diastolic blood pressure measurement consistently higher than an accepted normal value (this is above 129 mmHg or 139 mmHg systolic, 89 mmHg diastolic depending on the guideline). Other thresholds are used (135 mmHg systolic or 85 mmHg diastolic) if measurements are derived from 24-hour ambulatory or home monitoring. Recent international hypertension guidelines have also created categories below the hypertensive range to indicate a continuum of risk with higher blood pressures in the normal range. The *Seventh Report of the Joint National Committee on Prevention, Detection, Evaluation and Treatment of High Blood Pressure* (JNC7) published in 2003 uses the term prehypertension for blood pressure in the range 120 ~ 139 mmHg systolic or 80 ~ 89 mmHg diastolic, while European Society of Hypertension Guidelines (2007) and British Hypertension Society (BHS) IV (2004) use optimal, normal and high normal categories to subdivide pressures below 140 mmHg systolic and 90 mmHg diastolic. Hypertension is also sub-classified: JNC7 distinguishes hypertension stage Ⅰ, hypertension stage Ⅱ, and isolated systolic hypertension. Isolated systolic hypertension refers to elevated systolic pressure with normal diastolic pressure and is common in the elderly. The ESH-ESC Guidelines (2007) and BHS IV (2004) additionally define a third stage (stage Ⅲ hypertension) for people with systolic blood pressure exceeding 179 mmHg or a diastolic pressure over 109 mmHg. Hypertension is classified as resistant if medications do not reduce blood pressure to normal levels. In November 2017, the American Heart Association and American College of Cardiology published a joint guideline which updates the recommendations of the JNC7 report.

Children: Hypertension occurs in around 0.2% ~ 3% of newborns; however, blood pressure is not measured routinely in healthy newborns. Hypertension is more common in high risk newborns. A variety of factors, such as gestational age, postconceptional age and birth weight needs to be taken into account when deciding if a blood pressure is normal in a newborn.

Hypertension defined as elevated blood pressure over several visits affects 1% ~ 5% of children and adolescents and is associated with long term risks of ill-health. Blood pressure rises with age in childhood and, in children, hypertension is defined as an average systolic or diastolic blood pressure on three or more occasions equal or higher than the 95th percentile appropriate for the sex, age and height of the child. High blood pressure must be confirmed on repeated visits however before characterizing a child as having hypertension. Prehypertension in children has been defined as average systolic or diastolic blood pressure that is greater than or equal to the 90th percentile, but less than the 95th percentile. In adolescents, it has been proposed that hypertension and prehypertension are diagnosed and classified using the same criteria as in adults.

The value of routine screening for hypertension in children over the age of 3 years is debated. In 2004 the National High Blood Pressure Education Program recommended that children aged 3 years and older have blood pressure measurement at least once at every health care visit and the National Heart, Lung, and Blood Institute and American Academy of Pediatrics made a similar recommendation. However, the American Academy of Family Physicians supports the view of the US Preventive Services Task Force that the available evidence is insufficient to determine the balance of benefits and harms of screening for hypertension in children and adolescents who do not have symptoms.

5　Prevention

Much of the disease burden of high blood pressure is experienced by people who are not labeled as hypertensive. Consequently, population strategies are required to reduce the consequences of high blood pressure and reduce the need for antihypertensive medications. Lifestyle changes are recommended to lower blood pressure, before starting medications. The *British Hypertension Society Guidelines for hypertension management 2004 (BHS-IV)* proposed lifestyle changes consistent with those outlined by the US National High BP

Education Program in 2002 for the primary prevention of hypertension: maintain normal body weight for adults (e.g. body mass index $20 \sim 25$ kg/m^2); reduce dietary sodium intake to < 100 mmol per day (< 6 g of sodium chloride or < 2.4 g of sodium per day); engage in regular aerobic physical activity such as brisk walking (≥ 30 min per day, most days of the week); limit alcohol consumption to no more than 3 units per day in men and no more than 2 units per day in women; consume a diet rich in fruit and vegetables (e.g. at least 5 portions per day).

Effective lifestyle modification may lower blood pressure as much as an individual antihypertensive medication. Combinations of two or more lifestyle modifications can achieve even better results. There is considerable evidence that reducing dietary salt intake lowers blood pressure, but whether this translates into a reduction in mortality or cardiovascular disease remains uncertain. Estimated sodium intake ≥ 6 g/d and < 3 g/d are both associated with high risk of death or major cardiovascular disease, but the association between high sodium intake and adverse outcomes is only observed in people with hypertension. Consequently, in the absence of results from randomized controlled trials, the wisdom of reducing levels of dietary salt intake below 3 g/d has been questioned.

6　Management

According to one review published in 2003, reduction of the blood pressure by 5 mmHg can decrease the risk of stroke by 34%, of ischemic heart disease by 21%, and reduce the likelihood of dementia, heart failure, and mortality from cardiovascular disease.

Target blood pressure: Various expert groups have produced guidelines regarding how low the blood pressure target should be when a person is treated for hypertension. These groups recommend a target below the range $(140 \sim 160)$ mmHg / $(90 \sim 100)$ mmHg for the general population. Controversy exists regarding the appropriate targets for certain subgroups, including the elderly, people with diabetes, and people with kidney disease.

Many expert groups recommend a slightly higher target of 150/90 mmHg for those over somewhere between 60 and 80 years of age. The JNC-8 and American College of Physicians recommend the target of 150/90 mmHg for those over 60 years of age, but some experts within these groups disagree with this recommendation. Some expert groups have also recommended slightly lower targets in those with diabetes or chronic kidney disease with protein loss in the urine, but others recommend the same target as for the general population. The issue of what is the best target and whether targets should differ for high risk individuals is unresolved, but current best evidence supports more intensive blood pressure lowering than advocated in some guidelines.

Lifestyle modifications: The first line of treatment for hypertension is lifestyle changes, including dietary changes, physical exercise, and weight loss. Though these have all been recommended in scientific advisories, a Cochrane systematic review found no evidence for effects of weight loss diets on death, long-term complications or adverse events in persons with hypertension. The review did find a decrease in blood pressure. Their potential effectiveness is similar to and at times exceeds a single medication. If hypertension is high enough to justify immediate use of medications, lifestyle changes are still recommended in conjunction with medication.

Dietary changes shown to reduce blood pressure include diets with low sodium, the DASH diet, vegetarian diets, and green tea consumption.

Increasing dietary potassium has a potential benefit for lowering the risk of hypertension. The 2015 Dietary Guidelines Advisory Committee (DGAC) stated that potassium is one of the shortfall nutrients which are under-consumed in the United States.

Physical exercise regimens which are shown to reduce blood pressure include isometric resistance exercise, aerobic exercise, resistance exercise, and device-guided breathing.

Stress reduction techniques such as biofeedback or transcendental meditation may be considered as an add-on to other treatments to reduce hypertension, but do not have evidence for preventing cardiovascular disease on their own. Self-monitoring and appointment reminders might support the use of other strategies to improve blood pressure control, but need further evaluation.

Medications: Several classes of medications, collectively referred to as antihypertensive medications, are available for treating hypertension.

First-line medications for hypertension include thiazide-diuretics, calcium channel blockers, angiotensin converting enzyme inhibitors, and angiotensin receptor blockers. These medications may be used alone or in combination (ACE inhibitors and ARBs are not recommended for use in combination); the latter option may serve to minimize counter-regulatory mechanisms that act to revert blood pressure values to pre-treatment levels. Previously beta-blockers were thought to have similar beneficial effects when used as first-line therapy for hypertension. However, a Cochrane review that included 13 trials found that the effects of beta-blockers are inferior to that of other anti-hypertensive medications. Most people require more than one medication to control their hypertension. Medications for blood pressure control should be implemented by a stepped care approach when target levels are not reached.

Resistant hypertension: Resistant hypertension is defined as high blood pressure that remains above a target level, in spite of being prescribed three or more anti-hypertensive drugs simultaneously with different mechanisms of action. Failing to take the prescribed drugs, is an important cause of resistant hypertension. Resistant hypertension may also result from chronically high activity of the autonomic nervous system, an effect known as neurogenic hypertension. Electrical therapies that stimulate the baroreflex are being studied as an option for lowering blood pressure in people in this situation.

7　Epidemiology

Adults: As of 2014, approximately one billion adults or about 22% of the population of the world have hypertension. It is slightly more frequent in men, in those of low socioeconomic status, and it becomes more common with age. It is common in high, medium, and low income countries. The rates of raised blood pressure are highest in Africa, (30% for both sexes) and lowest in the WHO region of the Americas (18% for both sexes). Rates also vary markedly within WHO regions with rates as low as 3.4% (men) and 6.8% (women) in rural India and as high as 68.9% (men) and 72.5% (women) in Poland.

In Europe hypertension occurs in about 30% ~ 45% of people as of 2013. In 1995, it was estimated that 43 million people (24% of the population) in the United States had hypertension or were taking anti-hypertensive medication. By 2004 this had increased to 29% and further to 32% (76 million US adults) by 2017. In 2017, with the change in definitions for hypertension, 46% of people in the United States are affected. African-American adults in the United States have among the highest rates of hypertension in the world at 44%. It is also more common in Filipino Americans and less common in US whites and Mexican Americans.

Children: Rates of high blood pressure in children and adolescents have increased in the last 20 years in the United States. Childhood hypertension, particularly in pre-adolescents, is more often secondary to an underlying disorder than in adults. Kidney disease is the most common secondary cause of hypertension in children and adolescents. Nevertheless, primary or essential hypertension accounts for most cases.

8　Outcomes

Hypertension is the most important preventable risk factor for premature death worldwide. It increases the risk of ischemic heart disease, strokes, peripheral vascular disease, and other cardiovascular diseases, including heart failure, aortic aneurysms, diffuse atherosclerosis, chronic kidney disease, atrial fibrillation, and pulmonary embolism. Hypertension is also a risk factor for cognitive impairment and dementia. Other complications include hypertensive retinopathy and hypertensive nephropathy.

9　History

Measurement: Modern understanding of the cardiovascular system began with the work of physician William Harvey (1578–1657), who described the circulation of blood in his book *Demotu cordis*. The English clergyman Stephen Hales made the first published measurement of blood pressure in 1733. However, hypertension as a clinical entity came into its own with the invention of the cuff-based sphygmomanometer by Scipione Riva-Rocci in 1896. This allowed easy measurement of systolic pressure in the clinic. In 1905, Nikolai Korotkoff improved the technique by describing the Korotkoff sounds that are heard when the artery is auscultated with a stethoscope while the sphygmomanometer cuff is deflated. This permitted systolic and diastolic pressure to be measured.

Identification: The symptoms similar to symptoms of patients with hypertensive crisis are discussed in medieval Persian medical texts in the chapter of "fullness disease". The symptoms include headache, heaviness in the head, sluggish movements, general redness and warm to touch feel of the body, prominent, distended and tense vessels, fullness of the pulse, distension of the skin, coloured and dense urine, loss of appetite, weak eyesight, impairment of thinking, yawning, drowsiness, vascular rupture, and hemorrhagic stroke. Fullness disease was presumed to be due to an excessive amount of blood within the blood vessels.

Descriptions of hypertension as a disease came among others from Thomas Young in 1808 and especially Richard Bright in 1836. The first report of elevated blood pressure in a person without evidence of kidney disease was made by Frederick Akbar Mahomed (1849–1884).

Treatment: Historically the treatment for what was called the "hard pulse disease" consisted in reducing the quantity of blood by bloodletting or the application of leeches. This was advocated by the Yellow Emperor of China, Cornelius Celsus, Galen, and Hippocrates. The therapeutic approach for the treatment of hard pulse disease included changes in lifestyle (staying away from anger and sexual intercourse) and dietary program for patients (avoiding the consumption of wine, meat, and pastries, reducing the volume of food in a meal, maintaining a low-energy diet and the dietary usage of spinach and vinegar).

In the 19th and 20th centuries, before effective pharmacological treatment for hypertension became possible, three treatment modalities were used, all with numerous side-effects: strict sodium restriction (for example the rice diet), sympathectomy (surgical ablation of parts of the sympathetic nervous system), and pyrogen therapy (injection of substances that caused a fever, indirectly reducing blood pressure).

The first chemical for hypertension, sodium thiocyanate, was used in 1900 but had many side effects and was unpopular. Several other agents were developed after the Second World War, the most popular and reasonably effective of which were tetramethylammonium chloride, hexamethonium, hydralazine, and reserpine (derived from the medicinal plant Rauwolfia serpentina). None of these were well tolerated. A major breakthrough was achieved with the discovery of the first well-tolerated orally available agents. The first was chlorothiazide, the first thiazide diuretic and developed from the antibiotic sulfanilamide, which became available in 1958. Subsequently, beta blockers, calcium channel blockers, angiotensin converting enzyme (ACE) inhibitors, angiotensin receptor blockers, and renin inhibitors were developed as anti-hypertensive agents.

10　Society and Culture

Awareness: The World Health Organization has identified hypertension, or high blood pressure, as the leading cause of cardiovascular mortality. The World Hypertension League (WHL), an umbrella organization of 85 national hypertension societies and leagues, recognized that more than 50% of the hypertensive population worldwide are unaware of their condition. To address this problem, the WHL initiated a global awareness campaign on hypertension in 2005 and dedicated May 17 of each year as World Hypertension Day (WHD). Over the past three years, more national societies have been engaging in WHD and have been innovative in their activities to get the message to the public. In 2007, there was record participation from 47 member countries of the WHL. During the week of WHD, all these countries — in partnership with their local governments, professional societies, nongovernmental organizations and private industries — promoted hypertension awareness among the public through several media and public rallies. Using mass media such as Internet and television, the message reached more than 250 million people. As the momentum picks up year after year, the WHL is confident that almost all the estimated 1.5 billion people affected by elevated blood pressure can be reached.

Economics: High blood pressure is the most common chronic medical problem prompting visits to primary health care providers in USA. The American Heart Association estimated the direct and indirect costs of high blood pressure in 2010 as $76.6 billion. In the US, 80% of the people with hypertension are aware of their condition, 71% take some anti-hypertensive medication, but only 48% of people aware that they have hypertension and adequately control it. Adequate management of hypertension can be hampered by inadequacies in the diagnosis, treatment, or control of high blood pressure. Health care providers face many obstacles to achieving blood pressure control, including resistance to taking multiple medications to reach blood pressure goals. People also face the challenges of adhering to medicine schedules and making lifestyle changes. Nonetheless, the achievement of blood pressure goals is possible, and most importantly, lowering blood pressure significantly reduces the risk of death due to heart disease and stroke, the development of other debilitating conditions, and the cost associated with advanced medical care.

11　Research

A 2015 review of several studies found that restoring blood vitamin D levels by using supplements (more than 1000 IU per day) reduced blood pressure in hypertensive individuals when they had existing vitamin D deficiency. The results also demonstrated a correlation of chronically low vitamin D levels with a higher chance of becoming hypertensive. Supplementation with vitamin D over 18 months in normotensive individuals with vitamin D deficiency did not significantly affect blood pressure. There is tentative evidence that an increased calcium intake may help in preventing hypertension. However, more studies are needed to assess the optimal dose and the possible side effects.

Section 4　Words of TCM

1. 腠理 muscular interstices; striae; interstitial space

2. 癃闭 retention of urine

3. 八纲 the eight principal syndromes serving as guidelines in diagnosis

4. 八法 eight therapeutic methods

5. 八廓 the eight regions of the white of the eye

6. 脉象 pulse conditions; pulse pattern

7. 养生 health-cultivation

8. 病机总纲 general principle of pathogenesis or pathomechanism

9. 八纲辨证 analyzing and differentiating pathological conditions in accordance with eight principal syndrom

10. 治病求本 treating disease must concentrate on principle cause of disease

11. 舒肝和胃 soothing the liver and harmonizing the stomach

12. 清热泻火 clearing away heat and reducing fire

13. 补血养心 enriching blood to nourish the heart

14. 疏风泄热 dispelling wind and reducing heat

15. 行气消瘀 activating qi to resolve stagnation

16. 养血润肠 nourishing the blood and moistening the intestine

17. 祛虫消积 removing parasites to eliminate accumulation

18. 通腑泄热 purging fu-organs to eliminate heat

19. 燥湿化痰 drying dampness and resolving phlegm

20. 条达舒畅 free development

21. 安神醒脑法 mind-tranquilizing and brain-refreshing manipulation

22. 健脑益智法 mind-invigorating manipulation for improving intelligence

23. 宽胸理气法 chest-soothing and qi-regulating manipulation

24. 利肺益气法 lung-normalizing and qi-invigorating manipulation

25. 养心益神法 heart-nourishing and mind-benefiting manipulation

26. 健脾益胃法 spleen-strengthening and stomach-reinforcing manipulation
27. 消食导滞法 digestion-promoting and dyspepsia-removing manipulation
28. 壮腰强身法 waist-strengthening and constitution-enhancing manipulation
29. 补肾益精法 kidney-tonifying and essence-nourishing manipulation
30. 温补下元法 kidney-warming and -recuperating manipulation
31. 推拿按摩法 pushing, grasping, pressing and rubbing manipulation
32. 捏掐挤擦法 pinching, nipping, squeezing and scrubbing manipulation
33. 滚揉拍振法 rolling, kneading, patting and vibrating manipulation
34. 搓捻抖抹法 foulage, holding-twisting, shaking and wiping manipulation
35. 摇扳捣运法 rotating, pulling, pounding and arc-pushing manipulation
36. 点击、叩击法 digital-striking manipulation, tapping manipulation
37. 平直分合推法 flat-, straight-, parting- and meeting-pushing manipulation
38. 点按法 digital-pressing manipulation
39. 拔身法 traction and counter-traction manipulation
40. 一指禅 one-finger meditation

(Guo Yunliang, Ji Yaqing)

Chapter 15　Vitamins

Section 1　Vitamins

1　Vitamin A megadoses: boon or bust?

At least in the case of one fat-soluble vitamin — vitamin A — some people are making themselves sick trying to get healthy. Because the liver storage is large and is released very slowly, megadoses over time are unhealthy, even deadly. Although there are wise uses of moderate increases of certain vitamins, there is also abuse.

The public press constantly reminds us that food harvesting, storage, and processing methods are producing "empty-calorie" vegetables, not "half as nutritious as the ones our grandparents ate". Self-proclaimed nutrition "experts" tell us that even our grandparents' cooking could not provide the high amounts of nutrients we need today. So they claim we "must" take vitamins. This may actually be good advice in some individual cases of increased need or deficiency states. For example, the increased nutritional demands of pregnancy and lactation often require supplemental vitamins and minerals. Also, individuals whose eating habits are erratic may benefit from an appropriate intake of multi-vitamins. There is also evidence that certain vitamins offer protection against disease. Vitamin A apparently has some preventive association in the development of epithelial cancer in sites such as the lungs, larynx, esophagus, stomach, and urinary bladder. Studies have shown an inverse relationship between vitamin A (actually, beta-carotene) and the rate of lung cancer.

Unfortunately, such positive findings often fuel the fires of health faddists searching for "legitimate" reasons to take massive doses of various vitamins. This is never a good idea, of course, because it upsets the delicate balance of the 50-plus nutrients needed together to maintain good health. This is especially not a good idea in the case of fat-soluble vitamins, such as vitamin A, which are not rapidly excreted.

A growing number of people are inducing toxicity by taking readily available megadoses of vitamins. In the case of vitamin A, pills providing five times the recommended daily allowance (RDA) per capsule are becoming increasingly common. Some of the results are these: A 63-year-old man developed liver damage after 7 years of supplementing his diet with 7500 µg of vitamin A every day. His diet, which included generous portions of sweet potatoes, carrots, peaches, tomatoes, and desiccated beef liver, already provided $4500 \sim 9000$ µg of vitamin A per day. A 20-year-old female college student was hospitalized for the evaluation of wiat was thought to be a brain tumor after 2 year of supplementing her diet with $40\ 000 \sim 400\ 000$ IU of vitamin A. She had suffered severe headaches, loss of appetite, and dermatitis and had several abnormal neurologic findings.

Whether these individuals took vitamin A supplements specifically to ward off cancer is unknown. If that were the case, it would be ironic. Studies associating vitamin A with cancer prevention found that foods high in carotene are effective, not the carotene in pill form. Persons should learn that the most concentrated food sources of provitamin A (beta-carotene) are items such as mangos, carrots, cantaloupe, green cabbage, turnip greens, sweet potatoes, and kale. Each of these simple foods has substantially more than the recommended allowance for the whole day — plus many other interrelated nutrients — in just one moderate serving.

National US surveys show that about half of American adults consume vitamin and mineral supplements of some kind at some time. Approximately 23% take them daily. Doses of vitamin A in a subsampling of users in seven western states ranged from $(21\ 343 \pm 6945)$U to (9708 ± 2662)U. Sound public information is needed in the face of the self-medication trend with megadoses of nutrients. Since the potential for great harm exists in some instances, as it does with vitamin A, perhaps megadose supplements should have warning labels as cigarette packages do.

2   Vitamin B: Why is vitamin B important?

Do you ever wonder why doctors always tell you to eat a balanced diet? Say you love pineapple chicken, for example. Pineapples and chicken are both good for you, right? So why can't you just live off pineapple chicken? The reason is that the building blocks for good health come from a variety of foods, even if they are from the same family of nutrients. Such is the case with vitamin B, a key player in maintaining cell health and keeping you energized.

Not all types of vitamin B do the same thing. Additionally, the different types of vitamin B all come from different types of foods. vitamin B_{12}, for example, is found primarily in meat and dairy products. Vitamin B_7 and vitamin B_9 (and, to some degree, vitamin B_1 and vitamin B_2) are found in fruits and vegetables.

Deficiencies of any of these can lead to health problems. Sometimes a doctor will prescribe a supplement when they think you're not getting enough vitamin B. Certain groups, such as older adults and pregnant women, need larger amounts of some types of vitamin B. Certain conditions, such as Crohn's disease, Celiac disease, HIV, and misuse of alcohol can result in poor absorption of vitamin B.

Symptoms of a deficiency depend on what type of vitamin B you lack. They can range from fatigue and confusion to anemia or a compromised immune system. Skin rashes also can occur. Here's a rundown of the most common types of vitamin B: what they do, which foods contain them, and why you need them.

What it does: Vitamin B_{12} (cobalamin) helps regulate the nervous system. It also plays a role in growth and red blood cell formation.

Which foods contain it: Vitamin B_{12} is found primarily in meat and dairy products, so anyone on a strict vegan diet is at risk for deficiency. The only other dietary sources of Vitamin B_{12} are fortified foods. Some of the best sources of vitamin B_{12} include: eggs; cheese (one serving is the size of a domino); a glass of milk (1 cup); fish (a serving of any meat is the same size as a deck of cards); shellfish; liver; kidney; red meat. Try this recipe for a brunch version of ratatouille. Eggs and cheese make it a great source of vitamin B_{12}.

What happens if you don't get enough: Vitamin B_{12} deficiencies can lead to anemia and confusion in older adults. Psychological conditions such as dementia, paranoia, depression, and behavioral changes can result from a vitamin B_{12} deficiency. Neurological damage sometimes cannot be reversed. A vitamin B_{12} deficiency may cause the following symptoms: tingling in the feet and hands; extreme fatigue; weakness; irritability or depression.

3   Vitamin C: wonder drug of the 1990s?

When it comes to vitamin C, this question may well be gaining a more respectful answer of, "Well, maybe." At least researchers say that the climate in this controversial field is warming up as more information mounts on the antioxidant role of vitamin C in disease and health. Still others remain skeptical, disbelieving that vitamin C research can ever live down its checkered past that was littered with claims of cures for everything from cancer to the common cold. Who's right? Let's find out by taking a closer look at some of the problems this vitamin is supposed to solve.

(1) Cancer prevention: At least we sense a change in the wind by the fact that for the first time ever, in the fall of 1990, the National Cancer Institute (NCI) held a conference devoted entirely to vitamin C. And although the response to this initial conference was muted, at least there was response. The fact is established that "when you eat foods that are high in vitamin C you have a lower risk of cancer", as NCI's chief of prevention and control studies put it. NCI has several prevention trials underway testing the antioxidant capacities of vitamin C with supplements. At least now there are fewer skeptics.

(2) Prevention of colds: This has been the vitamin's main claim to fame, mainly through the work and writings of scientist Linus Pauling. Research subjects have reported less severe symptoms and shorter lengths of illness on megadoses. But vitamin C has not to show any ability to prevent a cold or control it to the point that it reduces its effect on sick time and works performance.

(3) Mental illness: Vitamin C is supposed to improve short-term memory, some claim, as well as "cure" schizophrenia and depression. Studies ruled out its effect on the former. However, in one study, large doses (3 g) of ascorbic acid were given to patients with depression, and an improved mental state followed. The investigators postulated that the vitamin inhibited vanadium, a rare metal that in toxic levels produces depression and melancholia. This does not mean that vitamin C is a "happy pill", however. Apparently vanadium levels that are toxic to persons suffering from depression fall within a range considered normal (1 ~ 2 mg/d) for everyone else. Thus megadoses of vitamin C may be helpful only to those individuals who are hypersensitive to vanadium.

(4) Stress: The adrenal glands respond to stress by producing epinephrine and other hormones. They respond best when their tissues are saturated with vitamin C. This does not require megadoses, however; intakes of 50 mg per day saturate half the tissues of the body. Thus person under a great deal of physiological and emotional stress may get by with as little as 60 ~ 100 mg per day.

(5) Heart disease: For some time there has been growing evidence that oxidation of low density lipoprotein (LDL) speeds the building up of the now familiar fatty plaques of atherosclerosis within artery walls. So scientists became excited about the effect of such strong antioxidants as vitamin C in preventing this build-up. And in their preliminary work this has indeed been the case. As they reported there was no oxidation damage to LDL as long as vitamin C was around.

(6) Wound healing: Wounds from scurvy heal on 4 ~ 8 mg per day. Wounds from surgery, which lowers the level of ascorbic acid in the blood, urine, and tissues, heal well at levels slightly above the RDA for vitamin C but no better than 1 ~ 2 g per day, thus eliminating another possible reason for megadoses. Apparently, there are many things the megadoses cannot do. What they can do is: (a) raise the risk for forming renal calculi, (b) reduce leukocyte activity against bacteria, and (c) cause gastrointestinal pain.

Obviously, the use of megadoses of vitamin C is not an entirely harmless practice. The public needs information with which they may recognize counterfeit claims, so as to avoid the potential dangers of self-medication in the absence of sound knowledge. This is true with any substance used in large amounts. Nonetheless, the sky seems to be brightening for vitamin C. On the basis of increasing knowledge of its antioxidant strength, especially in prevention of trouble rather than in treating it after it has happened, vitamin C may yet clear its name. It seems to be creeping closer to winning the respect it deserves.

Section 2   School of Watering Spleen

In traditional Chinese medicine spleen deficiency does not mean issues with the spleen as an anatomical organ. Spleen deficiency suggests an issue with the pancreas or with digestive function. Spleen prefers a dry environment; it is prone to conditions of dampness from climate and dietary factors. It is especially sensitive to cold, damp weather and cold or raw foods, both of which are fertile ground for the pathogenic factor of dampness. When the spleen functions properly, the body is strong and well nourished. Blood, fluids, and the organs are also in their proper places; thus there is no deficient-type bleeding (blood), edema (fluids), or prolapse (organs).

Spleen qi deficiency: When the qi of the spleen is deficient, the spleen is unable to perform its functions of digestion. In addition to the typical qi deficiency signs of fatigue and pale face and tongue, additional symptoms specific to the spleen include poor appetite, weight loss, fullness and sleepiness after eating, and loose stools. (Other conditions are associated with spleen qi deficiency, such as sagging organs and bleeding, but these are discussed as separate syndromes.) Some corresponding Western conditions are ulcers, gastritis, chronic fatigue, AIDS, chronic indigestion, and hepatitis. Treatment consists of tonifying spleen qi with herbs such as ginseng (renshen). The classic formula to tonify spleen qi is Four Gentlemen Decoction (Sijunzi Tang).

Spleen yang deficiency: This more severe version of spleen qi deficiency has the above-mentioned symptoms as well as cold signs such as cold hands and feet, edema, a desire for warm food and drinks, abdominal discomfort after eating cold food, and diarrhea with undigested food in the stools. Western diseases that fit this syndrome are chronic gastroenteritis, infection with Candida, food allergies, and chronic hepatitis. The treatment principle is to tonify spleen qi and yang and warm the interior with herbs such as ginseng (renshen), astragalus (huangqi), ginger (ganjiang), and black pepper (hujiao).

Spleen qi collapse or spleen qi sinking: Since spleen qi supports the organs with its uplifting energy, this aspect of deficient qi is associated with a prolapse (sagging) and a sensation of bearing down in the internal organs. Some organs affected are the stomach, transverse colon, uterus, and rectum. Hemorrhoids are also a condition of spleen qi collapse. In some cases, miscarriages can occur from lack of qi to hold things up, or retain the fetus with upward force. Treatment is to raise the middle qi with classic formulas such as Buzhong Yiqi Tang (decoction to tonify the middle burner and raise the vital energy). This formula contains herbs such as ginseng (renshen) and astragalus (huangqi) to build the spleen qi, along with herbs that have an uplifting energy such as bupleurum (chaihu) and cimicifuga (shengma).

Spleen not controlling the blood: Another function of spleen qi is to keep the blood flowing within the vessels. When this function is disturbed, standard symptoms of spleen qi deficiency occur along with bleeding under the skin (easy bruising), excessive menstrual bleeding, nosebleeds, and blood in the urine or stools. Since this bleeding is due to deficiency, the color of the blood is often lighter than might occur in excess bleeding disorders such as heat in the blood. Some of the western disease patterns that could fall into this pattern are any chronic bleeding diseases, hemophilia, bleeding hemorrhoids, bruising from vitamin deficiency, and periodontal disease. The treatment is to tonify spleen qi and tonify blood. The classic formula for this purpose, Eight Treasure Decoction (Bazhen Tang), combines the standard formulas for qi and blood tonification.

Cold and damp surrounding the spleen: This excess pattern arises when the dampness pernicious influence overwhelms the spleen. Symptoms include abdominal fullness and bloating, nausea, vomiting, watery stool, lack of thirst, sticky sensation and sweet taste in the mouth, dizziness, heavy feelings in the body, and a thick, greasy coat on the tongue. Some corresponding Western conditions are stomach flu, chronic gastritis, chronic colitis, ulcers, and hepatitis. The treatment involves the use of fragrant herbs that penetrate the dampness and wake up the spleen, such as patchouli (huoxiang).

Damp heat in the spleen: In this excess disharmony condition, the dampness symptoms combine with those of heat. They are: jaundice, yellow eyes, bitter taste in the mouth, nausea, vomiting, dislike of greasy food, burning urine and diarrhea, abdominal pain, bloating, and mouth sores. Some western diagnoses are hepatitis, gallbladder disease, and acute gastroenteritis. The treatment principle is to clear damp heat with herbs such as coptis (huanglian) and artemisia (yinchenhao).

Spleen yin deficiency is a common problem encountered in clinical practice and has been largely overlooked in the contemporary literature. Classically, the treatment of this pattern is based on the school of watering the spleen in the Yuan Dynasty. In Chinese medicine, it is called Hunger, yet no appetite — spleen yin deficiency. The other main signs and symptoms of this pattern include emaciation, dry lips and mouth, polydipsia, constipation, a thin, dry tongue coating, and a faint, rapid pulse.

Because of the dry climate of Xinjiang of China, a practitioner of traditional Chinese medicine in Xinjiang has had considerable experience in the diagnosis and treatment of spleen yin deficiency in his 23 years of clinical experience. He has found that this pattern is best treated by traditional Chinese dietary therapy, particularly in Xinjiang, the indigenous people's own dietary traditions which only need to be minimally modified.

Among the Moslems, the flat wheaten bread is baked in clay ovens. Tomatoes, which promote the secretion of body fluids, are grown here in profusion. Also, because of the high incidence of animal husbandry (sheep and goats), cheese is quite plentiful. In Chinese medicine, it is a well-known fact that dairy products are also extremely effective for promoting the secretion of body fluids and juice. If one cook tomatoes and cheese in a clay oven on top of the local flat bread one combines the moistening properties of the wheat, tomatoes, and cheese and arrives at an almost perfect food for the production of yin and water in the spleen. In the treatment of spleen yin deficiency, this combination should be eaten once per day. One course of treatment lasts for 30 days. Between courses, there should be a 5-day rest.

Because sugar and dairy secret body fluids help to hydrate the spleen so efficiently, the incidence of spleen yin efficiency is on the decline directly as a result of the improvement of living standard. Also, the Xinjiang people living and working in Shanghai as entrepreneurs have a lower incidence of this condition. The cuisine in Shanghai is based on the liberal use of cooking oil which therefore also moistens the spleen. In addition, the weather of Shanghai, unlike the Tarim Basin, is preponderantly damp. The combination of the Shanghai cuisine and Shanghai weather is well known in China for its ability to create plumper tongues with thicker coatings and a more sibilant pulse.

In conclusion, it seems safe to say that the spleen can be moistened by the judicious use of rationally selected foods based on traditional Chinese dietary therapy and that an understanding of the theories of the school of watering the spleen is one of the treasures of traditional Chinese medicine.

Section 3   Research Article

The protection of Bcl-2 over-expression on rat cortical neuronal injury caused by analogous ischemia-reperfusion in vitro

[Abstract] Recent studies have suggested that neuronal apoptosis in cerebral ischemia could arise from dysfunction of endoplasmic reticulum (ER) and mitochondria. B-cell lymphoma/leukemia-2 gene (Bcl-2) has been described as an inhibitor both in programmed cell death (PCD) and ER dysfunction during apoptosis, and the Bcl-2 family play a key role in regulating the PCD, both locally at the ER and from a distance at the mitochondrial membrane. However, its signal pathways and concrete mechanisms in endoplasmic reticulum initiated apoptosis remain incompletely understood. We therefore investigate whether ischemia-reperfusion (I / R) causes neuronal apoptosis in part via cross-talk between ER and mitochondria or not, and how the over-expression of Bcl-2 prevents this form of cell death. Here we show that analogous I/R-induced cell death occurs consequent to interactions of ER stress and mitochondrial death pathways. The participation of the mitochondrial pathway was demonstrated by the release of cytochrome C (Gyt C) from mitochondrial into cytoplasmic fractions and caspase-9 cleavage. The involvement of ER stress was further supported by the observable increase of glucose-regulated protein 78 (GRP78) / BiP expression and caspase-12 activity. Furthermore, prior to these changes, swelling of the ER lumen and dissociation of ribosomes from rough ER were detected by electron microscopy. Bcl-2 over-expression inhibits the release of Cyt C and the activation of caspase-9/caspase-8/caspase-3 but not caspase-12 based on the results of Western blot. These suggest that cross-talk between ER and mitochondria participate in neuronal damage after ischemia-reperfusion. Bcl-2 over-expression could suppress I/R-induced neuronal apoptosis via influencing mitochondrial integrity.

Keywords: cortical neuron; ischemia-reperfusion; endoplasmic reticulum stress; caspases; Bcl-2

1   Introduction

Cumulative evidence suggested that apoptosis plays a pivotal role in neuronal death in cerebral ischemic injury. Apoptotic signal involves both extrinsic and intrinsic stress induced pathways. The endoplasmic reticulum (ER) is an organelle that ensures the correction of protein fold and assembly via the expression of numerous molecular chaperones and other control system of protein quality (Hammond et al., 1994). Various conditions, such as glucose starvation, disturbance of intracellular calcium homeostasis, inhibition of protein glycosylation, as well as exposure to free radicals, unfolded proteins to accumulate in ER lumen, that is, a process named ER stress. ER stress could also be elicited in cell culture system by pharmacological agents, including tunicamycin (Tun), a protein inhibitor of N-glycosylation; brefeldin A (BFA), which blocks protein transportation from ER into Golgi; and thapsigargin (TG), which depresses ER uptake of calcium by inhibiting the sarcoplasmic endoplasmic Ca^{2+}-ATPase (SERCA) (Lee et al., 2001). Excessive ER stress induces cell death (Kadowaki et al., 2004). Caspase-12, a protease of caspase family, is localized in ER and specifically activated by ER stress (Nakagawa et al., 2000). And the activity of ER resident caspase-12 can ignite cytoplasmic caspase-3, but not mitochondria related caspase-9, during ER stress-induced apoptosis (Hitomia et al., 2003). Evidence also showed the cross-talk between ER and mitochondria. Bcl-2 family members have been considered as key mediators in either pro- or anti-apoptosis. Owing to the mitochondrial localization of many Bcl-2 family members, they are often assumed to play a direct biochemical effect in mitochondria. Recent work has demonstrated that in addition to maintaining mitochondrial integrity, pro- and anti-apoptotic members of Bcl-2 family also reside ER, where they regulate organelle homeostasis and cell death in response to signals impacting ER function (Oakes et al., 2006). Inhibition of I/R-induced cell death by antiapoptotic Bcl-2 family protein in vivo has been examined (Chien et al., 2007; Miao et al., 2007), nevertheless, the certain mechanisms of neuronal apoptosis underlying cerebral ischemia-reperfusion damage remains elusive. In the present study, we examined the involvement of ER stress and mitochondria and the effect of over-expression

Bcl-2 in rat neuronal apoptosis induced by analogous ischemia-reperfusion in vitro.

2   Materials and methods

2.1   Primary culture of cerebral cortical cells

Primary neuronal culture was performed as previously described (Wang et al., 2003). Briefly, cerebral cortex was isolated from 16 ~ 18 days old fetuses of Sprague-Dawley rats. After the removal of meninges and blood vessels, cerebral cortex was cut, digested with trypsin at 37.8 ℃ for 20 min, and filtered with a strainer to exclude tissue fragments. The filtrate was centrifuged at 300 g for 5 min and its sediment was washed twice with Hank's medium. Then cells were resuspended with DMEM medium containing 10% fetal bovine serum (FBS) and 10% horse serum (HS), adjusted to approximately 10^6 cell/mL, and plated into polylysine-coated plastic culture flasks and maintained at 37.8 ℃ in 5% CO_2 humid environment. At 24 h after initial plating, plate medium was completely replaced with neurobasal medium containing B27 supplements (Gibco, Rockville, MD, USA). After 4 days, half of medium was exchanged for glutamate free neurobasal medium. All experiments were performed on neurons after 7 ~ 10 days in culture.

2.2   Establishment of neuronal in vitro models of I/R

To mimic cerebral ischemia in vitro, I/R was performed with primary neuronal cultures as described previously (Meloni et al., 2001). Medium was first removed from the cultures, and then rinsed twice with phosphate buffered solution (PBS) without Ca^{2+}/Mg^{2+}. Cultures were subjected to ischemia in an anoxia chamber for 6 h by rinsing twice and covering with glucose-free Earles medium (143.8 mmol/L Na^+, 5.5 mmol/L K^+, 1.8 mmol/L Ca^{2+}, 0.8 mmol/L Mg^{2+}, 125.3 mmol/L Cl^-, 26.2 mmol/L HCO_3^-, 1.0 mmol/L $H_2PO_4^{2-}$, 0.8 mmol/L SO_4^{2-}, 0.01 mmol/L glycine, and 10 mmol/L HEPES at pH 7.4) pre-equilibrated with the atmosphere in the chamber (95% N_2 and 5% CO_2). Control cells were incubated in the same solution with glucose under normoxic conditions (in a CO_2 incubator). After ischemia cultures 6 h, glucose-free Earles medium was replaced by fresh neurobasal medium with B27 supplement. Finally, cultures were maintained in a CO_2 incubator for the next 48 h reperfusion, as mentioned above.

2.3   Plasmid

The pcDNA3-hBcl-2 was granted from Dr. Karen S. Poksay (Buck Institute for Age Research, Novato, California 94945 and the University of California, San Francisco, California 94143).

2.4   Transfection

All procedures were performed with the lipidosome 2000 transfection reagent (Invitrogen) following the manufacturer's protocols. Briefly, cells were seeded in the culture plates and cultured to achieve 50% of confluence. The cells were then transiently transfected using a mixture of plasmid and lipidosome 2000 in Optimem (Invitrogen). A lipidosome 2000 to DNA ratio of 3 mL : 2 mg was maintained for all experiments. Media was completely replaced with conditioned media 6 ~ 8 h after transfection, and neurons were undergone experiment 2 ~ 4 days after transfection.

2.5   Transmission electron microscopy (TEM)

The specimens were fixed in a mixture of 4% glutaraldehyde and 4% formaldehyde (freshly prepared from paraformaldehyde) buffered at pH 7.2 with 0.1 mol/L sodium cacodylate at room temperature for 16 ~ 20 h. After washings in 0.1 mol/L sodium cacodylate at pH 7.2, the specimens were transferred to cacodylate-buffered 1% osmium tetroxide at pH 7.2 for 1 h at room temperature. After treated with 0.5% uranyl acetate for 2 h, the specimens were dehydrated in gradient ethanol, rinsed in propylene oxide and then embedded in Araldite. Semithin sections stained with 1% toluidine blue were examined under a light microscope, and suitable regions were carefully selected for trimming of the blocks. Ultrathin sections were collected on collodion coated grids, stained in alcoholic 2% uranyl acetate and lead citrate and examined in a transmission electron microscope (Philips-CM 200).

2.6   Apoptosis assays

After subjected to ischemia-reperfusion, 10^6 cells were used to determine the translocation of phosphatidylserine to the outer surface of plasma membrane during apoptosis by using human phospholipids binding protein, annexin-V, conjugated with fluorescein isothiocyanate, according to the manufacturer's instructions (Bender Med. Systems). The percentage of apoptotic cells (annexin-V positive and propidium iodide negative) was determined by flow cytometric analysis (FACSCLSR, Becton-Dickton, USA). For fluorescent microscope, cells were incubated with Hochest 33258 with a final concentration of 5 mg/L.

2.7   Western blotting analysis

Total protein was extracted from cells in each group in accordance with kit operation of protein extraction, and explained by protein quantity kit. Western blot analysis was carried out by Shimokea et al. (2004), Shin et al. (2006), and Yokomaku et al. (2005). Briefly, total lysate (20 mg per lane) was subjected to SDS-PAGE, and blotted on a nitrocellulose membrane using a semi-dry blotter (Atto). After blocking with Block-Ace (Dainippon), anti-caspase-12 antibody (Stressgen), anti-bcl-2/cyt C antibody (Santa Cruz Biotechnology), anti-actin antibody

(Santa Cruz), anti-caspase-3/-8/-9 (Stressgen) or anti-GRP78 polyclonal antibody (Stressgen) was loaded to the membrane, followed by the HRP-conjugated secondary antibody, and the signal was enhanced using an ABC kit (Vector Laboratories). Immunoreactive proteins were detected with ECL detection system. The relative density of protein bands was quantified by Electrophoresis Documentation and Analysis System 120 (Eastman Kodak Com., Rochester, NY). The bands were visualized with a light capture system (Atto) using Immunostar reagents (Wako). Immunoreactivity was determined by Gel Documentation Systems (Bio-Rad). Data was normalized to a standard from one control group run on all gels.

2.8   Subcellular fractionation

Fractionation was performed as described previously (Rao et al., 2001; Cheung et al., 2006) with some modifications. Briefly, cells were resuspended and lysed in ice-cold hypotonic extraction buffer (10 mmol/L Tris-HCl, pH 7.4, 50 mmol/L KCl) using a B-type pestle. The lysate was immediately adjusted to 250 mmol/L sucrose, 1 mmol/L $MgCl_2$, 0.5 mmol/L ethylene glycol tetraacetate (EGTA), 1 mmol/L dithiothreitol (DTT), 0.1 mmol/L phenylmethylsulfonyl fluoride (PMSF), 5 mg/mL pepstatin A, 10 mg/mL leupeptin and aprotinin, and centrifuged at 750 g for 10 min at 4 ℃ so as to remove nuclei and cell debris. The supernatant was further centrifuged at 10 000 g for 30 min at 4 ℃ . The pellet containing mitochondrial fraction was resuspended in the buffer above. After re-centrifuged at 100 000 g for 60 min, the supernatant then contained soluble cytoplasmic fraction, and the pellet constituting ER enriched microsomal fraction was rinsed and resuspended as above. The quality of the fractionation experiments was controlled by assessing the distribution of mt-HSP70 for mitochondria, SREBP-1 for ER.

2.9   Statistical analysis

Statistical comparisons were made using an ANOVA with post hoc Tukey's HSD or Student's t-test.

3   Results

3.1   Primary culture of neurons

Cortical neurons were reacted with primary antibody NSE at 7 days after the culture. And these positive cells of NSE expression were accounted for (92.69 ± 4.1) % of the total cells. It was therefore deemed as pure neuron culture.

3.2   Mimic cerebral I/R in vitro induces ER stress and apoptosis

The induction of the ER chaperone GRP78 is an established marker for the presence of

ER stress (Gulow et al., 2002). To confirm induction of ER stress, protein levels of GRP78 were assessed by immunoblotting cell extracts with specific antibodies. As expected, GRP78 protein levels were elevated in neurons at I/R (6 h/48 h), supporting the induction of ER stress in these neurons in response to ischemia-reperfusion with or without transfection of pcDNA3-h-Bcl-2, but not in control cells (normal cultured). Neurons undergone I/R appeared typical morphological apoptotic changes, including nuclear fragmentation, chromatin condensation, pycnosis and cell shrinkage. Prior to these changes, swelling of the ER lumen and dissociation of ribosomes from rough ER were observed by electron microscopy. To determine whether ER stress resulted in apoptosis or not, we analyzed the apoptosis percentages by flow cytometry, which identifies the positive percentage of cells with annexin V-FITC without propidium iodide uptake. The apoptosis of normally cultured cortical neurons of rats notably increased after analogous I/R in vitro. The percentage of apoptotic cells was depressed after transfection of pcDNA3-h-Bcl-2. Furthermore, with Hochest 33258 stain, morphological alternation of apoptotic cells showed that the nucleus of living cell was uniformly stained blue while apoptotic cells were hyperchromatic.

3.3   The release of cytochrome C (Cyt C)

Recent studies indicate that the release of Cyt C from mitochondria is a critical step in apoptosis. We wonder whether I/R causes similar changes in the compartmentalization of Cyt C or not. In our previous study, we performed a detailed time course assessment of the concentration of Cyt C in cellular subfractions. There was only a negligible amount of Cyt C in the cytosolic fractions obtained from control cells. We found gradual appearance of Cyt C in the cytosol of neurons injured by I/R, which began at reperfusion 6 h, peaked at reperfusion 24 ~ 48 h, but mitochondrial outer membrane intact were observed by electron microscopy. In the present study, we found high expression of Cyt C in cytosolic and mitochondrial fractions of neurons injured by ischemia 6 h reperfusion 48 h, and the release of Cyt C from mitochondria to cytosol was significantly suppressed by overexpression of Bcl-2 (Figure 15-1).

3.4   Involvement of caspases in I/R induced neuronal apoptosis

Caspases are critical mediators of apoptosis in mammalian cells (Thornberry et al., 1998). Apoptosis can be activated through two distinct sets of cascades, which are the intrinsic or the extrinsic pathways. Intrinsic pathways involve either the ER stress response or mitochondrial-driven apoptosis. Cyt C is known to bind to dATP and apoptotic protease-activating factor-1 (Apaf-1) in order to form the apoptosome that activates caspase-9 (Li et al., 1997). Because caspase-12 is cleaved during ER stress (Nakagawa et al., 2000), and caspase-8 participates in ER stress-mediated apoptosis (He et al., 2002; Momoi, 2004; Sheikh et al., 1998), we investigated the expression of active-caspase-3, -8, -9, -12. The activity of caspase-3/-8/-9/12 were significantly high after ischemia 6 h reperfusion 48 h, and the levels of caspase-3/-8/-9 was obviously reduced by transfection of pcDNA3-h-Bcl-2, but not of caspase-12 (Figure 15-2).

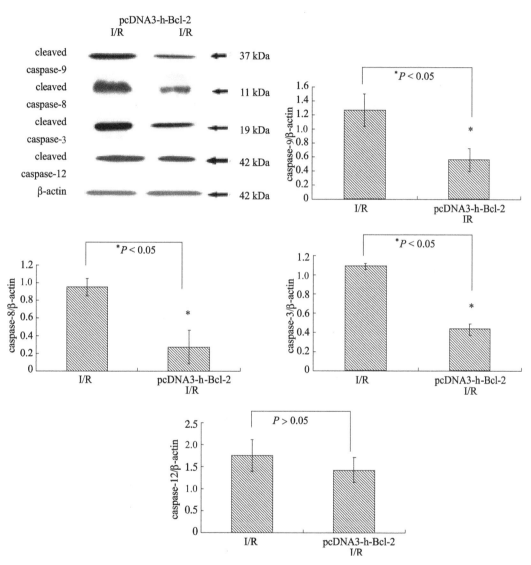

Figure 15-1 I/R induce early process of caspases

Neurons were exposed to ischemia 6 h reperfusion 48 h, and then cells were harvested and proteins extracted. Equal proteins were separated by SDS-PAGE and transferred to nitrocellulose for Western blotting with the indicated antibodies. After X-ray scanned slides with Bio-Rad 2000 gel imaging system, the absorbance (A) was determined by the application of Quantity One software. In the same specimen, the A value of beta actin, as an internal parameter, was also detected to calibrate the concentration of each target protein. Results are representative of those obtained in at least three different experiments. Western blotting showed that the expression level of capase-3, capase-8, capase-9 and capase-12 significantly increased at 48 h of reperfusion. The activity of capase-3, capase-8, capase-9 except capase-12 could be significantly depressed by transfection of pcDNA3-h-Bcl-2.

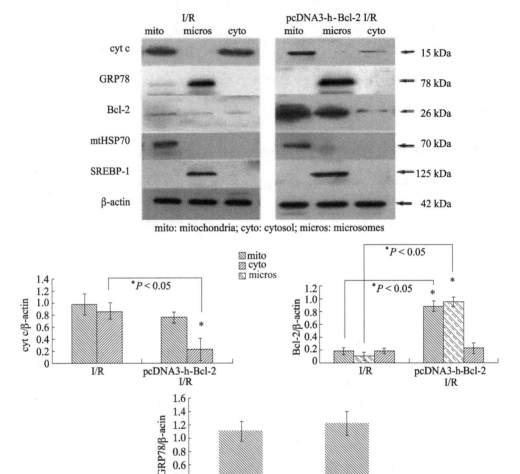

Figure 15-2 Over-expression of Bcl-2 cuts down the release of Cyt C

Proteins were separated by SDS-PAGE and transferred to nitrocellulose for Western blotting with the indicated antibodies. After X-ray scanned slides with Bio-Rad 2000 gel imaging system, the absorbance (*A*) was determined by the application of Quantity One software. In the same specimen, the value of beta actin, as an internal parameter, was also detected to calibrate the concentration of each target protein. Western blotting analysis of subcellular fractions samples showing that exogenous Bcl-2 located in both mitochondrial and microsomal fractions. After I/R (6 h/48 h), there was a significant release of CytC from mitochondria to cytosol and the release of Cyt C was obviously blocked by over-expression of Bcl-2. The expression level of GRP78 notably increased at 48 h of reperfusion, but the no observable change was detected after over-expression of Bcl-2. Data are expressed as (mean ± SE) from three independent experiments. The mtHSP70 and SREBP-1 are proteins localized to the mitochondria and the ER, and thus serve as markers of organelle specific preparations. mito: mitochondria; cyto: cytosol; micros: microsome.

3.5 Over-expression Bcl-2 prevents I/R induced cell death in cultured cerebral cortical neurons

Bcl-2 family members act as regulators in almost all known Q4 forms of programmed cell death (Cory et al., 2002). The Bcl-2 gene was firstly discovered as the first oncogene in inhibiting apoptosis. We examined the intracellular localization of Bcl-2 after plasmid pcDNA3-h-Bcl-2 transfection, the increased level of Bcl-2 was found in mitochondrial and microsomal fractions. Over-expressed Bcl-2 suppressed the activity of caspase-3/-8/-9 of neuronal injury and the release of Cyt C in cytosolic fraction after ischemia and reperfusion. GRP78, a calcium-binding chaperone protein, posseses cell-protective properties (Liu et al., 2000; Rao et al., 2002; Reddy et al., 2003), and has been used as a biomarker of ER stress. Over-expression and antisense approaches in cell systems show that GRP78 can protect against cell death caused by disturbance of ER homeostasis. But in this experiment over-expressed Bcl-2 did not up-regulate the level of GRP78.

4 Discussion

At the molecular level, several common features are often associated with apoptosis: mitochondrial dysfunction and Cyt C release, activation of caspases family, exposure of phosphatidyl serine to extracellular space, and DNA cleavage at internucleosomal regions (Thomenius et al., 2003). Mitochondria are of central importance in apoptotic process. The release of Cyt C from mitochondria triggers caspase activation. Currently, several pathways have been directly implicated in ER stress-induced apoptosis. The apoptosis signal of neuron caused by I/R is multiple. We report here that ER stress response and mitochondrial dysfunction are involved in neuronal apoptotic pathways induced by IR in vitro. Neurons showed typical apoptotic features, such as chromatin condensation, pycnosis and cell shrinkage. Prior to these changes, swelling of the ER lumen and dissociation of ribosomes from rough ER but mitochondria intact were observed by electron microscopy. Cyt C released to cytosolic fraction before mitochondrial swelling and disruption. Junichi et al. (2003) also found that ER stress inducers caused ER swelling prior to mitochondrial disruption, and the activation of ER resident caspase-12 caused activation of cytoplasmic caspase-3, but not mitochondria related caspase-9, during ER stress-induced apoptosis. Some results (Liu et al., 2006) report that intrinsic ER stress response pathways, not the extrinsic TNFα, cause caspase-8 activation in TS-infected cultured astrocytes. Caspase-12, one of the caspase family, is localized in ER and specifically activated by ER stress (Nakagawa et al., 2000). In spite of certain onset of caspase cascade initiated by I/R, we detected that caspase-8/caspase-9/caspase-3/caspase-12 were involved in neuronal apoptotic signals caused by I/R. Our results indicate that there is crosstalk between the ER and the mitochondria during I/R, as a result, induces neuronal apoptosis.

Bcl-2 has been described both as an inhibitor of programmed cell death and as an inhibitor of mitochondrial dysfunction during apoptosis. It has been demonstrated that in addition to controlling mitochondrial integrity, pro- and anti-apoptotic members of the Bcl-2 family are also distributed in the endoplasmic reticulum, where they regulate organelle homeostasis and cell death in response to signals that impact ER function. Generally, members of Bcl-2 family in cell death regulators are divided into three types based upon the four regions of homology (BH1-4) to the founding member Bcl-2. The different proteins within each subtype of the Bcl-2 family have distinct patterns of developmental expression, subcellular localization, and responsiveness to specific death stimuli (Danial et al., 2004). Bcl-2 in mitochondria was more protective than that in ER against serum withdrawal and etoposide treatment, and stimuli were slow in triggering mitochondrial disruption and cyt C release (Annis et al., 2001). In the present study, we found that exogenous over-expressional Bcl-2 localized both mitochondrial and ER fractions after ischemia and reperfusion. Meanwhile, the activity of Cyt C was decreased in cytosolic fraction. The subcellular distribution of Bcl-2 proteins undoubtedly plays a crucial role in the regulation of apoptosis. One potential way of Bcl-2 blocking the intrinsic death is to keep pro-apoptotic proteins at their action sites. It is more likely that Bcl-2 in ER can powerfully sequester BH3-only proteins from flowing into mitochondria. Therefore, Bax/Bak dependent mitochondrial dysfunction, Cyt C release, and caspase activation are inactive. The induction of glucose regulated proteins (GRPs) is commonly used as an indicator for the ER stress. Ramachandra et al. (2003) reported that without ER stress inducers, specific over-expression of GRP78 could block caspase-7 activation and further reduce apoptosis. They found that endogenous GRP78 constitutively associates with procaspase-7 but not with procaspase-3 and dATP releases procaspase-7 from GRP78, resulting in its activation. GRP78 is an ATP-binding protein and utilizes ATP for its chaperone function. Procaspase-7 interaction with GRP78 requires these specific residues within the ATP binding domain. In our early study, we did not detect cleaved caspase-7 in ER fractions (Zhang et al., 2008), and in the present study we did not find up-regulated expression of GRP78 after Bcl-2 over-expression. Perhaps, the loss of the ability of GRP78 to form a complex with procaspase-7 correlates with the loss of protection against I/R mediated apoptosis. Therefore, specific protective effect of Bcl-2 over-expression on cultured neurons in vitro maybe have no relation to GRP78.

5   Conclusion

In summary, this study provided that cultured neurons undergo caspase-3/-8/-9/-12-dependent apoptosis under analogous I/R circumstance and its mechanism might involve mitochondrial dysfunction and ER stress. Over-expression of Bcl-2 prevents this form of cell apoptosis in vitro via influencing mitochondrial integrity, thus we hypothesize that Bcl-2 over-expression might suppress ER stress-induced apoptosis from a distance. In the next experiment, we will further explore and verify the defined mechanism of ER-to-mitochondrion in neuronal apoptotic signals.

References

[1]   Annis M G, Zamzami N, Zhu W, et al. Endoplasmic reticulum localized Bcl-2 prevents apoptosis when redistribution of cytochrome c is a late event. Oncogene, 2001, 20(16): 1939-1952.

[2]   Cheung H H, Kelly N L, Liston P, et al. Involvement of caspase-2 and caspase-9 in endoplasmic reticulum stress-induced apoptosis: A role for the IAPs. Experimental Cell Research, 2006, 312(12): 2347-2357.

[3]   Chien C T, Shyue S K, Lai M K. Bcl-xL augmentation potentially reduces ischemia/reperfusion induced proximal and distal tubular apoptosis and autophagy. Transplantation, 2007, 84(9): 1183-1190.

[4]   Cory S, Adams J M. The Bcl-2 family: regulators of the cellular life-or-death switch. Nature Reviews Cancer, 2002, 2(9): 647-656.

[5]   Danial N N, Korsmeyer S J. Cell death : critical control points. Cell, 2013, 116(2): 205-219.

[6]   Gülow K, Bienert D, Haas I G. BiP is feed-back regulated by control of protein translation efficiency. Journal of Cell Science, 2002, 115(11): 2443-2452.

[7]   Hammond C, Helenius A. Quality control in the secretory pathway: retention of a misfolded viral membrane glycoprotein involves cycling between the ER, intermediate compartment, and Golgi apparatus. Journal of Cell Biology, 1994, 126(1): 41-52.

[8]   He Q, Dongik L, Rong R, et al. Endoplasmic reticulum calcium pool depletion-induced apoptosis is coupled with activation of the death receptor 5 pathway. Oncogene, 2002, 21(17): 2623-2633.

[9]   Hitomi J, Katayama T, Taniguchi M, et al. Apoptosis induced by endoplasmic reticulum stress depends on activation of caspase-3 via caspase-12. Neuroscience Letters, 2004, 357(2): 127-130.

[10]   Kadowaki H, Nishitoh H, Ichijo H. Survival and apoptosis signals in ER stress: the role of protein kinases. Journal of Chemical Neuroanatomy, 2004, 28(1-2): 93-100.

[11]   Lee A S. The glucose-regulated proteins: stress induction and clinical applications. Trends Biochem Sci, 2001, 26: 504-510.

[12]   Liu C Y, Schröder M, Kaufman R J. Ligand-independent Dimerization Activates the Stress Response Kinases IRE1 and PERK in the Lumen of the Endoplasmic Reticulum. Journal of Biological Chemistry, 2000, 275(32): 24881-24885.

[13]   Li P, Nijhawan D, Budihardjo I, et al. Cytochrome C and dATP-dependent formation of Apaf-1/caspase-9 complex initiates an apoptotic protease cascade. Cell, 1997, 91: 479-489.

[14]   Liu N, Scofield V L, Qiang W, et al. Interaction between endoplasmic reticulum stress and caspase 8

activation in retrovirus MoMuLV- ts 1-infected astrocytes. Virology, 2006, 348(2): 398-405.

[15] Meloni B P, Majda B T, Knuckey N W. Establishment of neuronal in vitro, models of ischemia in 96-well microtiter strip-plates that result in acute, progressive and delayed neuronal death. Neuroscience, 2001, 108(1): 17-26.

[16] Miao Y, Xia Q, Hou Z, et al. Ghrelin protects cortical neuron against focal ischemia/reperfusion in rats. Biochemical & Biophysical Research Communications, 2007, 359(3): 795-800.

[17] Momoi T. Caspases involved in ER stress-mediated cell death. Journal of Chemical Neuroanatomy, 2004, 28(1-2): 101-105.

[18] Nakagawa T, Yuan J. Cross-talk between two cysteine protease families: activation of caspase-12 by calpain in apoptosis. Journal of Cell Biology, 2000, 150(4): 887-894.

[19] Nakagawa T, Zhu H, Morishima N, et al. Caspase-12 mediates endoplasmic-reticulum-specific apoptosis and cytotoxicity by amyloid-beta. Nature, 2000, 403(6765): 98-103.

[20] Oakes S A, Lin S S, Bassik M C. The control of endoplasmic reticulum-initiated apoptosis by the BCL-2 family of proteins. Current Molecular Medicine, 2006, 6(1): 98-109.

[21] Rao R V, Ellerby HMBredesen D E. Coupling endoplasmic reticulum stress to the cell death program. Cell Death & Differentiation, 2004, 11(4): 372-380.

[22] Rao R V, Niazi K, Mollahan P, et al. Coupling endoplasmic reticulum stress to the cell-death program: a novel HSP90-independent role for the small chaperone protein p23. Cell Death & Differentiation, 2006, 13(3): 415.

[23] Reddy R K, Mao C, Baumeister P, et al. Endoplasmic reticulum chaperone protein GRP78 protects cells from apoptosis induced by topoisomerase inhibitors: role of ATP binding site in suppression of caspase-7 activation. Journal of Biological Chemistry, 2003, 278(23): 20915-20924.

[24] Sheikh M S, Burns T F, Huang Y, et al. p53-dependent and -independent regulation of the death receptor KILLER/DR5 gene expression in response to genotoxic stress and tumor necrosis factor alpha. Cancer Research, 1998, 58(8): 1593-1598.

[25] Shimokea K, Utsumia T, Kishia S, et al. Prevention of endoplasmic reticulum stress-induced cell death by brain-derived neurotrophic factor in cultured cerebral cortical neurons. Brain Res, 2004, 1028: 105-111.

[26] Shin W H, Park S J, Kim E J. Protective effect of anthocyanins in middle cerebral artery occlusion and reperfusion model of cerebral ischemia in rats. Life Sciences, 2006, 79(2): 130-137.

[27] Thomenius M J, Distelhorst C W. Bcl-2 on the endoplasmic reticulum: protecting the mitochondria from a distance. J Cell Sci, 2003, 116: 4493-4499.

[28] Thornberry N A, Lazebnik Y. Caspases: enemies within. Science, 1998, 281(5381): 1312-1316.

[29] Wang J F, Azzam J E, Young L T. Valproate inhibits oxidative damage to lipid and protein in primary cultured rat cerebrocortical cells. Neuroscience, 2003, 116(2): 485-489.

[30] Yokomaku D, Jourdi H, Kakita A, et al. ErbB1 receptor ligands attenuate the expression of synaptic scaffolding proteins, GRIP1 and SAP97, in developing neocortex. Neuroscience, 2005, 136(4): 1037-1047.

[31]   Zhang H, Liu X, Mei Y. The effect of silencing of cytochrome c on rat cortical neuronal injury caused by analogous ischemia/reperfusion in vitro. Stroke & Nervous Diseases, 2008, 15: 35-38.

Section 4   Words of TCM

1. 汤剂、煎剂、饮剂 decoction

2. 散剂 powder

3. 大丸剂、小丸药 bolus, pellet or pill

4. 蜜丸、水丸 honeyed bolus, water pellet

5. 糊丸、浓缩丸 paste pill, condensed pellet

6. 膏剂 paste; paste preparation; ointment; salve; plaster

7. 煎膏、软膏、硬膏 decocted paste, ointment, plaster

8. 浸膏、流浸膏 extract, liquid extract

9. 酒剂 medicinal wine

10. 茶剂 medicinal tea

11. 丹剂 pellet

12. 锭剂 lozenge; pastille; troche

13. 片剂 tablet

14. 栓剂 suppository

15. 针剂 injection

16. 引子 conductor

17. 胶囊剂 capsule

18. 糖浆剂、药露 syrup

19. 冲服剂 granule

20. 剂量、一服或一剂 dosage; portion

21. 大肠痈 acute appendictis

22. 大瘕泄 dysentery

23. 大结胸 large accumulation of phlegm-heat in the chest

24. 大头风 / 大头瘟 infection with swollen head

25. 大泻刺 drainage needling

26. 大周天 large circle of vital energy

27. 大眦漏 / 漏睛 dacryocystitis

28. 大肠滑脱 prolapse of rectum

29. 大眦脓漏 dacryocystitis with pyorrhea

30. 大风苛毒 most dangerous pathogenic factors

31. 上脘 shangwan; epigastrium
32. 口疳 aphthae in children
33. 口疳风 / 舌头泡 blisters of the tongue
34. 千日疮 verruca vulgaris
35. 千岁疮 / 流注疮 widespread scrofula
36. 久痔 / 肛漏 recto-anal fistula
37. 广疮 / 杨梅疮 syphilis
38. 丫刺毒 pustule in the web between the first and second metacarpals
39. 丁奚疳 infantile malnutrition due to excessive feeding
40. 吐虫 helminthemesis; vomiting worms

(Guo Yunliang, Wang Xiaolu)

Chapter 16　Influenza

Section 1　Avian Influenza

Avian influenza (Avian flu or Bird flu) has infected poultry stocks in a number of Asian countries of which a small number of people have contracted the avian flu virus from chickens. These events are concerned because it is feared that the avian flu virus could merge with a human flu virus to result in a new, highly infectious, rapidly fatal flu virus. Such a new virus would be transmitted rapidly from person to person with potentially devastating results. To keep the outbreak of avian flu virus under control, many of the Asian countries are culling their poultry stocks to prevent further spread of the virus.

Avian flu is used to describe the influenza viruses that infect birds — for example wild birds such as ducks and domestic birds such as chickens. In fact, birds appear to be a natural reservoir of flu viruses — 15 subtypes of influenza A virus are known to be circulating in bird populations. Many forms of avian flu virus cause only mild symptoms in the birds, or no symptoms at all. However, some of the viruses produce a highly contagious and rapidly fatal disease, leading to severe epidemics. These virulent viruses are known as highly pathogenic avian influenza and particularly concerned. One such avian flu virus is currently infecting chickens in Asian countries.

Until 1997 avian flu was believed to only infect birds; however, in 1997 it was discovered to infect occasionally people in close contact with live birds in markets or farms. This rare ability of avian flu viruses to infect humans throws up a worrying possibility. It is possible that a highly pathogenic avian flu virus could merge with a human flu virus and create a new virus that could be easily passed between humans and was rapidly fatal. If this happens, the result could be the next flu pandemic. When a new, highly infectious form of a flu virus is formed it can rapidly infect a large number of people. The result is an illness that rapidly spreads around the world and may cause widespread loss of life. An example is the Spanish flu pandemic of 1918–1919 which caused an estimated 40 ~ 50 million deaths worldwide.

There are two circumstances in which an avian flu virus could merge with a human flu virus to produce a new, highly infectious flu virus: (1) In humans, if a person who already has flu come into close contact with birds who have highly pathogenic avian flu, there is a tiny chance that the person could become infected with the avian flu virus. If this happens, the person would now be carrying both the human flu virus and the avian flu virus. The two viruses could meet in the person's body and swap genes with each other. If the new virus had the avian flu's genes that made it rapidly fatal and the human flu's genes to allow it to be passed from person to person, a flu pandemic could result. (2) In pigs, pigs are susceptible to both human and bird flu viruses. If a pig became infected with both viruses at the same time, it could act as a mixing vessel, allowing the two viruses to swap genes and produce a new virus.

Up to now, there is no evidence that the people who have been infected with avian flu have passed the disease on to other people. This suggests that a new, highly infectious, flu virus has not been produced yet. However, every time an avian flu virus jumps from a bird to a person, the risk of a new flu virus being produced increases. For this reason, governments are keen to prevent the spread of avian flu among birds and this is why they are culling their poultry stocks. When a bird is infected with avian flu, it sheds the flu virus in its feces, saliva and mucus. Other birds become infected by eating or inhaling the virus. Very rarely, the virus can infect people who are in close contact with infected birds — for example by people inhaling dried feces that have become trampled into dust. People cannot catch avian flu from eating cooked chickens. It is suggested that travelers to Asian countries affected by avian flu should avoid poultry markets and farms to minimize any risk of becoming infected.

What is being done to contain the spread of avian flu? In the countries that have been affected by avian flu, governments have begun to cull affected poultry stocks. They hoped the virus will be contained and removed from circulation by removing the potential for the virus to spread through the countries' chicken populations.

Avian flu appears to have a high mortality rate among people who get it. There have been a number of small outbreaks of avian flu since 1997. For example, Hong Kong 1997 — during this outbreak, 18 people were infected and 6 people died; Hong Kong 2003 — in a family that had visited southern China, there were two cases of the disease and one death; Far East 2004 — up to 10 deaths have been linked to this latest outbreak of the disease in a number of Asian countries.

Wild and farm birds often get a flu virus. Yet they usually are able to carry the virus without getting sick. In 1997, six people in Hong Kong died of a different kind of bird flu virus. It is called the H5N1 virus. The Hong Kong government quickly ordered to kill all farm birds there to control H5N1 spreading to people in Hong Kong. Yet the virus had already spread to other 16 countries of Asia between 2003 and 2006.

Section 2　Artemisinin

In 2011, Prof. Tu Youyou was awarded the prestigious Lasker-DeBakey Clinical Medical Research Award for her role in the discovery and development of artemisinin. On 5 October 2015, she was awarded half of the 2015 Nobel Prize in Physiology or Medicine for discovering artemisinin, a drug that has significantly reduced the mortality rates for patients suffering from Malaria. The other half of the prize was awarded jointly to William C. Campbell and Satoshi Ōmurafor discovering avermectin, the derivatives of which have radically lowered the incidence of River blindness and lymphatic filariasis, as well as showing efficacy against an expanding number of other parasitic diseases.

Artemisinin: Artemisinin and its semi-synthetic derivatives are a group of drugs used against Plasmodium falciparum malaria. It was discovered in 1972 by Tu Youyou, a Chinese scientist, who was awarded half of the 2015 Nobel Prize in Physiology or Medicine for her discovery. Treatments containing an artemisinin derivative (artemisinin-combination therapies, ACTs) are now standard treatment worldwide for P. falciparum malaria. Artemisinin is isolated from the plant Artemisia annua, sweet wormwood, a herb employed in traditional Chinese medicine. A precursor compound can be produced using genetically engineered yeast.

Chemical structure: Artemisinin is a sesquiterpene lactone containing an unusual peroxide bridge.This peroxide is believed to be responsible for the drug's mechanism of action. Few other natural compounds with such a peroxide bridge are known. Artemisinin and its endoperoxide derivatives have been used for the treatment of P. falciparum related infections but low bio-availability, poor pharmacokinetic properties and high cost of the drugs are a major drawback of their use. Use of the drug by itself as a monotherapy is explicitly discouraged by the World Health Organization, as there have been signs that malarial parasites are developing resistance to the drug. Therapies that combine artemisinin or its derivatives with some other antimalarial drug are the preferred treatment for malaria and are both effective and well tolerated in patients. The drug is also increasingly being used in *Plasmodium vivax* malaria.

Etymology: Artemisinin is an antimalarial lactone derived from qinghao (Artemisia annua or sweet wormwood). The medicinal value of this plant has been known to the Chinese for at least 2000 years. In 1596, Li Shizhen recommended tea made from qinghao specifically to treat malaria symptoms in his *Compendium of Materia Medica*. The genus name is derived from the Greek goddess Artemis and, more specifically, may have been named after Queen Artemisia Ⅱ of Caria, a botanist and medical researcher in the fourth century BC.

Discovery: Artemisia annua is a common herb found in many parts of the world, and has been used by Chinese herbalists for more than 2000 years in the treatment of malaria. The earliest record dates back to 200 BC, in the *Fifty-two Prescriptions* unearthed from the

Mawangdui. Its antimalarial application was first described in *Zhouhou Beiji Fang* (*The Handbook of Prescriptions for Emergencies*, Chinese), edited in the middle of the fourth century by Ge Hong; in that book, 43 malaria treatment methods were recorded. Images of the original scientific papers that record the history of the discovery, have been available online since 2006.

In 1967, a plant screening research program, under the name Project 523, was set up by the People's Liberation Army to find an adequate treatment for malaria; the program and early clinical work were ordered of Chairman Mao Zedong at the request of North Vietnamese leaders to provide assistance for their malaria-ridden army. In the course of this research, Tu Youyou discovered artemisinin in the leaves of Artemisia annua (annual wormwood; 1972). The drug is named qinghaosu in Chinese. It was one of many candidates tested as possible treatments for malaria by Chinese scientists, from a list of nearly 5000 traditional Chinese medicines. Tu Youyou also discovered that a low-temperature extraction process could be used to isolate an effective antimalarial substance from the plant. Tu says she was influenced by a traditional Chinese herbal medicine source *The Handbook of Prescriptions for Emergency Treatments* written by Ge Hong saying that this herb should be steeped in cold water. This book contained the useful reference to the herb: A handful of qinghao immersed with two litres of water, wring out the juice and drink it all. Tu's team subsequently isolated a useful extract. The extracted substance, once subject to purification, proved to be useful starting point to obtain purified artemisinin. A 2012 review reported that artemisinin-based therapies were the most effective drugs for treatment of malaria at that time; it was also reported to clear malaria parasites from patients' bodies faster than other drugs. In addition to artemisinin, Project 523 developed a number of products that can be used in combination with artemisinin, including lumefantrine, piperaquine, and pyronaridine.

Results were published in the *Chinese Medical Journal* in 1979. The research was met with skepticism at first, partly because the chemical structure of artemisinin, particularly the peroxide portion, appeared to be too unstable to be a viable drug.

In the late 1990s, Novartis filed a new Chinese patent for a combination treatment with artemether and lumefantrine, providing the first artemisinin-based combination therapies (ACTs)(Coartem) at reduced prices to the World Health Organisation. In 2006, after artemisinin had become the treatment of choice for malaria, the WHO called for an immediate halt to single-drug artemisinin preparations in favor of combinations of artemisinin with another malaria drug, to reduce the risk of parasites developing resistance.

Adverse effects: Artemisinins are generally well tolerated at the doses used to treat malaria. The side effects from the artemisinin class of medications are similar to the symptoms of malaria: nausea, vomiting, anorexia, and dizziness. Mild blood abnormalities have also been noted. A rare but serious adverse effect is allergic reaction. One case of significant liver inflammation has been reported in association with prolonged use of a relatively high-dose of artemisinin for an unclear reason (the patient did not have malaria). The drugs used in combination therapies can contribute to the adverse effects experienced by those undergoing treatment. Adverse effects in patients with acute P. falciparum malaria treated with artemisinin derivatives tend to be higher.

Resistance: Clinical evidence for artemisinin resistance in southeast Asia was first reported in 2008, and was subsequently confirmed by a detailed study from western Cambodia. Resistance in neighbouring Thailand was reported in 2012, and in Northern Cambodia, Vietnam and Eastern Myanmar in 2014. Emerging resistance was reported in Southern Laos, central Myanmar and North-Eastern Cambodia in 2014. The parasite's kelch geneon chromosome 13 appears to be a reliable molecular marker for clinical resistance in southeast Asia. In April 2011, the WHO stated that resistance to the most effective antimalarial drug, artemisinin, could unravel national, Indian malaria control programs, which have achieved significant progress in the last decade. WHO advocates the rational use of antimalarial drugs and acknowledges the crucial role of community health workers in reducing malaria in the region. Two main mechanisms of resistance drive Plasmodium resistance to antimalarial drugs. The first one is an efflux of the drug away from its action site due to mutations in different transporter genes (like pfcrt in chloroquine resistance) or an increased number of the gene copies. The second is a change in the parasite target due to mutations in corresponding genes. Resistance of Plasmodium falciparum to the new artemisinin compounds involves a novel mechanism corresponding to a quiescence phenomenon.

Section 3 Research Article

Neuregulin attenuates cerebral ischemic reperfusion injury via inhibiting apoptosis and up-regulating aquaporin 4

[Abstract] It has been demonstrated that neuregulin 1β (NRG1β) plays an active neuroprotective role in cerebral ischemic injury; however, its defined mechanisms and the perfect treatment window in rats following middle cerebral artery occlusion and reperfusion (MCAO/R) are still elusive. Therefore, we established the animal model of MCAO/R to evaluate neurological function score, infarction volume, cell apoptosis and the expression of aquaporin 4 (AQP4) in brain tissue. As a result, neurological function scores were decreased, and a small infarction focus could be detected in ischemic cortex in the control group at ischemic 0.5 h and reperfusion 24 h, along with the increased number of positive apoptosis cells and the elevated expression of AQP4 mRNA and protein. Accompanied with the ischemia time, neurological scores and infarction sizes obviously increased in the control group during ischemic 1.0 ~ 2.0 h. A large number of positive apoptotic cells were widespread in the cortex in the ischemic ipsilateral. Simultaneously, the expression of AQP4 mRNA and its protein increased to some extent. NRG1β treatment significantly improved the symptoms and signs of neurological function, decreased the infarction volume, and elevated the expression levels of AQP4 mRNA and its protein compared with that in the control group. The therapeutic effect of NRG1β was notable, especially in the ischemic 1.0 h subsection. These results demonstrate that NRG1β might play a neuroprotective effect on cerebral ischemic reperfusion by inhibiting mitochondrial apoptosis pathway and regulating the activation of AQP4. The perfect treatment window is at ischemic 1 h after MCAO.

Keywords: neuregulin; cerebral ischemia-reperfusion injury; apoptosis; AQP4; treatment time window; double fluorescence labeling; RT-PCR

It is well known that ischemia induces apoptosis or irreversible death of neurocyte, which in turns seriously influences the prognosis of cerebral ischemic damage. Thrombolytic therapy is considered as an efficient treatment method to acute ischemic stroke; however, its clinical application is largely restricted due to the limited treatment window and the urgent needs for high technological equipment conditions[1]. Other therapeutic methods only aim at some special target points and play an insignificant role in cerebral insult. Neuregulin 1β (NRG1β) is a member of growth factor family known to be involved in the survival and function of neuronal cells. NRG1β and its receptors, erbB receptors, are induced in neuronal cells following traumatic brain injury[2], and also in the peri-infarct (penumbral) region following permanent cerebral artery occlusion (MCAO) in rat[3-4]. It has been demonstrated that NRG1β displayed anti-inflammatory properties in the central nervous system both in vivo and in vitro, and might be involved in neuroprotection following ischemic stroke[5]. But the defined mechanism is still elusive. Here we investigate the neuroprotective mechanism of NRG1β in rats after MCAO/R and determine the best therapeutic time window for cerebral ischemic reperfusion insult.

Adult healthy male Wistar rats weighing 250 ~ 270 g, were granted by the Experiment Animal Center of Qingdao Drug Inspection Institute [SCXK(LU)20030010]. All surgical procedures were performed by sterile/aseptic techniques in accordance with institutional guidelines. The animal models of middle cerebral artery occlusion/reperfusion(MCAO/R) were performed with an intraluminal monofilament suture method as previously described[6]. Briefly, after animals were anesthetized intraperitoneally by 10% chloral hydrate (300 mg/kg), the left common carotid artery (CCA) was exposed through a midline incision and was carefully dissected free from surrounding nerves and fascia. The occipital artery branches of the external carotid artery (ECA) were then isolated, and the occipital artery and superior thyroid artery branches of the ECA were coagulated. The ECA was dissected further distally. The internal carotid artery (ICA) was isolated and carefully separated from the adjacent vagus nerve, and the pterygopalatine artery was ligated close to its origin with a 6.0 silk suture. Then, a 40 mm 3.0 surgical monofilament nylon suture (Harvard Apparatus, Holliston, Massachusetts) was coated with poly-L-Lysine with its tip rounded by heating near a flame. The filament was inserted from the ECA into the ICA and then into the circle of Willis to occlude the origin of the left middle cerebral artery (MCA). The suture was inserted 18 ~ 20 mm from the bifurcation of the CCA to occlude the MCA. Rats in the treatment group were immediately administrated 1.5% NRG1β (purity > 97%, R&D Systems, Inc, Catalog number: 396-HB) at a single dosage of 0.3 μg/kg from left external-internal carotid artery with a microsyringe at intervals 0 h, 0.5 h, 1.0 h, 1.5 h and 2.0 h after MCAO, while those in the control group were given the same dose of 0.1 mol/L phosphatase buffer solution (PBS)(containing 1.5% bovine serum albumin) at the same time-point. After the administration, the nylon suture was withdrawn and the ischemic brain tissue was reperfused for 24 h before sacrifice. Core body temperature was monitored with a rectal probe and maintained at 37 ℃ using a Homeothermic Blanket Control Unit (Wuhan Apparatus, China) during the surgery operation. Brain tissue were removed to prepare for paraffin sections, triphenyl tetrazolium chloride (TTC) stain or frozen in liquid nitrogen at −80 ℃ for RT-PCR.

Behavioral assessment was performed and scored at 24 h after ischemia and reperfusion according to the standard of Longa[7]. Rats in the control group present many symptoms and signs of neurological function, such as Horner sign, paralysis and weakness of the right limb, flexion, adduction and failure to extend right forelimb on lifting the whole body by tail, as well as circling to the contralateral on autonomic activities and even falling toward the right. After the treatment of NRG1β, the neurological symptoms were ameliorated and the scores were significantly decreased. There were statistical differences as compared to that in the vehicle control group ($P < 0.05$). Although the improvement of neurological score could be observed in every time-point in the treatment group, the outcome in the ischemic 1.0 h group was most notable (Table 16-1, $P < 0.01$).

Table 16-1   The comparison of neurological functional scores, infarction volume in different groups ($\bar{x} \pm s$, $n = 5$)

Group	n	Neurological scores		infarction volume/%	
		Control	Treatment	Control	Treatment
Ischemic 0 h	5	0.00 ± 0.00	0.00 ± 0.00	0.00 ± 0.00	0.00 ± 0.00
Ischemic 0.5 h	5	2.07 ± 0.51	1.43 ± 0.45	65.63 ± 5.1	61.50 ± 4.9
Ischemic 1.0 h	5	2.91 ± 0.44	1.72 ± 0.47*	72.76 ± 4.2	63.55 ± 4.1*
Ischemic 1.5 h	5	3.24 ± 0.49	2.44 ± 0.42	75.39 ± 4.8	70.82 ± 4.7
Ischemic 2.0 h	5	3.61 ± 0.39	3.02 ± 0.50	80.21 ± 4.2	74.91 ± 4.7

*$P < 0.01$ vs the control group.

To determine the infarction volume, five rats in each group were decapitated at given time after MCAO/R. The brain tissue was removed and successively sliced into 2.0 mm-thick coronal sections. The total of five brain slices were incubated in a 2% TTC solution for 10 min at 37 ℃ and then transferred into a 4% formaldehyde solution for fixation. The normal brain tissue appeared uniform red while the infarction region showed white. The infarction volumes were calculated in a blinded manner with Adobe PhotoShop CS analysis system. The data were expressed as the percentage of the cerebral infarction volume/the ipsilateral semisphere volume (%) at the coronal section of optic chiasma. As a result, the white infarction focus began to show in the cortex at ischemic 0.5 h in the vehicle control group. With the duration of ischemia, the infarction areas gradually spread to the adjacent striatum. The volume of infarction in the control group was about 60% ~ 80% of ipsilateral hemisphere (Table 16-1, Figure 16-1). The administration of NRG1β at various time-points decreased the infarction size to some extent as compared to that in the control group ($P < 0.05$), especially at ischemic 1.0 h ($P < 0.01$).

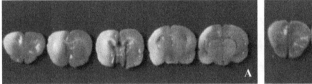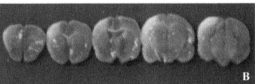

Figure 16-1　Four views were detected randomly in the cortex (green) and the striatum (yellow) of the confined areas from four serial slices in each rat

By TTC staining, the brain tissues appear red, and there is no infarction focus in the sham-operation group. With the duration of ischemia, the infarction sizes gradually increase in the control group. The administration of NRG1β significantly decrease the infarction volume compared with that in the control group.

Paraffin sections were prepared to detect cell apoptosis. In brief, brain samples were removed and post-fixed by 4% formaldehyde for 2 h, immersed in double distilled water for 4 h, dehydrated in gradient ethanol, transparented in dimethylbenzene and embedded in paraffin. Coronal sections of 6 μm thickness were cut successively with a microtome (Leica-RM2015, Shanghai Leica Instruments Corporation, China) from the posterior of the optic chiasma, adhered to the slides prepared with poly-L-Lysine, and finally stored at 4 ℃.

Terminal deoxynucleotidyl transference-mediated biotinylated deoxyuridine triphosphate nick end labeling technique (TUNEL) staining was performed according to protocol of DendEnd Fluorometric TUNEL Detection System (Santa Cruz Company). Some slides added DNase I at a dose of 1 μg/mL were regarded as positive control sample, and those treated without TdT as the negative ones. Under a fluorescent microscope (wavelength 488 nm), apoptotic cells were specifically labeled by fluorescein isothiocyanate (FITC) and appeared yellow-green fluorescence. Under a 400-fold fluorescent microscope, four views were detected randomly in the cortex of the confined areas from four serial slices in each rat (Figure 16-1). The absorbance (A) value of each view was determined in a blinded manner with LEICA QWin image processing and analysis system (Leica Company).

Few apoptotic cells could be observed in the ischemic 0 h group. Ischemia and reperfusion induced cell apoptosis. With the duration of ischemia, the number of apoptotic cells increased gradually in the control group. The color of these apoptotic cells deepened and the A value elevated accordingly. These positive signals were primarily distributed in the cortex and the striatum. After the administration of NRG1β, the quantity of positive cells decreased in the cortex, especially in the ischemic 1.0 h group. Compared with the vehicle control group, there were significant differences during ischemic 1.0 h to 2.0 h ($P < 0.05$, Table 16-2, Figure 16-2).

Table 16-2   The A value of XIAP and apoptosis in brain tissue in each group

Ischemic time	n	XIAP		Apoptotic cells	
		Control group	Treatment group	Control group	Treatment group
Ischemic 0 h	5	2.65 ± 0.21	2.76 ± 0.13	2.78 ± 0.15	2.54 ± 0.24
Ischemic 0.5 h	5	$12.68 \pm 1.76^{\Delta}$	$15.98 \pm 1.78^{\Delta*}$	$12.45 \pm 2.10^{\Delta}$	$10.65 \pm 2.47^{\Delta}$
Ischemic 1.0 h	5	$26.21 \pm 1.33^{\Delta}$	$30.56 \pm 4.50^{\Delta*}$	$16.34 \pm 2.03^{\Delta}$	$12.15 \pm 2.00^{\Delta*}$
Ischemic 1.5 h	5	$26.50 \pm 2.09^{\Delta}$	$30.75 \pm 4.31^{\Delta*}$	$18.62 \pm 2.12^{\Delta}$	$13.26 \pm 2.20^{\Delta*}$
Ischemic 2.0 h	5	$24.02 \pm 2.35^{\Delta}$	$28.54 \pm 3.76^{\Delta*}$	$20.46 \pm 2.38^{\Delta}$	$15.14 \pm 2.53^{\Delta*}$

$^{\Delta}P < 0.05$ *vs* the ischemic 0 h group; $^{*}P < 0.05$ *vs* the control group of the same time.

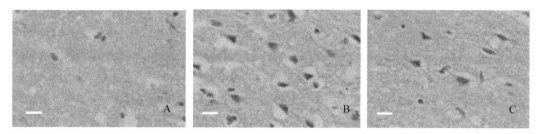

Figure 16-2   Positive apoptisis cells in different groups

Only a small quantity of positive apoptotic cells can be detected in cortex in the sham-operation group (A). The number of positive apoptotic cells obviously increases in the control group after MCAO/R (B). NRG1β reduces the amount of positive apoptotic cells (C). Scale bar is 30 μm.

To verify the defined effects of NRG1β on apoptosis pathway, we detected the expression of X-linked inhibitor of apoptosis protein (XIAP) in brain tissue after MCAO/R using immunofluorescent labeling analysis. XIAP monoclonal antibody, strept actividin-biotin peroxidase complex-fluorescein isothiocyanate (SABC-FITC) kit were purchased from Santa Cruz Company. All procedures were strictly performed in accordance with the manufacture directions. Under a 400-fold fluorescence microscope, a very small amount of XIAP positive cells were detected in the ischemia 0 h group, with light-green fluorescence, irregular shape and one or two short processes, scattered in brain tissue. The majority of positive signals distributed in cytoplasm around nuclear membrane, but none in dendrites and axons (Table 16-2). Ischemia induced the presence of XIAP protein. Accompanied with the ischemia, the number of XIAP-positive cells gradually increased in the control group and mainly located in cortex and striatum in ischemic penumbra, especially in cortex. But no positive cell can be seen in ischemic core area. After NRG1β treatment, XIAP positive cells significantly increased and the green fluorescence enhanced accordingly compared with that in the control group ($P < 0.01$). XIAP, an endogenous inhibitor of apoptosis proteins, is regarded as the most potent inhibitor of caspases[8]. Cumulative evidence reveal that XIAP does not only intervene the development of mitochondrial caspase pathway, but regulate the secondary activity of transcription factors associated with neuronal survival[3]. Our results show that at the early stage of cerebral ischemia (< 24 h), the number of apoptotic cells, along with XIAP protein expression, gradually increase in penumbra regions, but there is less correlation between them. This offers a potent evidence that a variety of factors are associated with the development of apoptosis. XIAP is only a checkpoint of caspase-3 activation in apoptosis pathway, not a key or rate-limiting enzyme. NRG1β inhibits the mitochondrial apoptosis pathway via up-regulating the activity of XIAP.

Then, paraffin sections were prepared as previously described to examine the presence of AQP4 protein in brain tissue after MCAO/R. AQP4 monoclonal antibody, SABC-FITC kit and water-solubility mounting reagent were granted by Santa Cruz Company. All immunofluorescent procedures were performed in accordance to the manufacturer's instruction. Four serial sections were observed under a 400-fold fluorescent microscope with laser excitation of 488 nm and reception of 510 ~ 530 nm wavelength. Four chosen views were detected randomly in the cortex and the striatum of the confined brain regions. And the measurement of A values have been described above. We found that AQP4 positive cells appeared light green fluorescence and irregular shape both in the sham-operation group and in the ischemia 0 h group. The distribution of positive signals was present both in cytoplasm and process. With the duration of ischemia, AQP4 positive cells gradually increased in the control group. The increased expression of AQP4 could also been seen after NRG1β treatment and its color has noticeably enhanced, especially at ischemic 1.0 h (Table 16-3). There exists statistical difference in contrast to the control group of the same time ($P < 0.05$). Using fluorescent double labeling, we found that some AQP4 positive cells also showed glial fibrillary acidic protein (GFAP)-immunoreaction both in the control group and in the treatment group after MCAO/R. GFAP is a direct evidence of the proliferation and function activation of astrocyte, which reflects an adaptive change on ischemic damage to neurons. These colocalization signals of AQP4 and GFAP strongly expressed in the surface of astrocyte around vessel and in the glial membrane formated by the endfoot of astrocyte closely enveloping capillary wall. However, not all of the AQP4-positive cells showed GFAP immune response, suggesting that AQP4 protein reside in the astrocytes, as well as other cell population (need to further elucidation).

Table 16-3　The A value comparison of the AQP4 protein in different regions($\bar{x} \pm s$, $n = 5$)

Group	n	cortex		striatum	
		control	treatment	control	treatment
Ischemic 0 h	5	4.36 ± 2.10	5.98 ± 2.10	4.14 ± 2.09	6.29 ± 2.12
Ischemic 0.5 h	5	6.55 ± 2.19	$14.45 \pm 2.11^{\Delta}$	5.87 ± 2.11	$12.66 \pm 2.10^{\Delta*}$
Ischemic 1.0 h	5	$16.49 \pm 2.23^{\Delta}$	$22.64 \pm 2.08^{\Delta*}$	$9.97 \pm 2.13^{\Delta*}$	$17.24 \pm 2.13^{\Delta*}$
Ischemic 1.5 h	5	$22.68 \pm 2.21^{\Delta}$	$29.73 \pm 2.03^{\Delta*}$	$16.47 \pm 2.12^{\Delta}$	$24.99 \pm 3.13^{\Delta*}$
Ischemic 2.0 h	5	$27.36 \pm 2.48^{\Delta}$	$36.87 \pm 1.76^{\Delta*}$	$24.25 \pm 2.07^{\Delta}$	$30.76 \pm 3.12^{\Delta*}$

$^{\Delta}P < 0.05$ vs the ischemic 0 h group; $^{*}P < 0.05$ vs the control group of the same time.

We also determined the expression level of AQP4 mRNA by RT-PCR. Total RNA was extracted from the tissue according to the manufacturer's suggestion. AQP4 primers were synthesized by Shanghai Biochemical Company. And the primer sequences were as follows: AQP4 primers: sense primer, 5'-TTGGACCATCATAGGCGC-3'; antisense primer, 5'-GCATGTTGATCGACATTGACC-3', expected product length 214 bp. As an internal parameter, GAPDH primers were synthesized: sense primer, 5'-TCCCATTCTTCCACCTTTGATG-3'; antisense primer, 5'-GTCCACCACCCTGTTGCTGTA-3', expected product length 111 bp. RT-PCR was then performed using a Thermo Hybaid thermal cycler. The PCR products were electrophoresed in 2.0% agarose gels buffered with TBE for 40 min, and visualized under ultraviolet illumination by ethidium bromide (EB) staining. The A value of each DNA band intensity in the same gel was captured and determined through Scion analysis software. In order to reduce the experiment error, the procedure of RT-PCR was performed twice in each rat. As a result, ten A values were obtained in each group and analyzed by SPSS 11.0. The relative A value of AQP4 mRNA were expressed as: the relative A value of AQP4 mRNA = the A value of AQP4 mRNA / the A value of GAPDH mRNA. As a result, AQP4 mRNA immunoreactive bands could be seen in left cerebral hemisphere in the sham operation group, with a low A value. The expression of AQP4 mRNA was ignited and quickly elevated at the early stage of ischemia (< 1.0 h), peaking at ischemic 1.0 h in the ischemic brain tissue in the control group. Along with the ischemic time prolonging (> 1.5 h), the relative A value gradually stabilized and kept at a higher level. Obvious differences could be shown among ischemic 1.0 h to 2.0 h groups compared with that in the ischemia 0 h group. NRG1β treatment increased the level of AQP4 mRNA expression, and there were statistical differences in contrast to the control group of the same time ($P < 0.01$).

With the discovery of biochemical and histological hallmarks of apoptosis, it has become increasingly evident that the intrinsic cellular suicide program not only is required for the development of normal central nervous system but also, if executed inappropriately, contributes to the pathology of stroke and neurodegenerative disorders[9-11].Two major apoptotic pathways have been identified: one activated via death receptor activation (death receptor pathway) and the other by stress inducing stimuli (the mitochondrial pathway). Apoptotic and antiapoptotic signaling pathways are activated after cerebral ischemia, and it is generally accepted that a shift in the balance between pro- and anti-apoptotic protein factors toward the expression of proteins that promote cell death may be one mechanism underlying apoptotic cell death[12]. To avoid disease and untimely cell death, apoptotic mechanisms must be closely regulated. XIAP has also recently been shown to bind and inhibit active caspase-9 and caspase-3 within the apoptosome complex[13]. Our study has shown that ischemia induced cell apoptosis and the expression of XIAP. As ischemic time went by, the number of apoptotic cells in cortex increased gradually in the control group, as well as the expression level of XIAP. NRG1β treatment significantly decreased the infarct size and number of apoptotic cells after MCAO/R, elevated the presence of XIAP protein, especially at ischemia 1.0 h, suggesting that NRG1β might inhibit the development of mitochondrial apoptosis pathway through up-regulating the activity of XIAP, and play a neuroprotective role against cerebral ischemia-reperfusion injury.

AQP4 was closely related to the occurrence of cerebral edema[14-15]. Overexpression of AQP4 after ischemia increased the membrane permeability of water and activated the transport function, resulting in the occurrence of cerebral edema. Thus the expression intensity of AQP4 was considered as a new indicator of brain edema[16]. Frydenlund et al.[17] insisted that although AQP4 was located in the astrocyte membrane around vascular and participated in the formation and dissipation process of brain edema, its expression patterns significantly varied in different brain regions. In the core area of striatum after ischemia-reperfusion 24 h, perivascular AQP4 level significantly decreased, and hence had no recovery tendency at all. In the ischemic core of cortex, however, the presence of AQP4 obviously reduced at 24 h and gradually recovered at 72 h after ischemic reperfusion to some extent. Its expression in cortex penumbra did not significantly reduce, but slightly increased.These show that AQP4 could regulate the fluid exchange between brain tissue and blood in the formation and dissipation of brain edema at different stages of cerebral ischemia-reperfusion. Suzuki et al.[18] argued that AQP1 and AQP4 co-expressed strongly in end-feet of astrocyte, and mainly located in the edema tissue, some of which wrapped around the capillaries in brain, thus played a crucial role in the formation and dissipation of brain edema. Our study also showed that the expression level of AQP4 gradually increased and had obvious regional selectivity in central nervous system accompanied with the extension of ischemic time. The majority of positive cells closely wrapped around capillary wall. This conforms to the result of Taniguchi[6,19], but slightly differs from Frydenlund's[17]. Besides, the colocalization signals of AQP4 and GFAP strongly expressed in the cortex and the striatum after MCAO/R. Thus we suspected that AQP4 mediating the transportation of water across cell membrane might be the key step of fluid removal induced by the secondary ischemic brain edema, and play various roles at different stages of the formation and dissipation in brain edema. In the early stage of cerebral infarction (< 2 h), the increased expression of AQP4 might take a self-protective effect so as to maintain the fluid balance of exterior and interior cells. Along with the aggravation of ischemia injury (> 24 h), the AQP4 level further elevates and might facilitate the formation and development of brain edema, that is to say, it plays a two-way regulatory role. This results are coincidence with Papadopoulos's[20], but disagree with Da T's[21]. The main reason resulting in the experiment differences is probably due to the chosen surgery procedure, the observed timepoints and injury areas.

NRG1β, as a neuroprotective reagent, was considered relating to neuronal survival and function, and played neuroprotective role through a variety of mechanisms, such as the regulation of two anti-apoptotic molecules Bcl-2 and Bcl-w expression[3], the inhibition of monocyte infiltration and astrocytes activation[22], the suppression of monocyte adhesion molecules and chemotaxis factor production on vessel endothelium, the induction of macrophage apoptosis or the promotion of monophosphoinositide-3-kinase/Akt signal transduction pathways in cell survival[5]. Our results show that there is no coexpression of AQP4 and GFAP in the sham-operation group and in the ischemic 0 h group. But the colocalization signals of the two protein expressed in the control group during ischemic 0.5 ～ 2.0 h after MCAO, and NRG1β treatment increased the expression level. It infers that the neuroprotective effect of NRG-1β might be related to the activation of AQP4 and GFAP. Because AQP4 protein may reside in the astrocytes, as well as other cell population, we can assume that NRG1β aims different target cells (need to further elucidation).

In addition, the present study has confirmed that the application of NRG1β at different ischemia (0.5 ～ 2.0 h) and reperfusion (24 h) timepoints could promote the recovery of neurological function, attenuate infarction volumn and cerebral edema, particularly in the ischemic 1.0 h group. Therefore, the most perfect therapeutic time of NRG1β might be at 1.0 h after ischemic stroke in rats. But before extensive clinical application, it still needs to be explored in nonhuman primates.

Acknowledgement

This work was supported by research grant Natural Science Fund of Shandong Province (Y2004C04, Z2007D05).

Reference

[1]　Bourekas E C, Slivka A P, Shah R, et al. Intraarterial thrombolyic therapy with 3 hours of the onset of stroke. Neurosurg, 2004, 54(1): 39-44.

[2]　Tokita Y, Keino H, Matsui F, et al. Regulation of neuregulin expression in the injured rat brain and cultured astrocytes. J Neurosci, 2001, 21(4): 1257-1264.

[3]　Xu Z, Ford B D. Upregulation of erbB receptors in rat brain after middle cerebral arterial occlusion. Neuroscience Letters, 2005, 375(3): 181-186.

[4]　Xu Z, Ford G D, Croslan D R, et al. Neuroprotection by neuregulin-1 following focal stroke is associated with the attenuation of ischemia-induced pro-inflammatory and stress gene expression. Neurobiol Dis, 2005, 19(3): 461-470.

[5]　Li Y, Xu Z, Ford G D, et al. Neuroprotection by neuregulin-1 in a rat model of permanent focal cerebral ischemia. Brain Res, 2007, 1184: 277-283.

[6]　Taniguchi M, Yamashita T, Kumura E, et al. Induction of aquaporin-4 water channel mRNA after focal cerebral ischemia in rat. Brain Res Mol Brain Res, 2000, 78(1-2): 131-137.

[7]　Longa E Z, Weinstein P R, Carlson S, et al. Reversible middle cerebral artery occlusion without craniectomy in rats. Stroke, 1989, 20(1): 84-91.

[8]　Zhu C, Wang X, Xu F, et al. The influence of age on apoptotic and other mechanisms of cell death after cerebral hypoxia-ischemia. Cell Death Differ, 2005, 12(2): 162-176.

[9]　Saito A, Hayashi T, Okuno S, et al. Interaction between XIAP and Smac/DIABLO in the mouse brain after transient focal cerebral ischemia. J Cereb Blood Flow Metab, 2003, 23(9): 1010-1019.

[10]　Trapp T, Korhonen L, Besselmann M, et al. Transgenic mice overexpressing XIAP in neurons show better outcome after transient cerebral ischemia. Mol Cell Neurosci, 2003, 23(2): 302-313.

[11]　Wang X, Zhu C, Wang X, et al. X-linked inhibitor of apoptosis (XIAP) protein protects against caspase activation and tissue loss after neonatal hypoxia-ischemia. Neurobiol Dis, 2004, 16(1): 179-189.

[12]　Saito A, Hayashi T, Okuno S, et al. Oxidative stress is associated with XIAP and Smac/DIABLO signaling pathways in mouse brains after transient focal cerebral ischemia. Stroke, 2004, 35(6): 1443-1448.

[13]　Srinivasula S M, Gupta S, Datta P, et al. Inhibitor of apoptosis proteins are substrates for the mitochondrial serine protease Omi/HtrA2. J Biol Chem, 2003, 278(34): 31469-31472.

[14]　Badaut J, Lasbennes F, Magistretti P J, et al. Aquaporins in brain: distribution, physiology, and pathophysiology. J Cereb Blood Flow Metab, 2002, 22(3): 367-378.

[15]　Venero J L, Vizuete M L, Machado A, et al. Aquaporins in the central nervous system. Prog Neurobiol, 2001, 63(3): 321-336.

[16]　Papadopoulos M C, Krishna S, Verkman A S. Aquaporin water channels and brain edema. Mt Sinai J Med, 2002, 69(2): 242-248.

[17]　Frydenlund D S, Bhardwaj A, Otsuka T, et al. Temporary loss of perivascular aquaporin-4 in neocortex after transient middle cerebral artery occlusion in mice. Proc Natl Acad Sci USA, 2006, 103(36): 13532-13536.

[18]　Suzuki R, Okuda M, Asai J, et al. Astrocytes co-express aquaporin-1, -4, and vascular endothelial growth factor in brain edema tissue associated with brain contusion. Acta Neurochir Suppl, 2006, 96: 398-401.

[19]　Chen C H, Xue R, Zhang J, et al. Effect of osmotherapy with hypertonic saline on regional cerebral edema following experimental stroke: a study utilizing magnetic resonance imaging. Neurocrit Care, 2007, 7(1): 92-100.

[20]　Papadopoulos M C, Manley G T, Krishna S, et al. Aquaporin-4 facilitates reabsorption of excess fluid in vasogenic brain edema. FASEB J, 2004, 18(11): 1291-1293.

[21]　Da T, Verkman A S. Aquaporin-4 gene disruption in mice protects against impaired retinal function and cell death after ischemia. Invest Ophthalmol Vis Sci, 2004, 45(12): 4477-4483.

[22]　Liu D, Smith C L, Barone F C, et al. Astrocytic demise precedes delayed neuronal death in focal ischemic rat brain. Brain Res Mol Brain Res, 1999, 68(1): 29-41.

Section 4　Words of TCM

1. 实热证 sthenic heat syndrome
2. 虚寒证 asthenic cold syndrome
3. 阳盛则热 excessive yang causing heat
4. 阴极生寒 extreme yin resulting in cold
5. 阴盛则寒 excessive yin leading to cold
6. 寒则气收 cold giving rise to qi contraction
7. 阳虚则寒 yang deficiency causing cold
8. 阴虚则热 yin deficiency causing heat
9. 阴中求阳 seeking yang within yin
10. 补其不足 curing the deficiency
11. 正虚邪实 asthenia of healthy qi and sthenia of pathogenic factors

12. 痰饮咳嗽 cough due to fluid retention; retention of phlegm

13. 实热蕴结 accumulation of sthenia-heat

14. 痰湿壅肺 accumulation of phlegm-dampness in the lung

15. 卫气不固 wei-energy fail to protect the body

16. 祛风散寒 dispelling wind and dispersing cold

17. 储血藏经 storing blood and essence

18. 天行瘟疫 pestilence

19. 肌肉消瘦 emaciation

20. 气滞腰痛 lumbago due to qi stagnation

21. 引经报使 guiding action

22. 伤寒 exogenous febrile disease (EFD)

23. 温病 seasonal febrile disease (SFD)

24. 夫精者，生之本也 essence is the basis of life; essence is essential to life

25. 肝主身之筋膜 the liver controls the tendons

26. 冲任不固 unconsolidation of thorough fare vessel (TV) and conception vessel (CV)

27. 月经来潮 menstrual onset

28. 宫寒不孕 hysterofrigic sterility; sterility caused by coldness of the uterus

29. 血枯经闭 amenorrhea due to blood exhaustion

30. 气虚滑胎 habitual abortion due to qi asthenia

31. 心肝血虚 asthenia / deficiency of heart and liver blood

32. 肝肾精血不足 insufficiency of liver and kidney essence and blood

33. 滋肾养肝 nourishing the kidney and liver

34. 滋阴降火 nourishing yin to lower/reduce fire

35. 滋水涵木 enriching water to nourish wood

36. 瘀血致泻 disease caused by blood stasis

37. 发热恶寒 fever and aversion to cold

38. 余热未尽 incomplete abatement of heat

39. 标本兼治 treatment focusing on relieving both secondary and primary symptoms

40. 辨证论治 treatment based on syndrome differentiation

41. 急则治其标 relieving the secondary symptoms first in treating acute disease

42. 缓则治其本 relieving the primary symptoms in treating chronic disease

(Li Yizhao, Ni Tongshang)

Chapter 17　Stroke

Section 1　Heart Attack or Stroke

Myocardial infarction (MI), commonly known as a heart attack or stroke, occurs when blood flow decreases or stops to a part of the heart, causing damage to the heart muscle. The most common symptom is chest pain or discomfort which may travel into the shoulder, arm, back, neck, or jaw. Often it occurs in the center or left side of the chest and lasts for more than a few minutes. The discomfort may occasionally feel like heartburn. Other symptoms may include shortness of breath, nausea, feeling faint, a cold sweat, or feeling tired. About 30% of people have atypical symptoms. Women more often have atypical symptoms than men. Among those over 75 years old, about 5% have had an MI with little or no history of symptoms. An MI may cause heart failure, an irregular heartbeat, cardiogenic shock, or cardiac arrest.

American researchers have developed a simple test to measure levels of a protein in the blood, which can tell if a person with heart disease is likely to suffer a heart attack. People with high levels of the protein are at high risk of heart attack, heart failure or stroke.

The researchers studied almost 1000 patients with heart disease for almost 4 years. During that time, more than 250 of the patients suffered a heart attack, heart failure or stroke and some of them died. They tested the heart disease patients for a protein called NTproBNP, which indicated that patients with the highest levels were nearly eight times more likely than those with the lowest levels to have a heart attack, heart failure or stroke. They found that patients with high levels of the protein were still more likely to have a health problem involving the heart. The presence of high levels of the protein in the blood shows the heart muscle is under pressure in some way. The study involved mostly men, so they could not say for sure that the results are true for women.

They also say the patients with the highest levels of NTproBNP were older and had other problems, like diabetes or high blood pressure. Such patients were more likely to be already taking medicine for their heart. But other researchers say more studies are needed to confirm if knowing the protein levels of a heart patient should affect that person's treatment. They also would like to know if more aggressive treatment would be able to reduce the patient's chance of suffering a heart attack or stroke.

Sometimes, small changes to your lifestyle can really cut your odds of having a heart attack or stroke. Try this step-by-step approach as following:

Exercise a little each day: Moderate physical activity lowers your chances of a heart attack. Shoot for 30 minutes of exercise that gets your heart pumping at least 5 days a week. Brisk walking or swimming are some good choices. On the other 2 days, do strength training, like lifting weights.

Set a reasonable weight: If you're overweight or obese, you don't have to get thin to reduce your risk for a heart attack or stroke. If you lose 5% ~ 10% of your weight, you'll improve your cholesterol numbers and lower your blood pressure and blood sugar levels.

Take your heart medicine: Many people don't take their medications the way their doctor told them to. Figure out what keeps you from taking your medicine — it could be side effects, cost, or forgetfulness — and ask your doctor for help.

Eat well: If you stick to a healthy diet, you could lower your odds of getting heart disease. Fill your plate with different kinds of fruits, veggies, whole grains, fish, lean meats, etc.. Stay away from processed or prepared foods that often are high in salt and added sugar.

Drink some alcohol but not too much: If you drink, any type of alcohol helps your heart, but don't drink too much. Too much raises your risk of high blood pressure, heart attack, and stroke.

Eat a little chocolate: Go for dark chocolate, and make sure the ingredients are at least 70% cacao. It's filled with nutrients that help protect your ticker.

Don't smoke: Smoking dramatically raises your risk of heart attacks and strokes. Talk to your doctor about how to quit. You'll also be doing your friends and family a favor, since secondhand smoke can also lead to heart disease.

Pay attention to your symptoms: See your doctor if you feel anything unusual, like shortness of breath, changes in your heart rhythm, or extreme tiredness. Also, watch for pain in your jaw or back, nausea or vomiting, sweating, or flu-like symptoms.

Section 2　Ligustrazine

Chuanxiong is a frequently used Chinese herb, commonly called ligusticum or cnidium. The latter name is the term most often used in the ITM literature, adopted from the common name offered by Oriental Healing Arts Institute (OHAI) in publications 30 years ago. The herb has been obtained from Ligusticum chuanxiong (Ligusticum wallichii) in China and from Cnidium officinale in Japan; the OHAI literature was heavily influenced by Japanese herb scholars. Recent evaluation of the genetic material of these two source materials has led to the suggestion that they are, in fact, the same plant, and that Cnidium officinale should be renamed as Ligusticum chuanxiong.

There are several active constituents in chuanxiong, but one of the most interesting is the alkaloid ligustrazine, which has the chemical name tetramethylpyrazine (because it is a pyrazine ring with four symmetrically placed methyl groups); it is sometimes simply called TMP. Isolated alkaloids from chuanxiong, and purified synthetic ligustrazine, have been used in China as medicinal agents for 30 years. The initial applications were based on traditional uses of the crude herb in decoctions and pills: for vitalizing blood circulation in the treatment of cardiovascular diseases and for treatment of headache and vertigo.

Applications: The applications of ligustrazine in China are many, and at first may appear quite diverse. However, upon examining the various applications, one can appreciate ligustrazine as providing a protective effect. The following are brief reviews of a few of the uses of ligustrazine.

Renal failure and dialysis: Ligustrazine has been used to slow or halt the progress of renal failure in Chinese patients. Experimental studies have been conducted to demonstrate this effect in laboratory animals. One of the proposed mechanisms is the superoxide scavenging effect, one type of antioxidant action. Salvia has also been used to protect against renal failure. Ligustrazine with salvia and tang-kuei have been used to aid patients undergoing renal dialysis. TMP is also used in conjunction with prednisone for patients with primary nephritic syndrome, which is said to function better than prednisone therapy alone. In the treatment of infants, ligustrazine was used to protect against the renal toxicity of gentamycin. Ferulic acid, possibly the primary active component of tang-kuei and one of the active components of chuanxiong, has shown benefits for treatment of patients with diabetic nephropathy.

Lung diseases with fibrosis: Ligustrazine is known to be a pulmonary vasodilator, but an area of particular interest is its action to protect against pulmonary fibrosis. Salvia and an active fraction of salvia have also been used for protection against pulmonary fibrosis, alone or with ligustrazine.

Neuroprotection for stroke: Chinese physicians have used chuanxiong and ligustrazine for treatment of stroke patients. Ligustrazine has been shown to have protective effects for the neurons, possibly based on anti-inflammatory activity. In clinical applications, ligustrazine in high dosage (480 mg/d) was found to lower fibrinogen and improve blood circulation in patients who suffered a stroke. Salvia is also known to confer neuroprotective effects in case of stroke. Ferulic acid or its sodium salt (sodium ferulate) is used in Chinese medicine to treat stroke patients; in laboratory studies, it was shown to limit damage and help reactivation of impaired nerve cells.

United Nations member states have agreed to reduce premature cardiovascular disease (CVD) mortality 25% by 2025. However, CVD is the major cause of death worldwide which is almost a third of all deaths globally in 2013. In low and middle income countries (LMIC), the situation is not optimistic similarly. The greatest burden of CVD is approximately 80% of cardiovascular deaths occurring in LMIC. The most of CVD deaths were from coronary heart disease (CHD). Unstable angina (UA) is a common manifestation of this disease. The three principal presentations of UA include rest angina, new-onset severe angina, and increasing angina. Unstable angina is a crucial phase of coronary heart disease with widely variable symptoms and prognoses. Thoracic pain may mark the onset of acute myocardial infarction. It typically occurs at rest and has a sudden onset, sudden worsening, and stuttering recurrence over days and weeks. UA which is a potentially life-threatening event is relatively more harmful than stable angina pectoris.

The objective of UA treatment is the improvement of symptoms, the relief of the progress of the disease, and the prevention of cardiovascular events, particularly myocardial infarction and death. Recently, conventional medicine has consisted of anti-platelet agents, anticoagulant agents, nitrates, beta-adrenergic blockers, calcium channel blockers, and inhibitors of the rennin angiotensin aldosterone system. Although these treatments are widely used in the acute relief of secondary angina pectoris and the long-term prophylactic management of angina pectoris, chuanxiong might also be useful for UA and for increased safety. Therefore, we contrasted chuanxiong with conventional medicine in this meta-analysis.

Traditional Chinese Medicine (TCM) is the result of Chinese civilization over 3000 years. The Chinese herb chuanxiong belongs to the Umbelliferae family. A book named *Shen Nong Ben Cao Jing*, which was published 2000 years ago, has been the original and existing writing record about chuanxiong. Ligustrazine is a principal ingredient of chuanxiong. It has been shown to play a critical role in cardiovascular treatments, mediated by inhibition of Ca^{2+} influx and by the release of intracellular Ca^{2+}. It significantly inhibits L-type calcium current in a concentration-dependent manner to make vasodilatory effect, to improve the situation of myocardium ischemia. It also suppressed calcium transient and contraction in rabbit ventricular myocytes under physiological and pathophysiological conditions. Besides, ligustrazine improves attenuation of oxidative stress. Treatment by ligustrazine decreased reactive oxygen species (ROS) production and enhanced cellular glutathione (GSH) levels. Ligustrazine treatment partially restored superoxide dismutase (SOD) activity, increasing in NO production. Recently, the oxidative stress has been shown to play a critical role in atherogenesis (AS). The PPAR signal pathway is involved in the molecular mechanism of ligustrazine in the treatment of AS. Although pharmacology research might indicate the cardiovascular protective effects of ligustrazine, the specific outcomes of the effectiveness of ligustrazine have not been elucidated.

Ischaemic diseases can be improved by the so-called complementary medicine in some report. Nevertheless, few relevant articles on ligustrazine for UA have been published in the English medical journals, and the situation reduces the evaluation of ligustrazine. Cao Suman's study was designed to compare the efficacy and safety of ligustrazine preparations and conventional medicine by including 16 RCTs and 1356 participants. There was a single study that mentioned the rate of cardiovascular events. Therefore, they were unable to summarize the effects of the routine use of antianginal treatment with ligustrazine on the reduction in incidence of acute myocardial infarction.

Nevertheless, the pooled analyses revealed that ligustrazine combined with conventional medicine appeared to have some benefits, such as increasing the rate of marked improvement of symptoms [RR =1.24, 95% CI (1.18, 1.30)] and the rate of marked improvement of ECG [RR = 1.32, 95% CI (1.21, 1.45)] when compared with conventional Western medicine alone. Additionally, the use of ligustrazine was associated with significant trends in the reduction of the consumption of nitroglycerin [MD = −0.14, 95% CI (−0.20, −0.08)] and the level of fibrinogen [MD = −0.78, 95% CI (−0.91, −0.65)] when compared with conventional Western medicine alone. Furthermore, in the meta-analysis of these four outcomes, no statistical heterogeneity was noted among the comparisons (all I2s = 0%). The outcomes of the time of the onset and the frequency of acute attack angina exhibited heterogeneity. Therefore, it should be careful in drawing conclusions about the efficiency of ligustrazine in the reduction of the time of onset or frequency of acute attack angina. There were no serious recorded adverse effects.

Although ligustrazine and conventional antianginal treatments that include ligustrazine exhibited some benefit, there are a number of limitations to this review. (1) The majority of the studies had small samples. (2) Only Chinese studies were found and included. (3) The included studies were of low methodological quality and used neither blinding nor allocation concealment. (4) The duration of treatment was insufficient in the majority of the studies (14 days). Limitations still contribute enlightenment to future studies. Researchers can improve the methodology, such as allocation concealment, blinding method, treatment duration, and long-term follow-up. Well-designed trials of ligustrazine in UA management will promote its application correctly.

Section 3   Research Article

Intra-ventricular infusion of rAAV1-EGFP resulted in transduction in multiple regions of adult rat brain: a comparative study with rAAV2 and rAAV5 vectors

[Abstract] Most gene transfer studies conducted in the central nervous system (CNS) with recombinant adeno-associated virus (rAAV) vectors have been carried out by direct intra-parenchymal injection. However, this delivery method usually results in transduction of cells in only a limited region and is quite invasive, which may hamper its potential clinical application. Injection of viral vectors into the cerebrospinal fluid (CSF) may provide an alternative strategy for widespread gene delivery to the CNS via the subarachnoid space. In this study we compared the transduction abilities of rAAV types 1, 2, and 5 when infused directly into the right lateral cerebral ventricle of adult rats. Multiple structures in the vicinity of the lateral ventricle were transduced by rAAV1, but not by rAAV2 or rAAV5 vectors. Double immunolabeling showed that the transduced cells included not only neurons, but also glia. Real-time quantitative reverse transcriptase polymerase chain reaction (RT-PCR) experiments demonstrated that rAAV1-mediated EGFP mRNA expression was significantly higher than that induced by either rAAV2 or rAAV5. Our data suggest that intra-ventricular infusion of rAAV1 vectors provides a useful method for broad gene delivery to cells in the adult rat CNS.

1　Introduction

Accumulating evidence implicates recombinant adeno-associated virus (rAAV) vectors as highly promising gene transfer vehicles for the central nervous system (CNS), owing to their properties of non-neurotoxicity, low immunogenicity and long-lasting gene expression. To date, 11 AAV serotypes have been identified (Gao et al., 2002; Mori et al., 2004; Passini et al., 2003), and several of these have been used in in vivo CNS transgene studies. Serotype 2 rAAV (rAAV2) vectors have been used in most of these studies and have been shown to strongly transduce neurons in several brain structures (Burger et al., 2005; Klein et al., 1998; McCown et al., 1996; Xu et al., 2003). AAV2 vectors have also been shown to have limitations in the CNS, such as low transduction efficiency and limited tropism among various cell types in the CNS. In addition, neutralizing antibodies to wild-type AAV2 vectors were found in a significant portion of the human population (Chirmule et al., 1999; Mastakov et al., 2002), which may further curb the application of rAAV2 vectors in clinical human gene therapy. Recent studies have demonstrated that other rAAV serotype vectors were able to transduce CNS cells with higher efficiency or broader cellular tropism than the rAAV2 serotype (Alisky et al., 2000; Burger et al., 2004; Cucchiarini et al., 2003; Davidson et al., 2000; Passini et al., 2003; Paterna et al., 2004; Vite et al., 2003; Wang et al., 2003). These other vectors may provide more promising approaches for widespread gene transfer in the CNS.

To date, most gene transfer studies with rAAV vectors in the CNS have been carried out by direct intra-parenchymal injection (Burger et al., 2004; Mastakov et al., 2002; Nomoto et al., 2003; Paterna et al., 2004; Wang et al., 2003). However, this delivery approach generally transduces cells in only a limited region and is invasive, which may hamper its potential clinical application. An alternative strategy for achieving widespread gene delivery is to inject viral vectors directly into the cerebral ventricles. By this route rAAV vectors may gain access to a multitude of locations in the CNS via the cerebrospinal fluid (CSF) flow in the subarachnoid space (Passini et al., 2001; Watson et al., 2005). Previous studies examining intraventricular injections into the brain with rAAV2, rAAV4 and rAAV5 vectors have failed to produce widespread CNS transduction in adult rodents (Davidson et al., 2000; Lo et al., 1999; Rosenfeld et al., 1997). This failure has largely been attributed to their high affinity for ependymal cells lining the ventricles. On the other hand, Passini et al. (2001) and Passini et al. (2003) have reported robust widespread transduction in neonate rodent brains following intra-ventricular rAAV vector injection. The authors suggested that this success may be due to the fact that, unlike adult brains, neonatal mouse brains are in a remodeling state, which may provide an advantageous environment for gene transfer. As of yet, it is not clear whether rAAV1 vectors can produce gene expression in adult rat brains following intra-ventricular injection. Therefore, being motivated by the important aim of achieving widespread gene transfer in the CNS, we asked whether, like in neonate brains, rAAV1 vectors are competent to mediate gene expression in the adult brains.

In the present study we compared the transduction efficiencies of rAAV1, rAAV2, and rAAV5, after being infused directly into the right lateral cerebral ventricle of the adult rats. We examined and compared the transduction efficiency of both neurons and glia following intra-ventricular infusion of the vectors. The implications of our findings for the utility of intraventricular infusion with the rAAV1 vector for gene delivery in the adult rat CNS, especially when broader gene expression is needed, are discussed.

2   Results

2.1   Multiple regions were transduced by rAAV1, but not rAAV2 or rAAV5, following direct intra-ventricular infusion

Confocal laser microscopy examination of 35 μm coronal sections using a FITC filter revealed EGFP expression in multiple regions of brain in the vicinity of the lateral cerebral ventricle in the group injected with rAAV1. Expression was distributed mainly in the caudate putamen, the corpus callosum, the dorsal part of the lateral septal nucleus, and the hippocampus. Both cell bodies and processes were clearly labeled. Interestingly, a few EGFP-positive cells were also present in the contralateral hemisphere, and some EGFP-labeled processes within the dorsal hippocampal commissure were also found to run across the midline. Furthermore, we found that there is a correlation between the distance to the lateral ventricle and the transduction of hippocampus, the nearer to the lateral ventricle, the stronger in EGFP expression. In some regions of the hippocampus, the estimated number of transduced pyramidal cells reaches 60% ~ 75%. However, only a few of sparse EGFP-positive cells were found near the ventricle wall in one of the four rats injected with rAAV5, and no detectable

EGFP fluorescence expression was observed in rats injected with rAAV2.

2.2 NeuN and GFAP double immunolabeling demonstrated rAAV1 vector transduction of neurons and glia

To assess cell tropism of rAAV1 in the rat brain, we performed double immunolabeling with monoclonal anti-NeuN and anti-GFAP antibodies in a series of coronal cryosections at an interval of 105 μm. Based on previous data showing that gene expression mediated by rAAV in vivo generally peaked after 3 weeks and lasted for at least 3 months to 1 year (Lo et al., 1999; McCown et al., 1996), all rat brains were collected for analysis 8 weeks after intra-ventricular injection. Confocal laser scanning microscopy examination showed that all of the EGFP-positive cells were NeuN-positive, which indicates that the primary tropism of rAAV1-EGFP is for neurons. Overlap between EGFP-positive cells and anti-GFAP labeling was also observed in some sections. However, the number of double-labeled EGFP and GFAP cells was small. This result indicates that some glial cells were also susceptible to rAAV1 vectors. These data support some previous works suggesting that AAV1 vectors are able to transduce both neurons and astrocytes (Vite et al., 2003; Wang et al., 2003).

2.3 Real-time quantitative PCR

To quantify transgene expression of the three rAAV vectors, we performed SYBR Green I real-time reverse transcriptase polymerase chain reaction (RT-PCR) analysis to detect the mRNA of EGFP in three regions of the brain: hippocampus, striatum, and cortex. The melting curves analysis of the PCR products showed that both of the 18 S RNA and the target genes were clear, without dimer and other contaminations, indicating that the samples were suitable for subsequent quantitative PCR. The amount of target gene expression was calculated from the respective standard curves, and quantitative expression of the target gene was normalized using the housekeeping gene 18 S. Consistent with the observation of native EGFP fluorescence, real-time quantitative PCR results showed that the amount of EGFP mRNA expression within regions differed among the rats injected with the three serotypes. The quantity of EGFP mRNA expression mediated by rAAV1 was significantly higher than that mediated by rAAV2 or rAAV5 in cortex, striatum, and hippocampus (ANOVA; $P < 0.01$).

3 Discussion

To date, several serotypes of rAAV vectors (rAAV1, rAAV2, rAAV4, rAAV5) have been tested in adult or neonate murine brains via intra-ventricular injections (Davidson et al., 2000; Liu et al., 2005; Lo et al., 1999; Passini et al., 2001; Passini et al., 2003; Watson et al., 2005). In adult rodents, rAAV2, rAAV4 and rAAV5 have not resulted in widespread CNS transduction following intra-ventricular injection, but rather mainly resulted in transduction of ependymal cells (Davidson et al., 2000; Liu et al., 2005; Lo et al., 1999). In neonatal mouse, however, Watson et al. (2005) recently showed that rAAV5 was capable of transducing both the choroid plexus and ependymal cells. Passini et al. compared the transduction profiles of AAV1 and AAV5 vectors after they were injected into cerebral lateral ventricles of mice at birth. Their findings showed that rAAV5 transduction is very limited, while injection of rAAV1 vectors resulted in robust widespread transduction in multiple structures (Passini et al., 2003). Studies illuminating whether rAAV vectors administered by intra-ventricular injection can transduce cells in adult brains as efficiently as in neonatal brains have not yet been reported. In the present work we showed that when rAAV1 vectors were infused into the adult cerebral ventricular system, they can produce widespread gene expression in multiple CNS structures. No EGFP expression was observed with injection of rAAV2, and within rAAV5 vectors injection group, only one section showed sparse cells being transduced.

In the current study, multiple brain regions near the cerebral ventricle were found to be transduced efficiently by rAAV1 vector. The EGFP-positive regions included the hippocampus, corpus callosum, caudate putamen, and the dorsal part of lateral septal nucleus, but tissues near the third ventricle and the dentate gyrus were not found to be transduced. The serial sections examination showed that the EGFP expression could spread at least 3 mm in the longitudinal direction (Bregma from −1.80 mm to −4.80 mm), and further, we observed that there is a correlation between the distance to the lateral ventricle and the transduction of hippocampus, the nearer to the lateral ventricle, the stronger in EGFP expression. In some region of the hippocampus, about 60% ~ 75% of the pyramidal cells were transduced. In addition, a few choroids plexus cells also expressed rAAV1-EGFP. However, this phenomenon was not observed in the rAAV2 or rAAV5 groups. rAAV2 did not transduce any structures, whereas rAAV5 infected a small number of cells near the cerebral ventricle wall. Observation of rAAV5 vector transduction of ependymal and choroid plexus cells throughout the ventricular system was previously reported (Watson et al., 2005). We did not detect these phenomena in the present study, with only a small number of cells adjacent to the lateral ventricle being found to be transduced by the rAAV5 vector.

Although the EGFP-positive cells in rAAV5 group seem to reside very close to the ventricle wall, we still suppose these cells are not ependymal cells, because the EGFP expression is merely near to the lateral ventricle wall, but not in the lateral ventricle wall. To quantitatively analyze the transduction efficiency of each serotype rAAV vectors, we further performed the real-time PCR experiments in different regions of the brain, and the result showed that EGFP-mRNA expression mediated by rAAV1 was significantly greater than that by rAAV2 or rAAV5. Because the real-time PCR is much higher in both sensitivity and specificity than direct observation by confocal microscopy, it should not be surprising that EGFP-mRNA was detected in all groups by real-time PCR assays. It is likely that EGFP gene expressions (i.e., the intensity of fluorescence) in both the rAAV2 and rAAV5 injection groups were below the threshold detectable by a fluorescence microscope. The use of different reporter genes and of examination methods with different detection sensitivities may be responsible for the distinction between the present data and some previous studies. Relatively lower titer in present study (5×10^{11} µg/mL in this study) might be another explanation for this discrepancy. In the literature, these phenomena were only observed in studies with high titer virus vector preparation, in which the vector titer is up to a grade of 10^{13} µg/mL. Future studies using AAV vectors with higher titers are needed to evaluate whether higher titers of virus have higher effective transduction in the CNS in serotype AAV2 and AAV5.

To exclude effects of serotype-specific inverted terminal repeats (ITRs) and promoters, the three kinds of vectors used in this study were designed with the same ITRs and promoter, and the only difference among them was the capsid. Therefore, we propose that the distribution of serotype-specific AAV receptors is likely divergent among different cell types and regions of CNS, and that receptor specificities may directly affect virion particle diffusion through the extracellular space. Heparan sulfate proteoglycans (HSPGs) (Summerford et al., 1998), integrin (Summerford et al., 1999), and fibroblast growth factor receptor (Qing et al., 1999) have been identified as important receptors for AAV-2. The receptors for AAV5 have been identified as N-linked sialic acid (Kaludov et al., 2001) and platelet-derived growth factor receptors (PDGFRs) (Di Pasquale et al., 2003). Receptors for AAV1 however have not yet been identified. It is well known that both HSPGs and PDGFRs are heavily expressed at the surface and in the extracellular matrix of neurons (Burger et al., 2004; Ding et al., 2005; Oumesmar et al., 1997). Therefore, both AAV2 and AAV5 particles would bind quickly to their receptors, thereby preventing spread into the parenchyma. Our findings indicate that divergent virus capsids and different receptor molecules may underlie, at least in part, the different gene expression patterns produced by serotyped 1, 2 and 5 rAAV vectors.

Another interesting finding in this study was that some cellular processes, rather than cell bodies, near the cerebral ventricle were strongly transduced. These EGFP-positive fibers were mainly present in the corpus callosum, hippocampus, and lateral septal nucleus. What is more, a few cells were found to be EGFP-positive in the contralateral hemisphere, and some EGFP-labeled processes of dorsal hippocampal commissure were also found to extend across the midline. This observation suggests that retrograde axonal transport may serve as a mechanism, at least in part, in gene transfer by the rAAV1 vector. Retrograde transport means a vector infects a neuron terminal first and then is transported to the cell body (Burger et al., 2004). Using cy3 labeled rAAV virions, Kaspar et al. (2002) and Passini and Wolfe (2001) have verified the existence of retrograde transport in the CNS. Both the lateral septal nucleus and hippocampus are adjacent to the lateral cerebral ventricle wall, and some of the cell processes in these structures are closer to the CSF than their somas. This arrangement places numerous neural fibers in good position to be transduced prior to the cell bodies. Thus our findings suggest that the transduction of multiple structures by rAAV1 is at least partly due to a retrograde axonal transport mechanism.

Consistent with previous reports (Burger et al., 2004; Passini et al., 2003), our EGFP double immunolabeling experiment with NeuN and GFAP showed that neurons were the predominant cell type that was transduced by the rAAV1 vectors. We also found some GFAP-positive glial cells that were susceptible to the rAAV1 vectors. Thus rAAV1 vectors appear to have a wider cell tropism than other vectors, affecting both neurons and glia. There are discrepancies in the literature about AAV serotype differences in cell tropism and transduction efficiency in the CNS. Davidson et al. (2000) described findings that rAAV5 transduced both neurons and astrocytes when injected directly into striatum, and had a much higher efficiency than did rAAV2. On the contrary, Burger et al. (2004) reported that all serotype 1, 2 and 5 rAAV vectors exhibited selective tropism to neurons. Nevertheless, rAAV1 vectors have been shown repeatedly to be promising gene transfer vehicles in the CNS (Passini et al., 2003; Rafi et al., 2005; Vite et al., 2003; Wang et al., 2003). Vite et al. (2003) reported in cats that rAAV2 vector transduced only the gray matter, rAAV1 affected both gray matter and white matter, and rAAV5 did not result in any detectable transduction. Wang et al. (2003) also reported that rAAV1 was capable of transducing not only neurons, but also glial and ependymal cells, and the transduction efficiency of rAAV1 vector was found to be 13- to 35-fold greater than that of the rAAV2 vector. This convergence of studies together suggest that rAAV1 may be a good gene transfer vehicle to the CNS.

In summary, our data demonstrated efficient transgene expression in multiple adult rat brain structures following rAAV1 intra-ventricular injection. Both cellular processes and cell bodies were transduced in multiple regions around lateral cerebral ventricle. Moreover our findings indicated that both neurons and glia were transduced by rAAV1 vectors. These results suggest that intra-ventricular rAAV1 vector infusion may have potential for gene therapy for some CNS diseases which need broad therapeutic gene expression. Many neurological disorders will require widespread gene transduction for successful treatment; however, one of the current challenges of rAAV-mediated gene therapy is achieving transduction of sufficient cells in the CNS to successfully treat these disorders (Burger et al., 2005; Passini et al., 2003). The current study showed that intra-ventricular administration of rAAV1 may bring us closer to meeting this challenge. Moreover, it is worth noting that intra-ventricular injection of gene vehicles is a relatively easy and less invasive route compared with intra-parenchymal injections. Thus this strategy may have good prospects for CNS disease gene therapy in the future.

4   Experimental procedures

4.1   rAAV vector preparation

The rAAV vector genome contained rAAV2 inverted terminal repeats (ITRs) flanking a transcription unit containing enhanced green fluorescent protein (EGFP) cDNA under the control of a cytomegalovirus (CMV) promoter. The vector plasmid was packaged into rAAV1, rAAV2 and rAAV5 capsid with AAVMax™ package system in a BHK-21 cell line (Wu et al., 2002). Briefly, a recombinant herpes simplex virus type 1 (HSV1-rc/ΔUL2), which is able to express adeno-associated virus Rep and Cap proteins, was used for rAAV replication and packaging. The rAAV proviral cell line (BHK/SG2) with EGFP gene expression cassette was established by transfecting BHK-21 cells with rAAV vector plasmid pSNAV-2-EGFP. The BHK/SG2 cells were infected with HSV1-rc/ΔUL2 to generate rAAV vectors. All vectors were purified by CsCl density gradient centrifugation. The rAAV titer was determined by dot blot assay expressed as vector genomes/mL (μg/mL) (Salvetti et al., 1998). Each rAAV vector serotype had a titer of 5×10^{11} μg/mL.

4.2   Animals and surgery

All animal studies were performed in accordance with the guidelines issued by the committee on animal research of Peking Union Medical College Hospital, and approved by the institutional ethics committee. Twenty-seven adult male Sprague-Dawley rats were divided randomly into three equal groups to be injected with titer and volume-matched rAAV1, rAAV2, and rAAV5-EGFP vectors. The rats were initially anesthetized with sodium pentobarbital (40 mg/kg) and all surgical procedures were performed using aseptic techniques. The stereotaxic brain coordinates used for right lateral ventricle injection were as follows: anterior-posterior (AP) −1.0 mm, lateral (Lat) +1.5 mm, dorsoventral (DV) −3.5 mm from dura. Small burr holes were made in the skull with a dental drill to expose the dura above the target. Injections were performed with a 10 μL Hamilton syringe fitted with a glass micropipette with an opening of approximately 60 ~ 80 μm. Ten microliters of rAAV vector solution (5×10^{9} μg) was injected into each rat's ventricle at a rate of 0.5 μL/min. The rate of injection was precisely controlled by piston-driven infusion pump. Following injections, the needle was left in place for 5 min prior to withdrawal to allow the injected solution to diffuse into the CSF.

4.3   Preparation of brains for histology

Eight weeks after surgery, four animals in each group were anesthetized with 2% sodium pentobarbital, and then perfused transcardially with chilled physiological saline (0.9%), followed by 4% paraformaldehyde in phosphate buffer (0.1 mol/L, pH 7.4). The rat brain samples were collected and fixed in 4% paraformaldehyde at 4 °C overnight, and then transferred to 30% sucrose in PBS for cryoprotection. Thirty-five micrometer coronal cryosections were cut with a freezing sliding microtome. For native EGFP fluorescence observation, a series of sections spaced 10^5 μm apart were mounted on poly-L-lysine-coated slides. Processed slides were later examined under an Olympus FV1000 confocal laser scanning microscope using a FITC filter.

4.4   Immunofluorescent labeling

For immunohistochemical analyses, free-floating sections were washed for 20 min in 0.1 mol/L PBS at pH 7.4 containing 0.2% Triton X-100, and then blocked with 5% normal donkey serum (Chemicon, Temecula, CA, USA) in PBS for 1 h. Mouse monoclonal IgG-specific anti-NeuN primary antibody (diluted 1 : 1000), which strongly stains neuronal cell nuclei and lightly stains neuronal cytoplasm was used to label neurons. Rabbit primary monoclonal antibody raised against GFAP (glial fibrillary acidic protein; diluted 1 : 800), an intermediate filament of astrocytes, was used to label glia. Cy3-conjugated donkey anti mouse IgG (diluted 1 : 400) and AMCA-conjugated donkey anti-rabbit IgG (diluted 1 : 100) were employed as secondary antibodies. All antibodies were obtained from Chemicon (Temecula, CA, USA). Sections were incubated overnight with both primary antibodies diluted in PBS with 3% BSA and 0.1% Triton X-100 at 4 °C, and then washed in PBS for 30 min at room temperature and incubated with secondary antibodies for 2 h at room temperature. The sections were mounted and coverslipped. Sections were examined under a confocal laser scanning microscope (Bio-Rad Olympus FV1000). Estimations of the number of EGFP-positive cells were automatically processed using an image-processing software Image-Pro Plus 5.02.

4.5   Real-time quantitative PCR

To quantify brain EGFP mRNA expression, we performed a real-time quantitative PCR assay, in which 18 S rRNA served as an internal reference. The cortex, striatum, and hippocampus ipsilateral to the injection in each group were dissected for PCR ($n = 5$). Total RNA from the brain tissue was prepared using Trizol® reagent (Gibco BRL, Gaithersburg, MD) according to the manufacturer's instructions. cDNA synthesis was conducted according to the RNA PCR kit protocol (TAKARA). Reverse transcription was performed using 5 μg of total RNA in 10 μL of the following solution: 2 μL MgCl$_2$, 1 μL 10× RT buffer, 1 μL dNTP, 0.25 μL RNase inhibitor, 0.5 μL AMV reverse transcriptase, 0.5 μL oligo dT primer and 3.75 μL RNase free ddH$_2$O. The reaction was incubated at 30 ℃ for 10 min, 42 ℃ for 50 min, 95 ℃ for 5 min, and 4 ℃ for 5 min. Primers for PCR were the following: EGFP forward 5'-GCA GAA GAA CGG CAT CAA GGT-3' and EGFP reverse 5'ACG AAC TCC AGC AGG ACC ATG 3', which was used to amplify a 203-bp fragment within the coding region of the EGFP genome. The 18 S rRNA forward primer was 5'-CTT AGA GGG ACA AGT GGC G-3', and the

18 S rRNA reverse primer was 5′-GGA CAT CTA AGG GCA TCA CA-3′. The housekeeping gene 18 S RNA was employed as a reference, and standard curves were generated for each group using purified PCR product. Briefly, PCR was performed using 10× diluted product of the reverse transcription as a template, target gene and housekeeping gene 18 S RNAprimers respectively, and HS Ex taqDNA polymerase (TAKARA). PCR products were examined by electrophoresis in a 2% agarose gel. Real-time PCR was performed using the Rotor Gene 3000™ Real-time DNA Detection System (Corbet Research), and was carried out with SYBR Premix Ex Taq (Perfect Real-time) kit (TAKARA) in a 25 μL volume of the following solution: 12.5 μL SYBR Premix Ex Taq, 0.5 μL PCR forward primer, 0.5 μL PCR reverse primer, 2.0 μL template, 2.0 μL 25 mmol/L $MgCl_2$, 7.5 μL ddH_2O, cycle conditions for EGFP PCR were 10 min at 95 ℃ followed by forty 5 s cycles of at 94 ℃, 30 s at 60 ℃, and 20 s at 72 ℃. During each extension step, SYBR green fluorescence was monitored and provided the real-time quantitative measurements of the fluorescence. Quantitation was carried out using an external standard curve. PCR results were analyzed using rotor-gene 5.0 software.

References

[1]   Alisky J M, Hughes S M, Sauter S L, et al. Transduction of murine cerebellar neurons with recombinant FIV and AAV5 vectors. Neuroreport, 2000, 11(12): 2669-2673.

[2]   Burger C, Gorbatyuk O S, Velardo M J, et al. Recombinant AAV viral vectors pseudotyped with viral capsids from serotypes 1, 2, and 5 display differential efficiency and cell tropism after delivery to different regions of the central nervous system. Molecular Therapy, 2004, 10(2): 302-317.

[3]   Burger C, Nash K, Mandel R J. Recombinant adeno-associated viral vectors in the nervous system. Human Gene Therapy, 2005, 16(7): 781-791.

[4]   Chirmule N, Propert K, Magosin S, et al. Immune responses to adenovirus and adeno-associated virus in humans. Gene Therapy, 1999, 6(9): 1574-1583.

[5]   Cucchiarini MRen X L, Perides G, Terwilliger E F. Selective gene expression in brain microglia mediated via adeno-associated virus type 2 and type 5 vectors. Gene Therapy, 2003, 10(8): 657-667.

[6]   Davidson B L, Stein C S, Heth J A, et al. From the Cover: Recombinant adeno-associated virus type 2, 4, and 5 vectors: Transduction of variant cell types and regions in the mammalian central nervous system. Proc Natl Acad Sci USA, 2000, 97(7): 3428-3432.

[7]   Di P G, Davidson B L, Stein C S, et al. Identification of PDGFR as a receptor for AAV-5 transduction. Nature Medicine, 2003, 9(10): 1306-1312.

[8]   Ding W, Zhang L, Yan Z, et al. Intracellular trafficking of adeno-associated viral vectors. Gene Therapy, 2005, 12(11): 873-880.

[9]   Gao G P, Alvira M R, Wang L, et al. Novel adeno-associated viruses from rhesus monkeys as vectors for human gene therapy. Proceedings of the National Academy of Sciences, 2002, 99(18): 11854-11859.

[10]　Kaludov N, Brown K E, Walters R W, et al. Adeno-associated virus serotype 4 (AAV4) and AAV5 both require sialic acid binding for hemagglutination and efficient transduction but differ in sialic acid linkage specificity. Journal of Virology, 2001, 75(15): 6884-6893.

[11]　Kaspar B K, Erickson D, Schaffer D, et al. Targeted Retrograde Gene Delivery for Neuronal Protection. Molecular Therapy the Journal of the American Society of Gene Therapy, 2002, 5(1): 50-56.

[12]　Klein R L, Meyer E M, Peel A L, et al. Neuron-specific transduction in the rat septohippocampal or nigrostriatal pathway by recombinant adeno-associated virus vectors. Experimental Neurology, 1998, 150(2): 183-194.

[13]　Lo W D, Qu G, Sferra T J, et al. Adeno-associated virus-mediated gene transfer to the brain: duration and modulation of expression. Human Gene Therapy, 1999, 10(2): 201-213.

[14]　During M J. Recombinant adeno-associated virus serotypes 2- and 5-mediated gene transfer in the mammalian brain: quantitative analysis of heparin co-infusion. Molecular Therapy, 2002, 5(4): 371-380.

[15]　Mastakov M Y, Baer K, Symes C W, et al. Immunological aspects of recombinant adeno-associated virus delivery to the mammalian brain. Journal of Virology, 2002, 76(16): 8446-8454.

[16]　Mccown T J, Xiao X, Li J, et al. Differential and persistent expression patterns of CNS gene transfer by an adeno-associated virus (AAV) vector. Brain Research, 1996, 713(1-2): 99-107.

[17]　Mori S, Wang L, Takeuchi T, et al. Two novel adeno-associated viruses from cynomolgus monkey: pseudotyping characterization of capsid protein. Virology, 2004, 330(2): 375-383.

[18]　Nomoto T, Okada T, Shimazaki K, et al. Distinct patterns of gene transfer to gerbil hippocampus with recombinant adeno-associated virus type 2 and 5. Neuroscience Letters, 2003, 340(2): 153-157.

[19]　Nait O B, Vignais L, Baron-Van E A. Developmental expression of platelet-derived growth factor alpha-receptor in neurons and glial cells of the mouse CNS. Journal of Neuroscience the Official Journal of the Society for Neuroscience, 1997, 17(1): 125-139.

[20]　Passini M A, Wolfe J H. Widespread gene delivery and structure-specific patterns of expression in the brain after intraventricular injections of neonatal mice with an adeno-associated virus vector. Journal of Virology, 2001, 75: 12382-12392.

[21]　Passini M A, Watson D J, Vite C H, et al. Intraventricular brain injection of adeno-associated virus Type 1 (AAV1) in neonatal mice results in complementary patterns of neuronal transduction to AAV2 and total long-term correction of storage lesions in the brains of β -glucuronidase-deficient mice. Journal of Virology, 2003, 77(12): 7034-7040.

[22]　Paterna J C, Feldon J, Büeler H. Transduction profiles of recombinant adeno-associated virus vectors derived from serotypes 2 and 5 in the nigrostriatal system of rats. Journal of Virology, 2004, 78(13): 6808-6817.

[23]　Qing K, Mah C, Hansen J, et al. Human fibroblast growth factor receptor 1 is a co-receptor for infectionby adeno-associated virus 2. Nature Medicine, 1999, 5(1): 71-77.

[24]　Rafi M A, Rao H Z, Passini M A, et al. AAV-Mediated expression of galactocerebrosidase in brain results in attenuated symptoms and extended life span in murine models of globoid cell leukodystrophy.

Molecular Therapy the Journal of the American Society of Gene Therapy, 2005, 11(5): 734-744.

[25]　Rosenfeld M R, Bergman I, Schramm L, et al. Adeno-associated viral vector gene transfer into leptomeningeal xenografts. J Neurooncol. 1997, 34(2): 139-144.

[26]　Salvetti A, Orève S, Chadeuf G, et al. Factors influencing recombinant adeno-associated virus production. Human Gene Therapy, 1998, 9(5): 695-706.

[27]　Summerford C, Samulski R J. Membrane-associated heparan sulfate proteoglycan is a receptor for adeno-associated virus type 2 virions. Journal of Virology, 1998, 72(2): 1438-1445.

[28]　Summerford C, Bartlett J S, Samulski R J. Alpha V beta 5 integrin: a co-receptor for adeno-associated virus type 2 infection. Nature Medicine, 1999, 5(1): 78-82.

[29]　Vite C H, Passini M A, Haskins M E, et al. Adeno-associated virus vector-mediated transduction in the cat brain. Gene Therapy, 2003, 10(22): 1874-1881.

[30]　Wang C, Wang C M, Clark K R, et al. Recombinant AAV serotype 1 transduction efficiency and tropism in the murine brain. Gene Therapy, 2003, 10(17): 1528-1534.

[31]　Watson D J, Passini M A, Wolfe J H. Transduction of the choroid plexus and ependyma in neonatal mouse brain by vesicular stomatitis virus glycoprotein-pseudotyped lentivirus and adeno-associated virus type 5 vectors. Human Gene Therapy, 2005, 16(1): 49-56.

[32]　Wu Z J, Wu X B, Cao H, et al. A novel and highly efficient production system for recombinant adeno-associated virus vector. Sci China C Life Sci, 2002, 45(1): 96-104.

[33]　Xu Y, Gu Y, Wu P, et al. Efficiencies of transgene expression in nociceptive neurons through different routes of delivery of adeno-associated viral vectors. Human Gene Therapy, 2003, 14(9): 897-906.

Section 4　Words of TCM

1. 暴饮暴食 crapulence
2. 外感六邪 six exogenous pathogenic factors
3. 内生五邪 five endogenous pathogenic factors
4. 风寒感冒 cold due to wind and cold
5. 风热头痛 anemopyretic headache
6. 感受寒邪 attack by pathogenic cold
7. 肺虚咳嗽 pneumasthenic cough; cough because of asthenia of the lung
8. 阳气衰退 decline of yang qi
9. 寒性凝滞 cold being coagulative- and obstructive-natured
10. 气血紊乱 disturbance of qi and blood
11. 湿邪困脾 pathogenic dampness blocking the spleen
12. 脾阳不振 insufficiency of spleen yang

13. 阴阳偏盛 relative predominance of yin or yang

14. 阴阳互损 mutual consumption of yin and yang

15. 五志过极 five extreme emotional changes

16. 五心烦热 feverish sensation of the five centers; dysphoria with feverish sensation of chest; palms and soles

17. 虚实夹杂 asthenia intermingled with sthenia

18. 邪正盛衰 superabundance or decline of pathogenic qi and healthy qi

19. 心肝火旺 exuberance of heart and liver fire

20. 心火亢盛 hyperactivity/exuberance of heart fire

21. 脉道不利 unsmoothness of vessels

22. 母病及子 disease of the mother-organ affecting the child-organ

23. 子病犯母 disease of the child-organ affecting the mother-organ

24. 方位配五行 correspondence of the directions to the five elements

25. 紫河车 ziheche; human placenta

26. 胆虚不得眠 insomnia due to gallbladder asthenia

27. 防御外邪入侵 preventing the invasion of exogenous pathogenic factor

28. 人中疔 boil on philtrum

29. 咬伤 human bite; bite by man

30. 入臼 joint reduction

31. 三陷证 three types of inward penetration of pyogenic agent

32. 三阴痉 convulsion with symptoms of three yin channels

33. 三阴疟 three-yin malaria

34. 三部九候 three portions and nine pulse-takings

35. 三阳合病 disease involving all three yang channels

36. 干疽 cellulitis at the anterolateral aspect of the shoulder

37. 干陷 dry type of inward penetration of pyogenic agent

38. 干癣 chronic eczema; neurodermatitis

39. 干血劳 emaciation due to blood disorders

40. 干胁痛 dry hypochondriac pain

(Cheng Baohe, Hu Guojie)

Chapter 18   Anxiety

Section 1   Anxiety and Fear

Fear and anxiety often occur together but these terms are not interchangeable. Even though symptoms typically overlap, a person's experience with these emotions differs based on their context. Fear relates to a known or understood threat, whereas anxiety follows from an unknown or poorly defined threat.

Anxiety is a diffuse, unpleasant, vague sense of apprehension. It is often a response to an imprecise or unknown threat. For example, imagine you're walking down a dark street. You may feel a little uneasy and perhaps you have a few butterflies in your stomach.These sensations are caused by anxiety that is related to the possibility that a stranger may jump out from behind a bush, or approach you in some other way and harm you. This anxiety is not the result of a known or specific threat. Rather it comes from your mind's interpretation of the possible dangers that could immediately arise.

Anxiety is often accompanied by many uncomfortable somatic sensations. Some of the most common physical symptoms of anxiety include: headaches; muscle pain and tension; sleep disturbances; tightness felt throughout the body, especially in the head, neck, jaw, and face; chest pain; ringing or pulsing in ears; excessive sweating; shaking and trembling; cold chills or hot flushes; accelerated heart rate; numbness or tingling; depersonalization and derealization; upset stomach or nausea; shortness of breath; feeling like you are going insane; dizziness or feeling faint.

Fear is an emotional response to a known or definite threat. If you're walking down a dark street, for example, and someone points a gun at you and says, "This is a stickup," then you'd likely experience a fear response. The danger is real, definite, and immediate. There is a clear and present object of the fear. Although the focus of the response is different (real *vs* imagined danger), fear and anxiety are interrelated. When faced with fear, most people will experience the physical reactions that are described under anxiety. Fear causes anxiety, and anxiety can cause fear. But, the subtle distinctions between the two will give you a better understanding of your symptoms and may be important for treatment strategies.

Anxiety and fear are common feelings that patients and families sometimes have when coping with cancer. These feelings are normal responses to the stress of cancer, and may be noticed more in the first week or two after diagnosis. Feeling of fear or anxiety (a feeling of worry or unease) may be due to changes in the ability to continue family duties, loss of control over events in life, changes in appearance or body image, uncertainty about the future, concerns about suffering, pain, and the unknown. Fears around loss of independence, changes in relationships with loved ones, and becoming a burden to others may overwhelm the patient, and complicate family life.

Family members may have these feeling because they feel uncertain about the future or angry that this person has cancer. They may notice guilt and frustration at not being able to "do enough". They may have stress due to problems with balancing work, childcare, self care, and other activities along with more responsibility at home.

Sometimes a person may become overly anxious, fearful, of depressed and may no longer cope well with his or her day-to-day life. If this happens, seeking help from a professional therapist or counselor is benefit to the patient and his family. The following items can be look for: feeling anxious; difficulty in thinking or solving problems; being nervous, agitated, irritable, or restless; feeling or looking tense; concern about losing control; uneasy sense that something bad is going to happen; trembling and shaking; headaches; being cranky or angry with others; tiredness or fatigue; trouble sleeping or restless sleep; denial of obvious tension or anxiety.

According to the adviser, the patient can: talk about feelings and fears that you or your family members maybe feel sad and frustrated; decide together with your family or caregiver what specific things you can do to support each other; avoid blaming yourself and others when you feel anxious and afraid. Instead, look for the cause (usually a thought or opinion about something) and talk about it; seek help through counseling and support groups; use prayer, meditation, or other types of spiritual support; try deep breathing and relaxation exercises several times a day (close eyes, breathe deeply, concentrate on one body part and relax it, starting with toes and working up to head. When relaxed, imagine being in a pleasant place, such as a beach in the morning or in a field on a spring day); consider asking for a referral to a counselor to work with you and your family; talk with your doctor about the possible use of medicine for anxiety.

The caregiver can: gently invite the patient to talk about his or her fears and concerns; avoid forcing the patient to talk before he or she is ready; listen carefully without judging the patient's feeling, or your own; decide together with the patient what specific things you can do to be supportive to each other; for severe anxiety, it is usually not helpful to try and reason with the patient. Instead, talk with the doctor about the symptoms and problems you notice; to reduce your own stress, try suggestions from the list above, and any others that have worked for you in the past; consider getting support for yourself, through groups or individual counseling.

It should be noted that some medicines or supplements cause or worsen anxiety symptoms. If anxiety gets worse after a new medicine is started, such as trouble breathing, sweating, and feeling very restless, you should talk with your doctor about it.

Section 2   Berberine

A compound called berberine is one of the most effective natural supplements available. It has very impressive health benefits, and affects your body at the molecular level. Berberine has been shown to lower blood sugar, cause weight loss and improve heart health, etc.. It is one of the few powerful supplements shown to be as effective as a pharmaceutical drug. This is a detailed review of berberine and its health effects.

1   What is berberine?

Berberine is a bioactive compound that can be extracted from several different plants, including a group of shrubs called Berberis. Technically, it belongs to a class of compounds called alkaloids. It has a yellow color, and has often been used as a dye. Berberine has a long history of use in traditional Chinese medicine, where it was used to treat various ailments. Now, modern science has confirmed that it has impressive benefits for several different health problems.

2   How does it work?

Berberine has now been tested in hundreds of different studies. It has been shown to have powerful effects on many different biological systems. After you ingest berberine, it gets taken in by the body and transported into the bloodstream. Then it travels into the body's cells. Inside the cells, it binds to several different molecular targets and changes their function. This is similar to how pharmaceutical drugs work.

Here is not going to get into much detail, because the biological mechanisms are complicated and diverse. However, one of the main actions of berberine is to activate an enzyme inside cells called AMP-activated protein kinase (AMPK).This enzyme is sometimes referred to as a metabolic master switch. It is found in the cells of various organs, including the brain, muscle, kidney, heart and liver. This enzyme plays a major role in regulating metabolism. Berberine also affects various other molecules inside cells, and may even affect which genes are turned on or off.

3   It causes a major reduction in blood sugar levels

Type 2 diabetes is a serious disease that has become incredibly common in recent decades, causing millions of deaths every year. It is characterized by elevated blood sugar (glucose) levels, either caused by insulin resistance or lack of insulin. Over time, high blood sugar levels can damage the body's tissues and organs, leading to various health problems and a shortened lifespan.

Many studies show that berberine can significantly reduce blood sugar levels in individuals with type 2 diabetes. In fact, its effectiveness is comparable to the popular diabetes drug metformin (glucophage). It seems to work via multiple different mechanisms: decreasing insulin resistance, making the blood sugar lowering hormone insulin more effective; increasing glycolysis, helping the body break down sugars inside cells; decreasing sugar production in the liver; slowing the breakdown of carbohydrates in the gut; increasing the number of beneficial bacteria in the gut.

In a study of 116 diabetic patients, one gram of berberine per day lowered fasting blood sugar by 20%, from 7.0 mmol/L to 5.6 mmol/L (126 mg/dL to 101 mg/dL), or from diabetic to normal levels. It also lowered hemoglobin A_{1c} by 12% (a marker for long-term blood sugar levels), and also regulated blood lipids like cholesterol and triglycerides. According to a big review of 14 studies, berberine is as effective as oral diabetes drugs, including metformin, glipizide and rosiglitazone.

It works very well with lifestyle modifications, and also has additive effects when administered with other blood sugar lowering drugs. If you look at discussions online, you often see people with sky-high blood sugars literally normalizing them just by taking this supplement. This stuff really works, in both the studies and the real world.

4   Berberine may help you lose weight

Berberine may also be effective as a weight loss supplement. So far, two studies have examined the effects on body weight. In a 12-week study in obese individuals, 500 mg taken three times per day caused about 5 pounds of weight loss, on average. The participants also lost 3.6% of their body fat. Another more impressive study was conducted in 37 men and women with metabolic syndrome. This study went on for 3 months, and the participants took 300 mg, 3 times per day. The participants dropped their body mass index (BMI) levels from 31.5

to 27.4, or from obese to overweight in only 3 months. They also lost belly fat and improved many health markers.

The researchers believe that the weight loss is caused by improved function of fat-regulating hormones, such as insulin, adiponectin and leptin. Berberine also appears to inhibit the growth of fat cells at the molecular level. However, more research is needed on the weight loss effects of berberine.

5　It lowers cholesterol and may reduce your risk of heart disease

Heart disease is currently the world's most common cause of premature death. Many factors that can be measured in the blood are associated with an increased risk of heart disease. As it turns out, berberine has been shown to improve many of these factors.

According to a review of 11 studies, it can: lower total cholesterol by 0.61 mmol/L (24 mg/dL); lower LDL cholesterol by 0.65 mmol/L (25 mg/dL); lower blood triglycerides by 0.50 mmol/L (44 mg/dL); raise HDL cholesterol by 0.05 mmol/L (2 mg/dL). It has also been shown to lower apolipoprotein B by 13% ~ 15%, which is a **very** important risk factor.

According to some studies, berberine works by inhibiting an enzyme called PCSK9. This leads to more LDL being removed from the bloodstream. Keep in mind that diabetes, high blood sugar levels and obesity are also major risk factors for heart disease, all of which seem to be improved with this supplement. Given the beneficial effects on all these risk factors, it seems likely that berberine could drastically reduce the risk of heart disease.

6　Other health benefits

Berberine may also have numerous other health benefits:

Depression: Rat studies show that it may help fight depression.

Cancer: Test tube and animal studies have shown that it can reduce the growth and spread of various different types of cancer.

Antioxidant and anti-inflammatory: It has been shown to have potent antioxidant and anti-inflammatory effects in some studies.

Infections: It has been shown to fight harmful microorganisms, including bacteria, viruses, fungi and parasites.

Fatty liver: It can reduce fat build-up in the liver, which should help protect against non-alcoholic fatty liver disease (NAFLD).

Heart failure: One study showed that it drastically improved symptoms and reduced risk of death in heart failure patients.

Many of these benefits need more research before firm recommendations can be made, but the current evidence is very promising.

7   Dosage and side effects

Many of the studies cited in the article used dosages in the range of 900 mg to 1500 mg per day. It is common to take 500 mg, 3 times per day, before meals (a total of 1500 mg per day). Berberine has a half-life of several hours, so it is necessary to spread your dosage to several times per day to achieve stable blood levels.

If you have a medical condition or are on any medications, then it is recommended that you speak to your doctor before taking it. This is especially important if you are currently taking blood sugar lowering medications. Overall, berberine has an outstanding safety profile. The main side effects are related to digestion, and there are some reports of cramping, diarrhea, flatulence, constipation and stomach pain.

8   Take home message

Berberine is one of very few supplements that are as effective as a drug. It has powerful effects on various aspects of health, especially blood sugar control.

If you want to try a berberine supplement, then there is a good selection of high-quality supplements available on Amazon. The people who stand to benefit the most are individuals with type 2 diabetes and metabolic syndrome.

However, it may also be useful as a general protection against chronic disease, as well as an anti-aging supplement. If you use supplements, then berberine may be one of the top ones to include in your arsenal.

Section 3   Research Article

Highdensity lipoproteins down-regulate CCL2 production in human fibroblastlike synoviocytes stimulated by urate crystals

[Abstract] Introduction: To investigate whether monosodium urate (MSU) crystals induce the production of CCL2 (monocytechemoattractant protein-1; MCP-1) in human fibroblast-like synoviocytes (FLS) and whether this mechanism would be affected by high-density lipoproteins (HDL). Methods: Human FLS isolated from synovial tissue explants were stimulated with MSU crystals ($0.01 \sim 0.5$ mg/mL) or interleukin (IL)-1β (10 pg/mL) in the presence or absence of HDL (50 μg/mL and 100 μg/mL). The production and expression of CCL2 was evaluated with ELISA, confocal microscopy, immunofluorescence microscopy, chemotaxis assay, and realtime quantitative PCR. **Results:** Exposure of FLS to MSU crystals induced CCL2 accumulation in culture medium in a dose- and time-dependent manner, reaching a plateau at 50 ~ 75 μg/ mL MSU crystals and 20 ~ 24 hours. Although low, the induced CCL2 levels were sufficient to trigger mononuclear cell migration. In resting FLS, CCL2 was localized in small cytoplasmic vesicles whose number diminished with MSU crystal stimulation. Concomitantly, MSU crystals triggered the induction of CCL2 mRNA expression. All these processes were inhibited by HDL, which cause a 50% decrease in CCL2 mRNA levels and a dose-dependent inhibition of the release of CCL2. Similar results were obtained when FLS were pretreated with HDL and washed before activation by MSU crystals or IL-1β, suggesting a direct effect of HDL on the FLS activation state. **Conclusions:** The present results demonstrate that MSU crystals induce FLS to release CCL2 that is stored in vesicles in resting conditions. This mechanism is inhibited by HDL, which may limit the inflammatory process by diminishing CCL2 production and, in turn, monocytes/macrophages recruitment in joints. This study confirms the anti-inflammatory functions of HDL, which might play a part in the limitation of acute gout attack.

1　Introduction

CCL2 (monocyte chemoattractant protein-1; MCP-1), a member of the C-C chemokine family, is a major monocyte chemoattractant[1]. CCL2 production is inducible in various types of cells, including synoviocytes[2-3]. In vivo studies suggest that CCL2 attracts monocytes to sites of inflammation in a variety of pathologic conditions, including atherosclerosis[4-5], pulmonary fibrosis and granulomatous lung disease[6], and degenerative and inflammatory arthropathies, including gout[7-9]. Gout is a consequence of elevated serum urate levels that lead to deposition of monosodium urate (MSU) crystals in joints, causing an acute inflammatory response[10]. MSU crystals are indeed potent inducers of inflammation, as demonstrated in vivo. When injected into the peritoneum or in the air pouch of animal models, MSU crystals induce an inflammatory response characterized by a cellular infiltrate rich in neutrophils and the production of proinflammatory cytokines, as well as other inflammatory mediators, including CCL2[11-13]. CCL2 has long been associated with crystal inflammation. Elevated levels of CCL2 were measured in synovial fluid of gout patients[14]. Besides, in gouty arthritis models, intraarticular injection of MSU crystals induces the rapid release of CCL2 within 1 hour after injection, reaching a maximum at 2 ~ 4 hours[7]. Thus, CCL2 might be involved in the recruitment of monocytes/macrophages at the site of inflammation.

Once infiltrated in the joints, MSU crystals trigger monocytes/macrophages to produce IL-1β, a mechanism highly relevant to gout, the acute form of which is effectively treated with the recombinant form of IL-1-receptor antagonist, a specific IL-1 inhibitor[15-16]. Although the presence of MSU crystal-specific receptor at the cell surface is unlikely, MSU crystals might stimulate cells through membrane lipid alteration[17].

By secreting CCL2, activated resident synoviocytes may display the ability to recruit monocytes into the joints and, in turn, to set in the inflammatory response that underlies the acute attack of gout. In most cases, the acute attack is self-limited by processes that remain largely unknown[18]. However, a number of plasma proteins and lipoproteins that suppress the MSU crystals deleterious effects have been identified in synovial fluids. Among them, apolipoprotein (Apo) B and Apo E inhibit crystal-induced neutrophil stimulation by binding to the surface of crystals[19-20]. In addition, low-density lipoproteins (LDL) and high-density lipoproteins (HDL) strongly inhibit calcium and MSU crystal-induced neutrophil cytolysis[21], and LDL contributes to the resolution of acute inflammatory attack induced by calcium crystals in the rat air-pouch model[22]. Recently, we demonstrated that HDL-associated Apo A-I can exert anti-inflammatory effects through the inhibition of cytokine production in monocytes/ macrophages on contact with stimulated T cells or with stimulated T cell-derived microparticles[23-24]. Together, these studies suggest that lipoproteins may act at several levels to dampen inflammation.

Because MSU crystals increase CCL2 expression in vascular smooth muscle and epithelial cells[25-26], this study was undertaken to assess whether MSU crystals might display similar activity toward fibroblast-like synoviocytes (FLS), and whether this activity might be modulated by HDL. The results show that FLS contain stores of CCL2 that are released on activation by MSU crystals. Furthermore, MSU crystals also induce CCL2 gene transcription to refurbish stores. Both these MSU-crystal activities are inhibited in the presence of HDL.

2　Materials and Methods

2.1　Human materials

Human synovial tissue from patients and blood from healthy volunteers was obtained with the approval of the Institutional Review Board of the University of Padova, which approved the study. An informed-consent form was signed by the patients and volunteers.

2.2　FLS isolation and culture

Synovial tissue specimens were obtained from three osteoarthritis patients undergoing surgical joint replacement. FLS were isolated from tissue explants, as previous described[27]. In brief, synovium samples were rinsed several times in PBS, minced into about 1 mm pieces, placed in T25 flasks (Falcon, Oxnard, CA, USA), and maintained in DMEM supplemented with 10% heat-inactivated fetal calf serum (FCS), 50 µg/mL streptomycin, 50 U/mL penicillin, and 2 mmol/L glutamine (10% FCS medium). At confluence, cells were harvested (trypsin/ EDTA) and seeded into new flasks. All experiments were carried out with passage 4 through 8

FLS. FLS were CD90$^+$, CD55$^+$, and were positive for prolyl-4-hydroxylase, as demonstrated by immunocytochemical staining with specific antibodies (Chemicon International, Temecula, CA, USA). FLS were seeded in 96-well culture plates at a density of 1×10^4 cells/well, unless otherwise stated. Cells were allowed to adhere for 24 h, and then the medium was exchanged for a medium supplemented with 2% FCS and the indicated concentration of MSU crystals and HDL. Cell viability was assayed with trypan blue exclusion staining and was found to be higher than 98% in basal conditions.

2.3   Isolation of HDL

Human serum HDL were isolated and quantified as previously described[23].

2.4   Synthesis of MSU crystals

MSU crystals were prepared as described by Denko and Whitehouse[28]. In brief, 4 g uric acid was dissolved in 800 mL of deionized water, heated to 60 ℃, adjusted to pH 8.9 with 0.5 N NaOH, and let crystallize overnight at room temperature. MSU crystals were recovered by centrifugation, washed with distilled water and dried at 40 ℃ for 24 h. Crystal shape and birefringence were assessed by compensated polarized light microscopy. MSU crystals were milled and then sterilized by heating at 180 ℃ for 2 h before each experiment. Less than 0.015 EU/mL endotoxin was measured in MSU crystal preparations by Limulus amebocyte lysate assay (E-toxate kit, Sigma-Aldrich SRL., Milano, Italy).

2.5   Cytokines production

FLS were stimulated by MSU crystals in DMEM supplemented with 2% heat-inactivated FCS, 50 μg/mL streptomycin, 50 U/mL penicillin, 2 mmol/L glutamine, 5 μg/mL polymyxin, and filtered before the use (2% FCS medium). HDL were added with or 1 h before stimulation by MSU crystals. Culture supernatants were harvested and stored at –20 ℃ before CCL2, IL-8, and IL-1β measurements by enzyme immunoassay (RayBiotech, Inc., Norcross, GA, USA). Cytotoxicity of MSU crystals and HDL was assessed with a colorimetric assay for cell proliferation and activity (MTT, Chemicon International, Temecula, CA, USA), which measures mitochondrial activity of cells. In some experiments, cells were pretreated with 10 μg/mL cycloheximide (CHX; Sigma-Aldrich SRL., Milano, Italy) for 30 min before stimulation. Alternatively, FLS were stimulated by IL-1β (Recombinant Human IL-1β; R&D systems, Minneapolis, MN, USA). Inhibition experiments were carried out with IL-1-receptor antagonist (IL-1Ra, R & D Systems, Minneapolis, MN, USA).

2.6   Confocal microscopy

FLS were grown in eight-well chamber slides at a density of 2×10^4 cells/well in 10%

FCS medium and then were incubated with MSU crystals (50 μg/mL) or HDL (50 μg/mL and 100 μg/mL) or both for 24 h in 2% FCS medium. Cells were washed 3 times in PBS, fixed with 4% paraformaldehyde for 10 min, and permeabilized with 0.1% Triton X-100 in PBS for 4 min at 4 ℃ . After washing and blocking with 2% BSA for 30 min at room temperature, cells were incubated for 1 h with anti-CCL2 mAb (R&D systems, Minneapolis, MN, USA) diluted 1 : 20 in blocking buffer. After washing, bound antibodies were detected by using Alexa Fluor 488 conjugated goat anti-mouse IgG secondary Ab (1 : 150; Invitrogen SRL., San Giuliano Milanese, Italy) for 30 min at room temperature in the dark. Samples were analyzed with confocal microscopy (2100 Multiphoton; Bio-Rad Laboratories, Inc., Italy), by using laser excitation at 488 nm.

2.7   Chemotaxis assay

Mononuclear cells were isolated from peripheral blood from healthy volunteers by density gradient centrifugation with Histopaque 1077 (Sigma-Aldrich S.r.l., Milano, Italy). The effects of MSU crystals and HDL on the chemotaxis of mononuclear cells were assessed by using a 48-well modified Boyden chamber (AC48; NeuroProbe, Bethesda, MD, USA). Culture supernatants of FLS stimulated by MSU crystals in the presence or absence of HDL were loaded in the bottom chamber, and mononuclear cells were added to the top chamber. DMEM was used as a negative control, and 10 ng/mL CCL2 (RayBiotech, Inc., Norcross, GA, USA) was used as a positive control. A polyvinylpyrrolidone-free polycarbonate 8 mm membrane with 5 μm pores, pretreated with 10 μg/mL fibronectin, was placed between the chambers. In brief, 28 μL aliquots of culture supernatants were dispensed into the bottom wells of the chamber. Fifty-microliter aliquots of mononuclear cells (1×10^6 cells/mL) resuspended in RPMI 1640 were added to the top wells. Chambers were incubated at 37 ℃ with 5% CO_2 for 2 h. The membrane was then removed, washed with PBS on the upper side, fixed, and stained with DiffQuik (Baxter Scientific, Miami, FL, USA). Cells were counted microscopically at ×1000 magnification in four fields per membrane. All assays were performed in duplicate.

2.8   CCL2 mRNA

FLS were grown to confluence in six-well culture dishes in 10% FCS medium and then incubated with MSU crystals (50 μg/mL) in the presence or absence of HDL (100 μg/mL) for the indicated time periods in 2% FCS medium. Supernatants were harvested for CCL2 measurements, and total FLS RNA was prepared by Tris-Reagent, as described by the provider (Sigma-Aldrich SRL., Milano, Italy). Quantitative real-time duplex PCR analysis (Taq-Man quantitative ABI PRISM 7300 Detection System, Applied Biosystems) was conducted after reverse transcription by Super-Script Ⅱ (Invitrogen SRL., San Giuliano Milanese, Italy). The levels of mRNA expression were normalized, with the expression of a housekeeping gene (18 S) analyzed simultaneously. CCL2 and 18 S probes were purchased from Applied Biosystems. All measurements were conducted in triplicate.

2.9　Statistical analysis

Data significance was assessed with students' t-test; $P < 0.05$ was considered significant.

3　Results

3.1　MSU crystals induce CCL2 release by human FLS

To evaluate the capacity of MSU crystals to induce CCL2 release, FLS were incubated for 24 h with increasing concentrations of MSU crystals. In the range of concentrations used, MSU crystals did not significantly affect cell viability, which was only slightly decreased at concentrations higher than 50 μg/mL (data not shown). In the absence of stimulus, FLS released low but significant levels of CCL2 amounting to (55 ± 20) pg/mL (Figure 18-1a). A similar pattern of CCL2 production was observed among FLS preparations, independent of the donor or cell passage, although the extent of CCL2 production varied between experiments, as indicated by the error bar dimension (Figure 18-1). MSU crystals induced a dose-dependent increase of CCL2 production in FLS, reaching a plateau at 50 ~ 75 μg/mL MSU crystals (Figure 18-1a). To determine the time required for maximal chemokine production, FLS were exposed to 50 μg/mL MSU crystals for increasing time periods. As depicted in Figure 18-1b, CCL2 production reached a plateau at 20 ~ 24 h. Therefore, in the experiments described later, FLS were activated for 24 h with an optimal dose of 50 μg/mL of MSU crystals. Because FLS might release IL-1, a potent stimulus of fibroblasts, FLS were stimulated by MSU crystals in the presence of the IL-1-specific inhibitor, IL-1Ra[29]. As shown in Figure 18-1c, the production of CCL2 induced by MSU crystals was not affected by 250 ng/mL IL-1Ra. In the same experiments, such an IL-1Ra dose abolished CCL2 production induced by 125 pg/mL IL-1β (Figure 18-1d). IL-1Ra per se had no effect on CCL2 production by FLS (Figure 18-1c and Figure 18-1d). These results demonstrate that the production of CCL2 was directly induced by MSU crystals, ruling out the participation of an autocrine loop of IL-1.

3.2　CCL2 is contained in small vesicles in FLS

Because CCL2 is constitutively contained in small storage granules within endothelial cell cytoplasm[30-31], the presence of such a compartment was assessed in FLS with confocal microscopy. In resting FLS, CCL2 was localized in small vesicles in cell cytoplasm (Figure 18-2a). Consistent with CCL2 release, after 24-hour stimulation with 50 μg/mL MSU crystals, a marked diminution of the number of CCL2-containing vesicles was observed as compared with unstimulated cells (Figure 18-2b). These data suggest that FLS contained intracellular pools of CCL2 that was stored in small vesicles and thus might be rapidly released on stimulation.

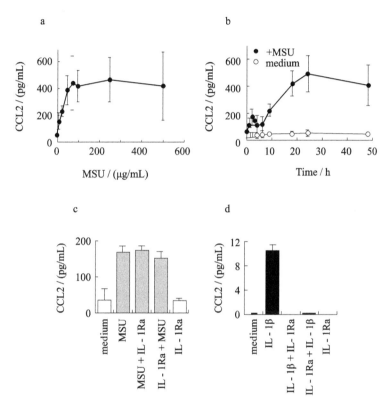

Figure 18-1   Effect of monosodium urate (MSU) crystals on CCL2 production in cultured fibroblast-like synoviocytes (FLS)

(a) FLS were treated with increasing concentrations of MSU crystals for 24 hours. (b) Synoviocytes were incubated in the presence (black circles) or absence (white circles) of 50 μg/mL MSU crystals for the indicated time. CCL2 was measured in culture supernatants with ELISA. (c) FLS were stimulated (grey columns) or not (white columns) for 24 hours with 50 μg/mL MSU crystals in the presence or absence of 250 ng/mL IL-1Ra. IL-1Ra was either added with MSU crystals (MSU + IL-1Ra) or added to FLS 1 hour before activation by MSU crystals (IL-1Ra + MSU). (d) FLS were stimulated (black columns) or not (white columns) for 24 hours with 125 pg/mL IL-1β in the presence or absence of 250 ng/mL of IL-1Ra. IL-1Ra was either added with IL-1β (IL-1β + IL-1Ra) or added to FLS 1 hour before activation by IL-1β (IL-1Ra + IL-1β). (c, d) Culture supernatants were analyzed for the production of CCL2. Results are presented as mean ± SD of three separate experiments.

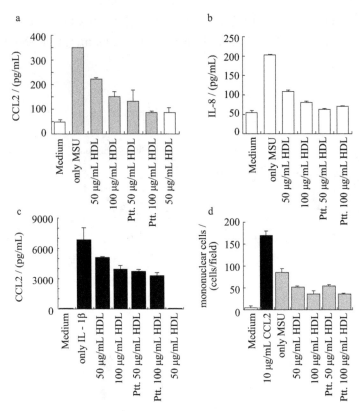

Figure 18-2　High-density lipoproteins (HDL) inhibit CCL2 production induced by monosodium urate (MSU) crystals in fibroblast-like synoviocytes (FLS)

　　(a, b) FLS were stimulated (grey columns) or not (white columns) for 24 hours with 50 μg/mL MSU crystals in the presence or absence of the indicated concentration of HDL. Alternatively, FLS were pretreated (Ptt.) with the indicated concentration of HDL, washed, and then stimulated for 24 hours with 50 μg/mL MSU crystals. Culture supernatants were analyzed for the production of CCL2 (a) and IL-8 (b). (c)FLS were stimulated (black columns) or not (white columns) with 10 pg/mL IL-1β for 24 hours. Culture supernatants were analyzed for the production of CCL2. (d) Culture supernatants of FLS, activated as in (a) and (b), were analyzed for their ability to induce mononuclear cell migration, as described in Materials and Methods. Migration induced by culture medium (white column), 10 ng/mL CCL2 (black column), and culture supernatants of FLS activated as in (a) and (b) (grey columns). Four fields were counted for the number of migrated cells.

3.3　HDL inhibit MSU crystal–induced CCL2 production in FLS

　　To assess the antiinflammatory activity of HDL, FLS were incubated with MSU crystals in the presence or absence of 50 μg/mL or 100 μg/mL HDL for 24 hours. HDL significantly decreased the MSU crystal-induced CCL2 production in a dose-dependent manner. This inhibition was not due to the formation of complexes between HDL and MSU crystals, because similar results were obtained when FLS were pretreated with HDL before activation by MSU crystals. In the latter setting, the inhibition of CCL2 production tended to be more pronounced when FLS were pretreated with HDL. To confirm that HDL directly affected the FLS stimulation state, we sought to assess the production of other cytokines and to test another FLS stimulus. The MSU crystals-induced production of IL-8 was inhibited in the presence of HDL and abolished when FLS were pretreated with HDL. When FLS were activated by IL-1β, the induced CCL2 production was inhibited in the presence of HDL in a dose-dependent manner, the inhibition being more pronounced when cells were pretreated with HDL. IL-1β was not detectable in MSU crystals-activated FLS supernatants (data not shown), thus ruling out a part of an autocrine loop of IL-1β, the induction of CCL2 or IL-8 production. Together, these results establish that HDL directly affected the FLS activation state. The amount of CCL2 induced by MSU crystals was very low as compared with that induced by IL-1β. However, CCL2 concentrations in supernatants of MSU crystals-activated FLS were sufficient to induce mononuclear cells migration. This effect was reduced when FLS were treated or pretreated with HDL.

The premise that HDL inhibited MSU crystal-induced CCL2 released by FLS was further confirmed by fluorescent microscopy. Intracellular CCL2 was drastically diminished in FLS after activation by MSU crystals, as compared with resting FLS. When FLS were activated by MSU crystals in the presence of HDL, their fluorescence intensity remained similar to that of resting FLS. To ascertain that all CCL2 recovered in FLS supernatants was provided by intracellular stores, the effect of cycloheximide (CHX; that is, an inhibitor of protein synthesis) was tested. CHX did not affect the production of CCL2 induced by MSU crystals, at least for a period of 48 h, demonstrating that protein neosynthesis was not required for optimal CCL2 release. This strengthened the premise that CCL2 release was a direct effect of MSU crystals and not due to an autocrine loop after the synthesis and secretion of a putative cytokine. Together, these results demonstrate that MSU crystal-activated FLS release CCL2 from cytoplasm stores, and that this release is inhibited in the presence of HDL.

3.4 MSU crystals induce CCL2 gene transcription, which is inhibited in the presence of HDL

Because MSU crystals induced the release of CCL2, it was important to assess whether cell stimulation induced CCL2 neosynthesis (that is, increased CCL2 mRNA levels), to replenish intracellular stores after activation. To investigate the effects of MSU crystals on CCL2 mRNA levels, FLS were incubated with MSU crystals, and CCL2 transcript levels were evaluated with real-time quantitative PCR. The induction of CCL2 gene transcription in FLS activated by MSU crystals was already detectable after 2 h stimulation and reached a maximum at 18 h, with enhancements varying between 3 and 13 times basal levels, depending on the experiment. MSU crystal induced expression of CCL2 mRNA was inhibited in FLS stimulated in the presence of HDL. In the absence of stimulus, HDL did not affect CCL2 mRNA levels. These results suggest that HDL directly acted on FLS to diminish MSU crystal-induced CCL2 production by inhibiting the release of vesicle content and by diminishing the neosynthesis of the chemokine.

4   Discussion

This study demonstrates that FLS contain intracellular stores of CCL2 which are released on activation by MSU crystals. CCL2 release is accompanied by the induction of gene transcription, suggesting that MSU crystals might also trigger CCL2 store refill. Both these processes are inhibited in the presence of HDL, confirming their anti-inflammatory activities and the part they might play in gout-attack limitation.

MSU crystals directly induced CCL2 production in FLS. Indeed, although MSU crystals were shown to activate the NALP3 inflammasome in mononuclear cells, resulting in IL-1β production[15], this mechanism does not apply to FLS in which MSU crystals activation does not induce the release of IL-1β. In addition to the premise that protein neosynthesis is not required for CCL2 production, our results strongly suggest that the effect of MSU crystals in FLS is not mediated by an autocrine loop of IL-1.

Intracellular stores of CCL2 were previously described in endothelial cells, where it is stocked in granules different from intracellular stores of other chemokines[30-31]. Endothelial cells are known to contain small intracellular granules that may release several inflammatory factors, including CCL2, more rapidly than the content of Weibel-Palade bodies[31-32]. Our results suggest that such a process may occur in FLS. To our knowledge, it is the first time that chemokine secretory granules were observed in FLS. The premise that CCL2 is immediately available in joints subjected to attacks of inflammatory agents suggests that in gout, monocytes may precede neutrophil infiltration. This was previously suggested in the rat air-pouch model, in which monocyte/macrophage number increases as early as 2 h after MSU crystal injection, whereas neutrophils peak at 4 h and 24 h[33]. Thus, the presence of intracellular stores of CCL2 might participate in the rapid response of joint cells to MSU crystals, attracting monocytes/macrophages into the tissue in an attempt to eliminate the inflammatory agent rapidly.

In addition to the release of CCL2 from intracellular granules, MSU crystals induced CCL2 gene transcription in human FLS. Noticeably, CCL2 mRNA transcription was slow and peaked at 18 h, displaying a 3-fold to 13-fold increase, as compared with basal levels in resting FLS. However, the enhancement of CCL2 was not accompanied by the enhancement of granule numbers at 24 h. Because the production of CCL2 was not enhanced after 24 h activation, these results suggest that the CCL2 transcript is not traduced immediately, and that longer periods are required to replenish storage granules.

The anti-inflammatory role of HDL has been widely described in in vitro as well as in in vivo models of atherosclerosis[34-35]. In addition, HDL-associated Apo A-I display anti-inflammatory effects in other inflammatory disorders in which T cell contact-induced cytokines production in monocytes/macrophages is likely to play a part[23, 36]. HDL also potently reduce radical oxygen species production induced in neutrophils on contact with stimulated T cells. Recently we demonstrated that Apo A-I, HDL, and total cholesterol levels are decreased in plasma, whereas Apo A-I is increased in the synovial fluid of patients with inflammatory arthritis. The correlation between synovial fluid/serum Apo A-I ratio and both local and systemic inflammatory indexes suggests the involvement of HDL in the synovial inflammatory process. The mechanisms of HDL antiinflammatory effects were partly identified. For instance, HDL might hamper the binding of LPS to its receptor at the cell surface, as reviewed by Wu et al. [37]. Similarly, it is likely that HDL impede the interaction between stimulated T cells and monocytes[23]. Here we demonstrate that HDL display anti-inflammatory properties in MSU crystal-induced inflammation by decreasing the production and expression of CCL2 in human FLS. Although this study does not elucidate the mechanism of HDL action, the premise that cell preincubation with HDL resulted in an increased inhibition of CCL2 production and expression suggests that HDL may act directly on FLS either by blocking putative MSU crystal receptors/sensors or by changing the threshold of FLS response to crystals. The latter hypothesis suggests that HDL could directly signal FLS, rendering them less sensitive to inflammatory agents. Apolipoproteins, either Apo B or Apo E, were shown to dampen crystal-induced neutrophil activation, a mechanism that might be relevant to gout attack resolution[19-20]. Here we show that FLS activated by MSU crystals produce CCL2 and thus may attract monocytes/macrophages into the joint. Because they inhibit this process, HDL might contribute to limit a gout attack at its very beginning by acting on resident FLS, which play a major part in chronic inflammation and the destruction of joint tissues.

References

[1]   Boring L, Gosling J, Chensue S W, et al. Impaired monocyte migration and reduced type 1 (Th1) cytokine responses in C-C chemokine receptor 2 knockout mice. Journal of Clinical Investigation, 1997, 100(10): 2552-2561.

[2]   Rollins B J. MCP-1, MCP-2, MCP-3, MCP-4, and MCP-5: in cytokine reference. London: Academic Press, 2000: 1145-1160.

[3]   Berckmans R J, Nieuwland R, Kraan M C, et al. Synovial microparticles from arthritic patients modulate chemokine and cytokine release by synoviocytes. Arthritis Research & Therapy, 2005, 7(3): R536-R544.

[4]   Combadière C, Potteaux S, Rodero M, et al. Combined inhibition of CCL2, CX3CR1, and CCR5 abrogates Ly6C(hi) and Ly6C(lo) monocytosis and almost abolishes atherosclerosis in hypercholesterolemic mice. Circulation, 2008, 117(13): 1649-1657.

[5]　Kusano K F, Nakamura K, Kusano H, et al. Significance of the level of monocyte chemoattractant protein-1 in human atherosclerosis. Circulation Journal, 2004, 68(7): 671-676.

[6]　Chensue S W, Warmington K S, Ruth J H, et al. Role of monocyte chemoattractant protein-1 (MCP-1) in Th1 (mycobacterial) and Th2 (schistosomal) antigen-induced granuloma formation: relationship to local inflammation, Th cell expression, and IL-12 production. Journal of Immunology, 1996, 157(10): 4602-4608.

[7]　Matsukawa A, Miyazaki S, Maeda T, et al. Production and regulation of monocyte chemoattractant protein-1 in lipopolysaccharide- or monosodium urate crystal-induced arthritis in rabbits: roles of tumor necrosis factor alpha, interleukin-1, and interleukin-8. Lab Invest, 1998, 78: 973-985.

[8]　Villiger P M, Terkeltaub R, Lotz M. Monocyte chemoattractant protein-1 (MCP-1) expression in human articular cartilage. Induction by peptide regulatory factors and differential effects of dexamethasone and retinoic acid. Journal of Clinical Investigation, 1992, 90(2): 488-496.

[9]　Villiger P M, Terkeltaub R, Lotz M. Production of monocyte chemoattractant protein-1 by inflamed synovial tissue and cultured synoviocytes. Journal of Immunology, 1992, 149(2): 722-727.

[10]　So A. Developments in the scientific and clinical understanding of gout. Arthritis Research & Therapy, 2008, 10(5): 1-6.

[11]　Martin W J, Walton M, Harper J. Resident macrophages initiating and driving inflammation in a monosodium urate monohydrate crystal-induced murine peritoneal model of acute gout. Arthritis & Rheumatology, 2009, 60(1): 281-289.

[12]　Esteban Ortiz-Bravo M D, Sieck M S, Jr H R S. Changes in the proteins coating monosodium urate crystals during active and subsiding inflammation: immunogold studies of synovial fluid from patients with gout and of fluid obtained using the rat subcutaneous air pouch model. Arthritis & Rheumatology, 1993, 36(9): 1274-1285.

[13]　Ryckman C, Mccoll S R, Vandal K, et al. Role of S100A8 and S100A9 in neutrophil recruitment in response to monosodium urate monohydrate crystals in the air-pouch model of acute gouty arthritis. Arthritis & Rheumatology, 2003, 48(8): 2310-2320.

[14]　Harigai M, Hara M, Yoshimura T, et al. Monocyte chemoattractant protein-1 (MCP-1) in inflammatory joint diseases and its involvement in the cytokine network of rheumatoid synovium. Clinical Immunology & Immunopathology, 1993, 69(1): 83-91.

[15]　Martinon F, Pétrilli V, Mayor A, et al. Gout-associated uric acid crystals activate the NALP3 inflammasome. Nature, 2006, 440(7081): 237-241.

[16]　So A, Smedt T D, Revaz S, et al. A pilot study of IL-1 inhibition by anakinra in acute gout. Arthritis Research & Therapy, 2007, 9(2): R28.

[17]　Ng G, Sharma K, Ward S, et al. Receptor-independent, direct membrane binding leads to cell-surface lipid sorting and Syk kinase activation in dendritic cells. Immunity, 2008, 29(5): 807-818.

[18]　Terkeltaub R A. What stops a gouty attack. Journal of Rheumatology, 1992, 19(1): 8-10.

[19]　Terkeltaub R, Martin J, Curtiss L K, et al. Apolipoprotein B mediates the capacity of low density

lipoprotein to suppress neutrophil stimulation by particulates. J Biol Chem, 1986, 261: 15662-15667.

[20] Terkeltaub R A, Dyer C A, Martin J, et al. Apolipoprotein (apo) E inhibits the capacity of monosodium urate crystals to stimulate neutrophils. Characterization of intraarticular Apo E and demonstration of Apo E binding to urate crystals in vivo. Journal of Clinical Investigation, 1991, 87(1): 20-26.

[21] Burt H M, Jackson J K, Rowell J. Calcium pyrophosphate and monosodium urate crystal interactions with neutrophils: effect of crystal size and lipoprotein binding to crystals. Journal of Rheumatology, 1989, 16(6): 809-817.

[22] Kumagai Y, Watanabe W, Kobayashi A, et al. Inhibitory effect of low density lipoprotein on the inflammation-inducing activity of calcium pyrophosphate dihydrate crystals. Journal of Rheumatology, 2001, 28(12): 2674-2680.

[23] Hyka N, Dayer J M, Modoux C, et al. Apolipoprotein A-I inhibits the production of IL-1beta and tumor necrosis factor-alpha by blocking contact-mediated activation of monocytes by T lymphocytes. Blood, 2001, 97(8): 2381-2389.

[24] Scanu A, Molnarfi N, Brandt K J, et al. Stimulated T cells generate microparticles, which mimic cellular contact activation of human monocytes: differential regulation of pro- and anti-inflammatory cytokine production by high-density lipoproteins. J Leukoc Biol, 2008, 83: 921-927.

[25] Kanellis J, Watanabe S, Li J H, et al. Uric acid stimulates monocyte chemoattractant protein-1 production in vascular smooth muscle cells via mitogen-activated protein kinase and cyclooxygenase-2. Hypertension, 2003, 41(6): 1287-1293.

[26] Umekawa T, Chegini N, Khan S R. Increased expression of monocyte chemoattractant protein-1 (MCP-1) by renal epithelial cells in culture on exposure to calcium oxalate, phosphate and uric acid crystals. Nephrol Dial Transplant, 2003, 18(4): 664-669.

[27] Scanu A, Oliviero F, Braghetto L, et al. Synoviocyte cultures from synovial fluid. Reumatismo, 2007, 59(1): 66-70.

[28] Denko C W, Whitehouse M W. Experimental inflammation induced by naturally occurring microcrystalline calcium salts. Journal of Rheumatology, 1976, 3(1): 54 -62.

[29] Burger D, Chicheportiche R, Giri J G, et al. The inhibitory activity of human interleukin-1 receptor antagonist is enhanced by type II interleukin-1 soluble receptor and hindered by type I interleukin-1 soluble receptor. J Clin Invest, 1995, 96: 38-41.

[30] Oynebraten I, Barois N, Hagelsteen K, et al. Characterization of a novel chemokine-containing storage granule in endothelial cells: evidence for preferential exocytosis mediated by protein kinase A and diacylglycerol. Journal of Immunology, 2005, 175(8): 5358-5369.

[31] Oynebraten I, Bakke O, Brandtzaeg P, et al. Rapid chemokine secretion from endothelial cells originates from 2 distinct compartments. Blood, 2004, 104(2): 314-320.

[32] Zupancic G, Ogden D, Magnus C J, et al. Differential exocytosis from human endothelial cells evoked by high intracellular Ca^{2+} concentration. Journal of Physiology, 2002, 544(Pt 3): 741-755.

[33] Schiltz C, Lioté F, Prudhommeaux F, et al. Monosodium urate monohydrate crystal-induced

inflammation in vivo: quantitative histomorphometric analysis of cellular events. Arthritis & Rheumatism, 2002, 46(6): 1643-1650.

[34]　Navab M, Reddy S T, Lenten B J V, et al. The role of dysfunctional HDL in atherosclerosis. Journal of Lipid Research, 2009, 50(Suppl): S145-S149.

[35]　Shao B, Heinecke J W. HDL, lipid peroxidation, and atherosclerosis. Journal of Lipid Research, 2009, 50(4): 599-601.

[36]　Burger D, Dayer J M, Molnarfi N. Cell contact dependence of inflammatory events. Abingdon, UK: Taylor & Francis Books Ltd, 2007: 85-103.

[37]　Wu A, Hinds C J, Thiemermann C. High-density lipoproteins in sepsis and septic shock: metabolism, actions, and therapeutic applications. Shock, 2004, 21(3): 210-221.

Section 4　Words of TCM

1. 津液输布 transportation and distribution of body fluids
2. 伤津脱液 consumption of body fluid
3. 脾散津功能 splenic function of transmiting nutrients
4. 刺痒脏腑 moistening and nourishing viscera
5. 水液停聚 retention of body fluid
6. 水湿困脾 body fluid troubling the spleen
7. 湿邪内盛 excessive internal pathogenic dampness
8. 脾虚水肿 edema due to asthenia of the spleen
9. 润滑关节 lubricating joints; smooth movement of joints
10. 人痘接种 human variolation
11. 四气五味 four properties and five tastes
12. 辛味药 pungent-flavored drugs; drugs (prescriptions) with pungent
13. 甘味药 sweet-flavored drugs; drugs (prescriptions) with sweet
14. 酸味药 sour-flavored drugs; drugs (prescriptions) with sour flavor
15. 苦味药 bitter-flavored drugs; drugs (prescriptions) with bitter
16. 咸味药 salty-flavored drugs; drugs (prescriptions) with salty
17. 煎药法 drug-decocting methods
18. 煎药用水 drug-decocting water
19. 煎药用具 drug-decocting utensils
20. 煎药火候 drug-decocting fire
21. 干眼症 xerophthalmia
22. 土风疮 popular urticaria

23. 沙眼 trachoma
24. 土喜温燥 earth prefers warmth and dryness
25. 土郁夺之 dampness accumulated in the spleen(earth) should be removed
26. 下疳 chancre
27. 下膈 intake of food in the morning and vomiting in the evening
28. 下乳 / 催乳 lactogenesis
29. 下丹田 lower elixir field
30. 下马痈 acute pyogenic infection of right
31. 下石疽 indurated mass of knee
32. 下注疮 eczema of shank
33. 下腹胀气 flatulence in the lower abdomen
34. 下汲肾阴 consumption of the kidney-yin by the excessive heart fire
35. 下焦如渎 lower-jiao resembling water passages
36. 下厥上竭 exhaustion of blood with cold limbs
37. 下利清谷 diarrhea with undigested food in the stool
38. 下胎毒法 dispelling toxic heat and meconium gathered at the fetus for the new born
39. 下利赤白 dysenteric diarrhea
40. 镜面舌 mirror-like tongue

(Ye Xuemin, Wang Yue)

References

[1]   Bani-Sadr F, Teissiere F, Curie I, et al. Anti-infection prophylaxis after sexual assault. Experience of the Raymond Poincaré-Garches Hospital. Presse Med, 2001,30(6): 253-258.

[2]   Mathis D, Shoelson S E. Immunometabolism: an emerging, frontier. Nature Reviews Immunology, 2011, 11(2): 81-84.

[3]   Binbin C, Yinglu F, Juan D, et al. Upregulation effect of ginsenosides on glucocorticoid receptor in rat liver. Horm Metab Res, 2009, 41: 531-536.

[4]   Chen H H, Song H Y, Liu X, et al. Buyanghuanwu Decoction alleviated pressure overload induced cardiac remodeling by suppressing Tgf-β /Smads and MAPKs signaling activated fibrosis. Biomed Pharmacother, 2017, 95: 461-468.

[5]   Chen Y, Zhang M Z, Li Q, et al. Interfering effect and mechanism of neuregulin on experimental dementia models in rats. Behavioral Brain Research, 2011, 222(2): 321-325.

[6]   Feng Y L, Ling C Q, Zhai X F, et al. A New way: alleviating postembolization syndrome following transcatheter arterial chemoembolization. J Alternat Compl Med, 2009, 15(2): 175-181.

[7]   Feng Y L, Zheng G Y, Ling C Q, et al. Investigation on correlation between metabolic syndrome and constitution types in senior military ex-service personnel of the People's Liberation Army. Chin J Integr Med, 2012, 18(7): 485-489.

[8]   Frankenstein Z, Alon U, Cohen I R. The immune-body cytokine network defines a social architecture of cell interactions. Biology Direct, 2006, 1(1): 32.

[9]   Gu N, Ge K, Hao C, et al. Neuregulin1 β effects on brain tissue via ERK5-dependent MAPK pathway in a rat model of cerebral ischemia-reperfusion injury. J Mol Neurosci, 2017, 61(4): 607-616.

[10]   Guo Y L, Xu X Y, Li Q, et al. Anti-inflammation effects of picroside Ⅱ in cerebral ischemic injury rats. Beha Brain Funct, 2010, 6(1): 43-53.

[11]   Guo Y L, Wang X J, Pan Y X, et al. ZJXG Decoction promotes the expression of bone morphogenetic protein-7 to enhance fracture healing in rats. J Trauma Treat, 2012, 1(1): 1-4.

[12]   Hotamisligil G S. Inflammation, metaflammation and immunometabolic disorders. Nature, 2017, 542(764): 177-185.

[13]   Hiroyasua S, Sniraishi M, Koji T, et al. Analysis of FAS system in pulmonary injury of GHVD after rat intestinal transplantation. Transplantation, 1996, 8(7): 33-38.

[14]   Ji Y Q, Teng L, Zhang R, et al. NRG1 β exerts a neuroprotective effect via the JNK signaling pathway to prevent ischemia reperfusion-induced injury in rats. Neurosci, 2017, 362: 13-24.

[15]   Li B S. The treatment of hundreds of disease with vinegar & eggs. Shanghai: Shanghai Science & Technology Publishing Co., 1992.

[16]   Li Q, Li Z, Mei Y W, et al. Neuregulin attenuated cerebral ischemia-reperfusion injury via inhibiting apoptosis and upregulating aquaporin-4. Neurosci Lett, 2008, 443(3): 155-159.

[17]   Li Q, Li Z, Xu X Y, et al. Neuroprotective properties of picroside II in rat model of focal cerebral ischemia. Int J Mol Sci, 2010, 11(11): 4580-4590.

[18]   Li S, Wang T T, Zhai L, et al. Picroside II plays a neuroprotective effect by inhibiting mPTP permeability and EndoG release after cerebral ischemia/reperfusion injury in rats. J Mol Neurosci, 2018, 64(1): 144-155.

[19]   Li X D, Ning C, Zhou Z, et al. Zhuang Jin Xu Gu decoction improves fracture healing in rats by augmenting the expression of NPY. Int J Pharmacol, 2014, 10(3): 175-181.

[20]   Li S F, Wang R Z, Meng Q H, et al. Intra-ventricular infusion of rAAV1-EGFP resulted in transduction in multiple regions of adult rat brain: a comparative study with rAAV2 and rAAV5 vectors. Brain Res, 2006, 1122(1): 1-9.

[21]   Li Y A. Innovation medical English textbook. Shanghai: Shanghai Science & Technology Publishing Co., 2008.

[22]   Liu G Y, Song J M, Guo Y L, et al. Astragalus injection protects cerebral ischemic injury by inhibiting neuronal apoptosis and the expression of JNK3 after cerebral ischemia reperfusion in rats. Beha Brain Funct, 2013, 9(9): 36-43.

[23]   Liu X J, Zheng X P, Zhang R, et al. Combinatorial effects of miR-20a and miR-29b on neuronal apoptosis induced by spinal cord injury. Int J Exp Pathol, 2015, 8(4): 3811-3818.

[24]   Long S H, Yu Z Q, Shuai L, et al. The hypoglycemic effect of the kelp on diabetes mellitus model induced by alloxan in rats. Int J Mol Sci, 2012, 13(3): 3354-3365.

[25]   Pei H T, Su X, Zhao L, et al. Primary study for the therapeutic dose and Time window of picroside II in treating cerebral ischemic injury in rats. Int J Mo Sci, 2012, 13(2): 2551-2562.

[26]   Pi W L. School of watering the Spleen and traditional Chinese dietary therapy. Am J of Acupunct, 1988, 16(4): 4-5.

[27]   Qiu L M. New uses of Bu Zhong Yi Qi Tang. Sichuan J Tradit Chin Med, 2000(6): 57.

[28]   Scanu A, Oliviero F, Gruaz L, et al. High-density lipoproteins downregulate CCL2 production in human fibroblast-like synoviocytes stimulated by urate crystals. Arthritis Research & Therapy, 2010, 12: R23.

[29]   Surapaneni KM, Venkataramana G. Status of lipid peroxidation, glutathione, ascorbic acid, vitamin E and antioxidant enzymes in patients with osteoarthritis. Indian J Med Sci, 2007, 61(1): 9-14.

[30]   Wang T T, Zhai L, Zhang H Y, et al. Picroside II inhibits the MEK-ERK1/2-COX2 signal pathway to prevent cerebral ischemic injury in rats. J Mol Neurosci, 2015, 57(8): 335-351.

[31]   Xu X Y, Yu Z Q, Guo Y L, et al. The effect of kelp on serum lipids of hyperlipidemia in rats. J Food Biochemistry, 2011, 35(6): 1-7.

[32]　Zhang H, Li Q, Li Z, et al. The protection of Bcl-2 overexpression on rat cortical neuronal injury caused by analogous ischemia/reperfusion in vitro. Neurosci Res, 2008, 62(2): 140-146.

[33]　Zhang H Y, Zhai L, Wang T T, et al. Picroside II exerts a neuroprotective effect by inhibiting the mitochondria cytochrome C signal pathway following ischemia reperfusion injury in rats. J Mol Neurosci, 2017, 61(2): 267-278.